Blackwell Scientific Publications
Editorial offices:
Three Cambridge Center, Cambridge,
Massachusetts 02142, USA
Osney Mead, Oxford OX2 0EL, England
25 John Street, London, WC1N 2BL,
England
23 Ainslie Place, Edinburgh, EH3 6AJ,
Scotland
54 University Street, Carlton, Victoria 3053,
Australia

Other editorial offices:
Arnette SA, 2 rue Casimir-Delavigne, 75006
Paris, France
Blackwell-Wissenschaft, Meinekestrasse 4,
D-1000 Berlin 15, Germany
Blackwell MZV, Feldgasse 13, A-1238
Wien, Austria

Distributors:
USA and Canada
  Mosby-Year Book, Inc.
  11830 Westline Industrial Drive
  St. Louis, Missouri 63146
  (Orders: Tel. 800-633-6699)
Australia
  Blackwell Scientific Publications
  (Australia) Pty Ltd
  54 University Street
  Carlton, Victoria 3053
  (Orders: Telephone: 03-347-0300)
Outside North America and Australia
  Blackwell Scientific Publications, Ltd.
  Osney Mead
  Oxford OX2 0EL
  England
  (Orders: Telephone: 011-44-865-240201)

Typeset by Modern Graphics, Inc.
Printed and bound by The Maple-Vail Book
Manufacturing Group

© 1991 Blackwell Scientific Publications
Printed in the United States of America
91 92 93 94 5 4 3 2 1

**Library of Congress Cataloging in
Publication Data**

Cornblath, Marvin.
    Disorders of carbohydrate metabolism
in infancy / Marvin Cornblath, Robert
Schwartz.—3rd ed.
        p. cm.
    Includes bibliographical references and
index.
    ISBN 0-86542-137-4
    1. Carbohydrate metabolism disorders
in infants. 2. Carbohydrate metabolism
disorders in pregnancy. I. Schwartz,
Robert, 1922–   . II. Title.
    [DNLM: 1. Carbohydrate Metabolism
Inborn Errors. WD 205.C2 C812d]
RJ399.C3C67   1991
618.9'2399—dc20
DNLM/DLC
for Library of Congress   90–14531
                                      CIP

DISORDERS OF

CARBOHYDRATE

METABOLISM

IN INFANCY

THIRD EDITION

Marvin Cornblath

Lecturer in Pediatrics
The Johns Hopkins University School of Medicine
Clinical Professor, Department of Pediatrics
University of Maryland School of Medicine
Baltimore, Maryland

Robert Schwartz

Professor of Pediatrics and Medical Science
Department of Pediatrics
Brown University Program in Medicine
Formerly, Director of the Division of Pediatric Metabolism and Nutrition
Rhode Island Hospital
Providence, Rhode Island

Boston

BLACKWELL SCIENTIFIC PUBLICATIONS

Oxford   London   Edinburgh   Melbourne   Paris   Berlin   Vienna

DISORDERS OF

CARBOHYDRATE

METABOLISM

IN INFANCY

HYPOGLYCEMIC INFANTS

SGA	AGA	LGA
Symptomatic Transient	Asymptomatic	Symptomatic Persistent (Hyperinsulinemic)

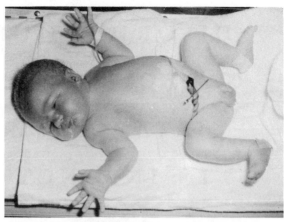

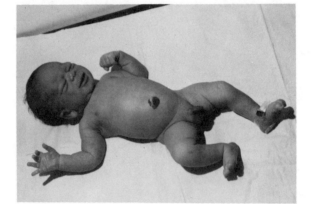

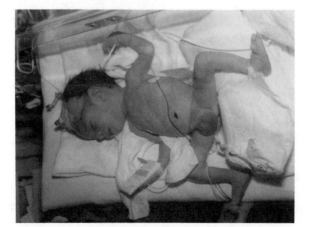

MOTHERS

Hypertensive	Insulin-Dependent Controlled	Normal

Affectionately dedicated to our families, especially our wives Joan and Joyce, and to our children and grandchildren

CONTENTS

PREFACE

TO THE
FIRST EDITION

. . . our first encounters with Nature's own chemical error rarely lack an element of disbelief or even indignation. Only as the fantastic complexity of our genetic-metabolic make-up dawns on us do we begin to wonder that her slips are so few. And even more slowly do we realize that they are, in fact, not nearly so few as we had imagined.

Editorial, The Lancet, September 1963, p. 619.

The disorders of carbohydrate metabolism exemplify the intimate relationship between the clinical and basic sciences. The pathogenesis of these disturbances has been elucidated and effective therapy often introduced as a result of investigations initiated in the laboratory and extended to the bedside. Unsuspected and puzzling clinical manifestations likewise have stimulated investigators to clarify and reinterpret metabolic pathways and physiological observations.

In the past three decades, this relationship has resulted in a better understanding of the genetics, biochemistry, physiology, and clinical findings of a number of diseases. New disorders have been discovered and have provided a stimulus for further research.

In this monograph, we have attempted to present our own current concepts of the normal and abnormal physiology of carbohydrate metabolism in the fetus, the pregnant mother, the neonate, and the infant. In citing references to the literature we have tried to be selective rather than comprehensive. We have tried to emphasize known facts and to relate them to the management of clinical problems of the infant as they present to the physician. Certain prejudices will be apparent in both interpretation and treatment; we hope these will serve as a stimulus to research into the many unsolved problems that yet remain.

Since each of us has followed a different path in training, we hope that the combination of our backgrounds has resulted in a comprehensive approach to the problems of carbohydrate metabolism in the newborn and infant. One of us (M. C.) became interested in these problems under the tutelage and stimulation of Alexis F. Hartmann, Carl F. Cori, Harry H. Gordon, Victor A. Najjar, and C. R. Park. The other (R. S.) was guided by Daniel C. Darrow, L. Emmett Holt, James L. Gamble, William M. Wallace, Charles S. Davidson and Charles A. Janeway; the M. D. Seminar luncheons of A. Baird Hastings were also a major stimulus. Any advance or success which results from the merging of these two pathways of training and inspiration can be attributed to the excellence of our teachers.

The pioneering investigations of Professor S. Van Creveld have been the model for all further studies and continue to stimulate research in every phase of carbohydrate metabolism. His contributions to this field over four decades have been monumental.

The authors are grateful to many for permission to use published and unpublished data. Any error in interpretation is solely our responsibility.

We wish, first, to thank Dr. Irving Schulman and Dr. Frederick C. Robbins, our department chairmen, whose encouragement and forbearance enabled us to take the time and devote the effort necessary to complete this task. Several conferences with Doctors Robert A. Ulstrom and Henry S. Sauls were invaluable in our attempt to unravel the mysteries of hypoglycemia in infancy and to present a rational approach to diagnosis and therapy. Grateful appreciation is expressed to Professors Andrea Prader and Niilo Hallman and to Doctors E. R. Froesch, S. Auricchio, R. Gitzelmann, and Robert E. Greenberg for use of their manuscripts. Thanks are also due to Doctors Sydney Segal, Giorgio Semenza, and Ira M. Rosenthal for reviewing selected chapters and to Doctors L. Stanley James, Melvin M. Grumbach, James W. Farquhar, Lula O. Lubchenco, John W. Gerrard, and W. A. Cochrane; Professors J. H. Hutchison and R. Zetterström; and Dr. M. G. Hardinge for allowing us to reproduce data and pictures and charts of their patients, some of which have not been published before.

Much of our own work that is reported in this book has been made possible through the collaboration of a number of research associates, trainees, and fellows. For their loyalty and effort we wish to thank Doctors Ephraim Y. Levin, Dimitrios Nicolopoulos, Gloria S. Baens, Susan H. Wybregt, Salomon H. Reisner, Audrey E. Forbes, Russell Snow, Paula B. Mulligan, Malcolm Bowie, Harold Gamsu, Chiung H. Chen, Michael L. McCann and Peter A. J. Adam. Their interest, stimulation, penetrating questions and enthusiasm were always important.

We gratefully acknowledge the expert secretarial assistance and devotion of Mrs. De Lores Stratten and Mrs. Marian Perez. Our thanks are expressed to Mrs. Jane Squires and Miss Gretchen Kruissink of the department of medical illustration at the University of Illinois for preparing the charts and tables. Miss Bernita A. Youngs provided the therapeutic diets in the appendix, and Miss Barbara Millar verified each reference in the bibliography. Finally, we thank Dr. Alexander Schaffer and the Saunders Company for inviting us to participate in this series of monographs.

The research studies of M. C. reported in the monograph were supported in part by a research grant (HD 00235-04) and a training grant (HD 88-02) from the National Institute of Child Health and Human Development and a research grant (6015-04) from the National Institute of Arthritis and Metabolic Disease, National Institutes of Health, United States Public Health Service, as well as by research grants from The National Foundation and the Psychiatric Training and Research Fund of the Illinois Department of Mental Health. The research of R. S. was supported by a research grant (AM 06795-02) and a training grant (TI-AM 5356-03) from the National Institute of Arthritis and Metabolic Diseases, by a Public Health Service Research Career Program Award (K3HD 1488-02) of the National Institute of Child Health and Human Development, and by grants from the Association for Aid to Crippled Children and the Cleveland Diabetes Fund.

MARVIN CORNBLATH
ROBERT SCHWARTZ
1966

PREFACE

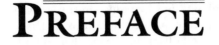

TO THE
THIRD EDITION

In the past 15 years since the second edition, there have been extraordinary advances in developmental biology, molecular physiology, molecular genetics, and microanalytic methodology. The improvements in obstetrical and neonatal care have been dramatic, resulting in the frequent, but not guaranteed, intact survival of "the micropreemie," very low birth weight infants and high-risk sick neonates of gestational ages ranging from 24 to 45 weeks. In addition, there have been major modifications in society, behavior, and attitudes toward research. As a result, this edition, while retaining many of the characteristics of the previous ones, has undergone significant changes.

Emphasis has been placed on the neonate and infant in whom disorders of carbohydrate metabolism occur significantly more frequently than in the toddler, older child, or adolescent. With less data available from human studies, more emphasis has been placed on animal data than was previously the case. In so doing, we have limited the discussion to the specific issues involved. We have not comprehensively reviewed all species whose metabolic regulation has been studied developmentally.

There have been a number of significant changes in the text. The section on methods for analyzing plasma glucose concentrations for both screening and diagnosis has been revised considerably, along with definitions of normal, low, and high plasma glucose values. The previously suggested classification for neonatal hypoglycemia has been discarded. The sections on neonatal hypopituitarism, congenital optic nerve hypoplasia, and hyperinsulinism, as well as that on hyperglycemia, have been expanded significantly. Disorders of fatty acid and amino acid metabolism now have their own chapter in view of the advances in knowledge about those areas. The sections on glycogen storage disease, galactosemia, and hereditary fructose intolerance have been updated, with emphasis on new therapeutic approaches and understanding of their precise genetic mechanisms. More illustrative cases have been added. Another new addition is Appendix I, which addresses those factors that interfere in the analysis of blood glucose concentrations by glucose oxidase methods.

Only a few areas involving the older infant and child have changed. The most dramatic change is the disappearance of such entities as ketotic hypoglycemia unless a specific endocrine deficiency is present. The only area in which there has been a significant problem is the increasing frequency of iatrogenic hypoglycemia involved in the care of the infant or child with insulin-dependent diabetes mellitus (IDDM). The care of the IDDM has been addressed elsewhere and is beyond the scope of this edition. The chapter on disorders of carbohydrate absorption and digestion has been removed as well.

Working on this book has been exciting for us because of the enormous interest of our colleagues throughout the world who have been most generous in sharing their thoughts. We have benefited from and been influenced by their contributions. Many have provided specific useful suggestions and unpublished manuscripts. We are grateful to each and every one of you.

Finally, we wish to express our gratitude to Dr. Derek J. Chadwick, Director of The Ciba Foundation in London, and his excellent staff for assisting us in having a limited-size international conference on Hypoglycemia in Infancy: The Need for a Rational Definition, held in October 1989. This opportunity to discuss problems with basic and clinical scientists provided an added dimension to this monograph.

We both have been fortunate in having the support of the National Institutes of Health throughout our careers, as well as that of a number of local, national, and international organizations and private foundations. We also wish to express our appreciation to the excellent students, residents, fellows, trainees, and colleagues who are and have been so important to us throughout the years. We wish to thank Dr. Robert B. Tudor for sending us his ongoing current updates of the literature related to hypoglycemia.

Finally, we acknowledge with deep appreciation and admiration the expert secretarial assistance and devotion of Ms. Donna Berger.

MARVIN CORNBLATH
ROBERT SCHWARTZ

NOTICE

DISORDERS OF

CARBOHYDRATE

METABOLISM

IN INFANCY

C H A P T E R   1

THE
METABOLISM
OF CARBOHYDRATE

The primary function of carbohydrate in man is to provide energy for cellular metabolism. Specific organs and tissues vary in their glucose requirement, depending upon their energy needs and their ability to utilize other substrates as sources of energy. A variety of controlling mechanisms, including the circulation, transmembrane glucose transport, hormonal interrelationships, and intracellular metabolism also determine the needs of specific organs for glucose. The liver is unique in its ability both to store glucose as glycogen and to provide free glucose, depending upon the availability of carbohydrates and glucose precursors and the needs of the peripheral tissues. In contrast, the brain usually requires a constant supply of glucose, although other substrates such as ketones, glycerol, and lactate can also support a major portion of cerebral metabolism. The level of glucose in the blood reflects a dynamic equilibrium between the glucose input from dietary sources, plus that released from the liver and kidney, and the glucose uptake that occurs primarily in brain, muscle, adipose tissue, and blood elements.

In the fetus, neonate, and young infant, the rapid rate of differentiation, maturation, and growth, along with the increased basal energy requirements and variable physical activity, contribute to the relatively greater caloric requirements during this dynamic period of life. In order to better explain the carbohydrate disorders of infancy, a brief discussion of the general aspects of carbohydrate metabolism is presented. More detailed discussions are available in recent review articles and texts [1–5].

• Sources of Carbohydrate

The fetus receives glucose by continuous infusion transplacentally from the mother; this glucose is probably its major source of energy and its only source of carbohydrate. The precise contributions of alternative energy sources (e.g., free fatty acids, amino acids, ketones) have not been elucidated in the human. At birth, this glucose supply is abruptly terminated, and the newborn must rely on (1) the availability of hepatic glycogen stores and (2) the net hepatic glucose synthesis from amino acids and other precursors (gluconeogenesis). After birth, there is a transition to the utilization of other fuels as well, including free fatty acids, ketones, and additional substrates provided by feeding. The latter include proteins, fat, and complex sugars. The breast-fed infant ingests mainly lactose, while the formula-fed infant may be offered the disaccharide maltose and the polysaccharide dextrin in addition. With the introduction of solid foods, the disaccharide sucrose and another polysaccharide, starch, is provided; the latter ultimately becomes the major source of dietary carbohydrate.

Digestion

Although the human fetus at 3 months' gestation has well-developed digestive enzymes and continually swallows and absorbs amniotic fluid, the relative importance of gastrointestinal absorption in utero as a source of energy is undetermined but is probably not significant [6]. Lactose may supply half of the required carbohydrate in the neonate [7], whereas in the older infant and adult, oligo- and complex polysaccharides in the form of starch are the major sources of carbohydrate. Starch is initially degraded by salivary amylase and later by pancreatic amylase to the disaccharides maltose (glucose-glucose 1,4) and isomaltose (glucose-glucose 1,6), maltotriose and glucose. Maltose, isomaltose, maltotriose, and dietary sucrose (glucose-fructose) are further degraded to free monosaccharides by disaccharidases present in the intestinal brush border (Fig. 1-1). In addition, lactose, a disaccharide of galactose-glucose, is hydrolyzed by the specific enzyme lactase also located in the intestinal brush border. Normally, the activities of the disaccharidases are not rate-limiting for the absorption of disaccharide in the infant [6].

The monosaccharides (glucose, galactose, and fructose) are transported across the intestinal cells to the portal circulation. Glucose and

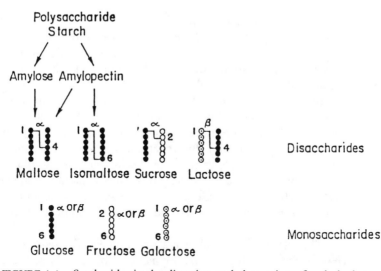

FIGURE 1-1. Saccharides in the digestion and absorption of carbohydrates. (Adapted from Prader, Auricchio, and Semenza. *Monatsschr Kinderheilkd.* 1964; 112:177.)

galactose are actively transported across the cell membrane by specific glycoprotein transporters utilizing an energy-dependent process that involves a phosphorylation-dephosphorylation step. However, fructose and a variety of other sugars (e.g., ribose, xylose) are transported either by facilitated diffusion or by passively crossing the intestinal surface [8]. The relative rates of sugar transport are generally found to be: galactose > glucose > fructose > mannose > xylose.

Distribution

Of the monosaccharides absorbed intact into the portal circulation, almost all the galactose and a major portion of the fructose are removed by the liver [9]. The extent of glucose uptake by the liver varies greatly and depends upon the nutritional status of the individual, the quantity of glucose absorbed, and a variety of hormonal factors [10,11]. Disaccharides, as such, may be absorbed in trace quantities in young infants and appear in the urine [6,12].

The distribution of glucose, whether derived from diet or from the liver via glycogenolysis or gluconeogenesis, is determined by its rate of delivery to tissues by the circulation. Organs rapidly perfused at high blood flow rates include the brain, liver, kidney, and heart. The brain extracts a given amount of glucose per unit time independent of the concentration of glucose in the perfusate as long as a minimum concentration is provided [13]. Glucose enters the liver and kidney in proportion to the extracellular-to-intracellular concentration ratio. Insulin does not appear to control entry of glucose into the cells of the brain or the liver [11]. Uptake may itself be a limiting factor [13].

In contrast, two important tissues, muscle and adipose tissue, are perfused at slower and more variable rates. These tissues extract glucose from the blood at rates dependent upon membrane permeability as influenced by insulin, oxygenation, and substrate concentration. The cellular blood constituents (red cells, white cells, platelets) also play a significant role in the utilization of plasma glucose [11]. Other, more slowly perfused, tissues and organs such as bone and connective tissue do not appear to be quantitatively important in glucose metabolism.

The relative and absolute masses of the various tissues in the body change significantly with development (Table 1-1, Figs. 1-2 and 1-3). The size and proportion of the major organs controlling glucose metabolism, i.e., brain, liver, muscle, and adipose tissue, differ in the fetus and neonate from those in the older child and adult. Friis-Hansen [14] has presented data on total body adipose tissue during human development. During the third trimester of gestation, the amounts of fat and muscle tissue begin to develop significantly. At term, total body fat is approximately 12 percent of the body weight, and total body water is 73 percent; brain, muscle, and liver represent about 12, 25, and 5 percent of body weight, respectively [15].

Following birth, the dramatic changes from the fetal to the extrauterine type of circulation result in a redistribution of the perfusion of substrates. In addition, the availability of multiple substrates and their relationships to hormonal response and metabolic adaptation result in further modification of glucose utilization. Precise requirements of specific organs have not been defined. Isotope dilution studies with labeled dideutero-glucose indicate that basal hepatic glucose production is 4–6 mg/kg/min [16], as contrasted to 2–4 mg/kg/min in the adult [17].

Cahill and his associates [11,18] have calculated that in the normal adult (70 kg) man, under postabsorptive conditions, the brain consumes the largest fraction of total glucose (~50 percent), while the blood elements and muscles both consume about 15 percent. Assuming rates of glucose utilization comparable to that of the adult brain, the newborn brain would require about 6.5 mg/kg/min [19].

Cerebral metabolism in the subhuman newborn primate, baboon, has been studied by Levitsky et al [20] using measurement of cerebral blood flow and arterio-venous (A-V) differences of major substrates, including glucose, acetoacetate, D-betahydroxybutyrate, glycerol, and

TABLE 1-1. Estimation of percent basal metabolic rate (BMR) contributed by brain metabolism (BrMR), liver metabolism (LMR), and muscle metabolism (MMR) at different body and organ weights*

BODY WEIGHT (KG)	TOTAL BMR	BRAIN WEIGHT (KG)	BrMR (KCAL/DAY)	LIVER WEIGHT (KG)	LMR (KCAL/DAY)	MUSCLE MASS (KG)	MMR (KCAL/DAY)	PERCENT TOTAL BMR AS		
								BrMR	LMR	MMR
5.5	300	0.65	192	0.19	55	1.21	21	64	18	7
11.0	590	1.05	311	0.37	107	2.57	45	53	18	8
19.0	830	1.24	367	0.64	186	6.65	117	44	22	14
31.0	1160	1.35	400	0.94	272	11.59	204	35	23	18
50.0	1480	1.36	403	1.17	339	21.20	373	27	23	25
70.0	1800	1.40	414	1.65	478	28.3	500	23	27	28

*Total organ metabolic rates (kcal/day) were derived utilizing the following constant rates in kilocalorie per kilogram organ weight per day: BrMR = 296; LMR = 290; MMR = 17.6. (Modified from Holliday. *Pediatrics* 1971; 47:169.)

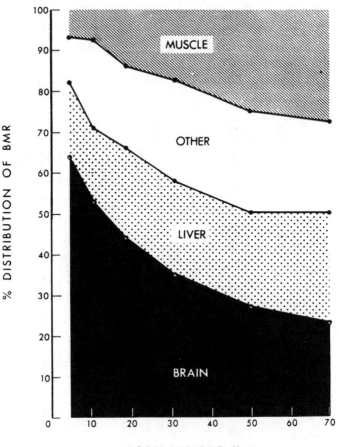

FIGURE 1-2. The changing contribution to basal metabolic rate (BMR) derived from brain, liver, and muscle as percent total BMR as growth proceeds. (See Table 1-1.) (Modified from Holliday. *Pediatrics.* 1971; 47:169.)

lactate. In the first 50 hours of life, uptake of both ketone bodies and lactate occurred.

More recently, Nehlig [21] has studied rats aged 10 days to adult sequentially with the Sokoloff [22] technique of quantitative autoradiographic imaging of 2-¹⁴C-deoxyglucose to evaluate local cerebral metabolism and of ¹⁴C-antipyrine for cerebral blood flow. Average glucose utilization per 100 gm brain weight was low at 10 days (less than half the adult rate) and increased progressively to 35 days. Local cerebral glucose metabolism varied from region to region and progressed at different rates. In contrast, cerebral blood flow was also

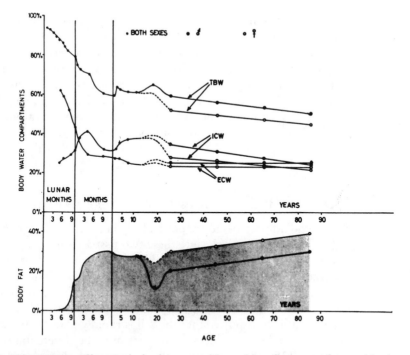

FIGURE 1-3. Changes in body composition with reference to fat, total body water (TBW), extracellular water (ECW), and intracellular water (ICW) from early fetal life to old age. (Modified from Friis-Hansen. *Pediatrics.* 1971; 47:264.)

initially low but achieved adult rates by 17 days, indicating a transient uncoupling between cerebral glucose utilization and cerebral blood flow in the rat. Studies of D-betahydroxybutyrate, measured semi-quantitatively, indicated a high rate of utilization during the suckling period which was maximal at 14 days, but a progressive decrease after weaning until the low rates were found in the adult [23]. Thus, it is apparent that several species have the capacity to metabolize substrate other than glucose in the newborn period.

Recent studies by Chugani et al. [24] using positron emission tomography (PET) with 2-deoxy-2-[^{18}F]-fluoro-D-glucose quantified glucose metabolic rates in specific brain areas. For infants from birth to 1 year, the rates in the cerebral hemisphere were 20.4 ± 1.8 (SD) μM/min/100 gm compared to those in adults at 24.3 ± 1.1 (SD) μM/min/100 gm with a ratio of 0.84. When the infant data are corrected for cerebral mass (335 gm at birth or 925 gm at 1 year), cerebral glucose utilization is estimated to be 20.35 μM/min/100 gm × 335 gm × 180 μg/μM or 12.8 mg/min for 3.5 kg body weight equivalent to 3.66 mg/kg/min. For the adult, comparable glucose utilization estimates are 24.27 μM/min/100 gm × brain weight (1,500 gm) divided by 70 kg body weight equivalent to 0.94 mg/kg/min. When compared to the total body glucose metabolism (see above) of 4–6 mg/kg/min, it is apparent that the newborn has a high glucose requirement because of the large brain mass rather than high glucose consumption per unit tissue. When the source of dietary carbohydrate is limited, as in starvation, the rate of uptake of glucose by muscle, adipose tissue, and the heart is essentially nil, so that the major recipient of the hepatic glucose output is the brain [11,18].

Uptake of Glucose by Muscle and Adipose Tissue

Muscle and adipose tissue are particularly important in the regulation of the blood glucose level, since these two tissues represent the largest portion of the body mass and readily extract glucose from plasma. The transport of glucose across muscle and adipose tissue cell membranes is dependent upon saturation kinetics, competition with other monosaccharides, stereospecificity, and countertransport. Since the glucose that is transported into the cell is rapidly phosphorylated and does not remain free, glucose transport must be differentiated from utilization [25]. Physiologically, the transport of glucose and not its phosphorylation limits glucose uptake [26]. Studies with the nonmetabolizable analogues, 2-deoxyglucose and 3-O-methylglucose, have helped to clarify the specific control mechanisms.

One of the exciting scientific discoveries of the past decade has been the isolation and characterization of a family of specific glucose transporter cDNAs from human tissues. Mueckler et al. [27] initially cloned the glucose transporter cDNA that codes for a 55,000 kd. protein with 12 putative membrane-spanning helices. Presently, four different glucose transport systems are recognized in mammalian cells [28,29]. These are: (1) the constitutively active, facilitative carrier characteristic of human erythrocytes, human hepatoma cells, and rat brain; (2) the sodium-dependent active transporter of kidney and small intestine; (3) the facilitative carrier of rat liver; and (4) the specific insulin-dependent carrier of muscle, heart, and adipose tissue. In resting cells, the insulin-dependent transporter resides primarily in an intracellular compartment and is translocated to the cell surface upon cellular insulin exposure. The cDNAs encoding the major human insulin-responsive glucose transporter have been isolated. This transporter from heart, skeletal muscle, and adipose tissue is a 509-amino acid protein having 65.3, 54.3, and 57.5 percent identity with the erythrocyte/hepatoma liver, and fetal muscle glucose transporters, respectively. The gene was mapped to the short arm p11-p13 of chromosome 17. Current studies are concerned with how glucose and other signals activate the transporter gene and its products as well as what biochemical controls exist for modifying transporter action.

Insulin stimulates glucose transfer across the cell membrane by translocating glucose transporters from the intracellular compartment to the cell surface where their number is increased [30]. In the presence of insulin, the rate of glucose transport is maximal, free glucose may accumulate intracellularly, and phosphorylation of glucose becomes rate-limiting in both muscle [26] and adipose tissue [31]. In adipose tissue, even low concentrations of insulin have a profound effect [32,33]. In muscle, insulin may also stimulate phosphorylation of glucose, but this effect is slower and less pronounced than that on transport [26].

Under normal conditions, muscle and adipose tissue provide sites for the removal and disposal of plasma glucose as controlled primarily by the concentration of circulating insulin and its cellular actions. The biochemical basis of insulin action has rapidly emerged with the isolation and characterization of the cellular insulin receptor [34]. The insulin receptor is a membrane glycoprotein composed of two alpha and two beta subunits joined by three disulfide bonds. When activated by insulin coupling, autophosphorylation occurs, as does increased tyrosine kinase activity, resulting in the presumed phosphorylation of specific target proteins.

Relationship between Glucose and Other Substrates

With the ingestion of food, the blood glucose concentration rises, insulin is released, the hepatic output of glucose is inhibited, and glycogen is stored in liver, muscle, and adipose tissue. Fat synthesis occurs simultaneously. The secretions of growth hormone, glucocorticoids, epinephrine, and glucagon are suppressed (Fig. 1-4).

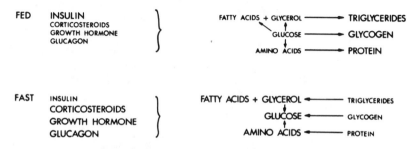

FIGURE 1-4. Substrate-hormone interrelationships in fed and fasted man.

Although a role for gut factors in influencing blood glucose concentration was postulated at the turn of the century, it has only been during the past 20 years that specific hormones and neural mechanisms have been defined (Fig. 1-5) [35]. Unger [36] proposed the term "enteroinsular axis" to encompass (1) endocrine transmission, (2) neurotransmission, and (3) substrate transmission from gut to pancreas. Insulinotropic regulatory gastrointestinal peptides include: gastrin, secretin, cholecystokinin (CCK), vasoactive intestinal peptide (VIP), gastrin releasing peptide (GRP), enteroglucagons, and gastric inhibitory peptide (GIP). Gastrin and secretin do not have insulin stimulation properties at physiological levels, while CCK effects are variable. VIP and GRP are primarily neurotransmitters. The physiologic role of glucagonlike peptides (enteroglucagons) in insulin secretion is presently obscure. Gastric inhibitory peptide has emerged as an important insulin secretory hormone. Oral glucose is a strong stimulus for GIP release, following cellular entry and/or intracellular metabolism in GIP cells of the gut. While galactose and saccharose can also stimulate GIP release, fructose and monosaccharides do not. It has been demonstrated in vivo and in vitro that physiologic concentrations of GIP are insulinotropic and that this effect is glucose-dependent.

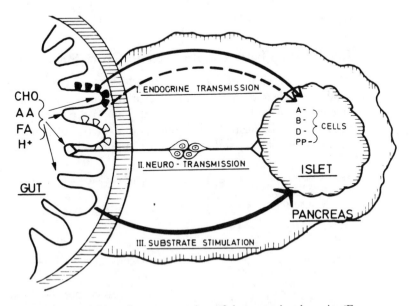

FIGURE 1-5. Schematic representation of the enteroinsular axis. (From Creutzfeldt W. The incretin concept today. *Diabetologia.* 1979; 16:75, with permission.)

In starvation, blood glucose concentrations slowly decrease, with concomitant decreases in the serum insulin levels and elevations of growth hormone, glucagon, and glucocorticoids [18,37]. The increased rate of lipolysis in adipose tissue results in elevated plasma-free fatty acid concentrations which are available for uptake and catabolism by liver, heart, and muscle. The liver metabolizes free fatty acids to ketone bodies, which serve as a major fuel for heart and muscle. During prolonged starvation, the adult brain may obtain some of its energy requirements from ketones [11]. All the enzymes necessary for ketone metabolism are present in the brain at birth [38,39]. In animals, increased supplies of ketone bodies induce the activities of rate-limiting, ketone-utilizing enzymes [40,41]. In the newborn rat, ketones support cerebral metabolism in addition to glucose [23]. Ketone metabolism also affects glycolysis and amino acid metabolism in the developing brain [42,43]. A simultaneous cessation of fatty acid synthesis occurs.

Tissue glycogen stores are depleted, and gluconeogenesis in the liver and kidney increases to provide glucose for the brain, erythrocytes, and renal medulla. Gluconeogenic amino acids in muscle are transaminated to pyruvate, thus providing alanine for gluconeogenesis, i.e., glucose-alanine cycle. Glycerol from lipolysis and lactate from muscle glycolysis also serve as precursors. In addition, the pathways for glucose catabolism in liver, muscle, and adipose tissue are markedly depressed [11,18]. Clearly, the type of diet, number of calories ingested, degree of activity, and overall metabolic requirements of the individual organs are factors influencing the concentration of glucose in the blood.

A close relationship exists between the metabolism of glucose and free fatty acids. Glucose may be the precursor of fatty acids and of glycerol in adipose tissue in the formation of depot triglycerides. Glucose exerts a profound effect on fatty acid mobilization as well [44, 45]. Glucose, directly through metabolism and indirectly by stimulating insulin secretion, suppresses fatty acid catabolism and ketogenesis in both adipose tissue and liver [46]. Hepatic cellular control of triglyceride synthesis versus ketone formation is provided by malonyl CoA which in high concentrations inhibits carnitine acyltransferase I (CAT I) in the mitochondrial membrane and stimulates fatty acid synthesis in the presence of high insulin concentrations [47]. Conversely, increased glucagon and diminished insulin result in decreased malonyl CoA formation with resultant disinhibition of CAT I and production of ketones. A decrease in ketone body production results from a diminished supply of acetyl-CoA, since beta-oxidation of fatty acids is decreased. Glucose also affects fatty acid biosynthesis beyond the simple provision of substrate [45]. One finding suggests that the metabolism of glucose increases the production of alpha-glycero-phosphate, which reacts with fatty acid-CoAs to form triglyceride. This reduces the concentration of fatty acid-CoAs that inhibit acetyl-CoA carboxylase, the rate-limiting step [48,49] in malonyl CoA synthesis which is the committed step in promoting fatty acid synthesis [50].

The effects of free fatty acids on carbohydrate metabolism appear to be more complex and controversial. Randle and his associates have suggested that the rate of glucose catabolism in muscle is decreased by free fatty acids [51,52]. Their experiments have demonstrated both diminished glucose uptake by heart and diaphragm muscle and changes in the levels of glycolytic intermediates. Acetyl-CoA accumulates and then inhibits the pyruvate dehydrogenase complex. Citrate derived from the acetyl-CoA inhibits phosphofructokinase. Glucose-6-phosphate accumulates after phosphofructokinase inhibition and in turn inhibits hexokinase. However, the studies by Kipnis [53] have questioned the significance of these results and their relation to skeletal muscle. In the liver, there is an apparent increase in gluconeogenesis and a decrease in glucose catabolism in the presence of free fatty acids. The alterations in the levels of intermediates and their effects on enzyme activity promote glycogenolysis and decrease glycolysis [52]. Thus, an increase in glucose production by the liver and a reduction in glucose utilization in muscle are synergistic in maintaining the substrate supply to the brain.

• Availability of Hormones in the Fetus and Neonate

The presence of certain hormones in the human fetus and neonate has been studied extensively [54,55]. Some of the major hormones related to the regulation of carbohydrate metabolism are briefly described.

Insulin in the Fetus

Although the ultrastructure of the islets of Langerhans and the mechanism of insulin secretion, as well as the diverse biochemical and physiologic control factors, are summarized carefully in the *Handbook of Physiology* [56], minimal reference is made to the developmental aspects of the human endocrine pancreas. Since the advent of immunochemical techniques, significant advances in the understanding of fetal endocrine control have been made.

The original histologic observations of Robb [57], which described the sequential changes in the human islet beginning with budding from acinar elements at about 10 weeks' gestation and progressing through mantle islets and finally mature islets, have been supplemented by more detailed ultrastructural analyses by Hellman [58] and Orci [59], as well as the histochemical studies by Van Assche [60,61]. At least four types of cells have been identified: (1) B or beta cells, (2) A or alpha cells (segregated into A_1 and A_2 cells by Hellerström and Hellman [62]), (3) D cells that produce gastrin and somatostatin, and (4) PP cells that produce pancreatic polypeptide. Insulin is produced in beta cells, while glucagon is produced in the alpha (A_2) cells. The initial stages of embryogenesis of the pancreas involve formation from the gut of a pancreatic diverticulum, which has a high number of glucagon-containing cells (A cells), before B cell differentiation occurs. During a transition phase described by Pictet and Rutter [63], a dramatic increase in both exocrine and endocrine beta cells occurs. Thereafter, varying cell number and hormone concentrations occur until a mature islet is formed.

Adesanya, Grillo, and Shima [64] found immunologically identified insulin in the human pancreas as early as 12 weeks' gestation, but not at eight weeks. Similar data have been reported by Rastogi [65], Schaeffer [66], Kaplan [67], and Milner [68]. Insulin has been found in human fetal plasma as early as 12 weeks' gestation [69]. Since free maternal insulin does not cross the placenta, fetal plasma insulin must be of fetal origin [70,71].

The biosynthesis of insulin has been elegantly elucidated by Steiner [72], who first described "big" insulin or proinsulin (Figs. 1-6 and 1-7). The initial single-chain molecule of 86 amino acids consists of a continuum from alpha to beta chains with a C-peptide link. During secretion or shortly thereafter, the C-peptide of 31 amino acids is cleaved from the interlinked (S-S) alpha and beta chains. Both C-peptide and insulin can be immunologically identified in the circulation. Proinsulin, the storage form of insulin, has been isolated from the human fetal pancreas [73].

Fetal plasma insulin levels normally do not differ under basal, i.e., short-fasting, conditions from maternal or adult levels [74]. The true fetal plasma insulin levels of the human are currently being determined by cordocentesis (see page 16). Comparisons of fetal umbilical vein and maternal vein plasma glucose and insulin levels after an overnight fast and anesthesia are given in Table 1-2 for early gestation (13 to 18 weeks) compared to full-term after labor and delivery.

Early in gestation, the human fetal pancreas is relatively insensitive to glucose infused to the mother for several hours [75]. At term, however, the fetus in utero is responsive to a continuous glucose stimulus (Fig. 1-8), but there is a delay in the response to an acute glucose load [76–78].

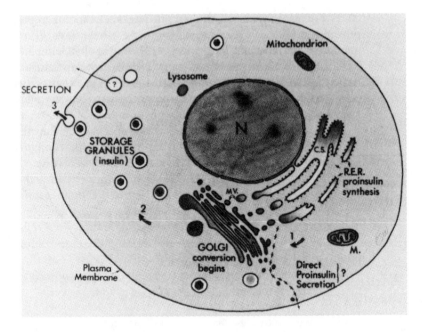

FIGURE 1-6. Subcellular organization (schematic) of the insulin biosynthetic machinery of the B cell. The biosynthesis of proinsulin occurs in the ribosomes in the rough endoplasmic reticulum (RER). The newly formed polypeptide rapidly folds to assume its normal conformation before or during its transit to the Golgi region via the cisternae of the RER and the microvesicles. New secretion granules are formed from the periphery of the Golgi apparatus. Evidence suggests that the transformation of proinsulin to insulin begins to occur in the Golgi apparatus or during the subsequent phase of granule maturation. The transforming enzymes may be added or activated in the Golgi apparatus, or they may be located on the inner surface of the membrane that surrounds the immature secretory granules. As this process occurs, the granules undergo changes in morphology. After about 1 hour, new granules begin to be secreted from the cell by emiocytosis. (From Steiner et al. The biosynthesis of insulin. In: Greep RO, Astwood EB, eds. *Handbook of Physiology,* Section 7, vol. 1. Baltimore: Williams & Wilkins Co., 1972, with permission.)

Arginine administration to the mother either in the second trimester or at term did not elicit a fetal insulin response. However, analysis of the maternal-to-fetal arginine concentration gradient indicated that an adequate fetal insulinogenic arginine concentration may not have been achieved [79].

Milner [80] has studied in vitro fragments of human fetal pancreas obtained from fetuses of 14 to 24 weeks' gestation at hysterotomy. He found glucose to be a poor stimulus for insulin release. However, the beta cell was functional, since insulin release occurred

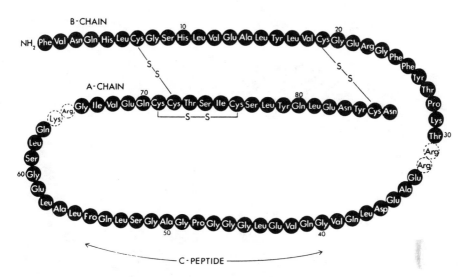

FIGURE 1-7. Amino acid sequence of human proinsulin based on the known structure of human insulin, and of the human C peptide. The basic residues indicated in open circles have been assigned as they are known to occur in bovine and porcine proinsulin. (From Steiner et al. The biosynthesis of insulin. In: Greep RO, Astwood EB, eds. *Handbook of Physiology*, Section 7, vol. 1. Baltimore: Williams & Wilkins Co., 1972, with permission.)

TABLE 1-2. Maternal-fetal glucose and insulin values*

		MATERNAL	FETAL
Early pregnancy	Glucose (mg/100 ml)	70.8 ± 3.3*†	55.5 ± 3.4
(n = 29)	Insulin (μU/ml)	3.7 ± 0.75	4.1 ± 0.47
Term pregnancy	Glucose (mg/100 ml)	91.7 ± 4.0	79.5 ± 3.5
(n = 22)	Insulin (μU/ml)	13.3 ± 2.2	8.0 ± 1.1

*Data of R. Schwartz and associates.
†Values are given as mean ± standard error of the mean.

during incubation with ionic stimuli, potassium or barium [68]. Furthermore, glucagon, theophylline, and dibutyryl adenosine 3':5'-cyclic monophosphate, all of which increased intracellular cyclic-AMP, resulted in insulin secretion into the medium. Finally, leucine acted as an effective insulinogenic stimulus, while arginine did so only in tissue from older fetuses. Milner [81] proposed that normal fetal development and growth depend upon amino acid transport and protein synthesis, which are insulin dependent, whereas glucose homeostasis is achieved by maternal control. Hence, the fetal beta cell is relatively

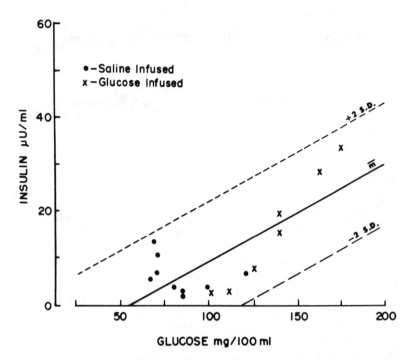

FIGURE 1-8. Relation of blood glucose and plasma insulin in the fetus at term delivery. Mothers were infused with either saline or glucose. (From Obenshain et al. Reprinted, by permission of *The New England Journal of Medicine,* 283;566, 1970.)

insensitive to glucose but is responsive to selected amino acids. Whether the pattern or concentrations of amino acids are sufficient to stimulate insulin release in vivo is unknown. It is more likely that a relatively constant basal level of insulin is maintained which permits glycogenesis, lipogenesis, and protein synthesis to proceed during the second and third trimester.

The advent of the technique for in utero fetal blood sampling without maternal anesthesia has made possible more precise analysis of fetal blood gases, substrates, and hormones. In 1989, Economides et al. [82] reported fetal plasma insulin concentrations in umbilical cord blood from 68 fetuses between 17 and 36 weeks' gestation and with suspected, but later unconfirmed, genetic abnormalities. Mean fetal insulin concentration was 4.5 μU/ml (27 pM) with a range of 1–20 μU/ml (6–120 pM), while simultaneously sampled umbilical venous plasma glucose was 67.9 mg/dl (3.77 mM) with a range of 43–92 mg/dl (2.4–5.1 mM) (see Fig. 1-9). The insulin to glucose ratio was 0.07 and increased with gestation.

AVAILABILITY OF HORMONES IN THE FETUS AND NEONATE

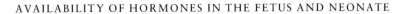

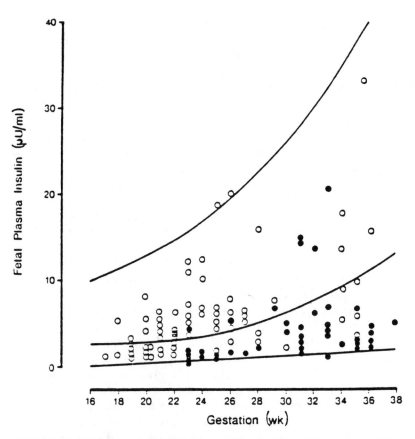

FIGURE 1-9. Reference ranges (mean and 95 percent confidence intervals) of fetal plasma insulin (microunits per milliliter) with gestation. Individual values of AGA (o) and SGA (●) fetuses are also shown. (From Economides DL et al. *Am J Obstet Gynecol.* 1989; 160: 1091, with permission.)

Fetal Glucagon

Glucagon-producing alpha cells develop in the primitive gut and in the early pancreatic anlage by 8 weeks of gestation. The earliest islets have a predominance of alpha over beta cells; however, with maturation, the adult ratio of 3 to 9:1 is approached. The glucagon concentration of the human pancreas has been studied by Assan [83] and found to vary from 1.28 μg/g at eight weeks' gestation to 7.15 μg/g at 25 weeks; this is contrasted with the adult pancreas concentration of 1,000–3,000 μg/g. Although glucagon has been identified in umbilical plasma from term infants [84,85], there is a paucity of data from more immature fetuses; however, three fetuses, ages 15, 25, and

26 weeks, were found to have values in plasma comparable to adults, i.e., 80, 240, and 90 pg/ml [83]. In the human fetus, intraperitoneal arginine had no effect on plasma glucagon concentration [83]. Wise et al. [86] have given intravenous alanine to women in labor at term and prior to delivery and found a significantly elevated value of glucagon in umbilical venous plasma as compared to samples of plasma from control subjects whose mothers received saline. Epstein et al. [87] could not demonstrate fetal alpha cell responsiveness to intravenous alanine or to maternofetal insulin induced hypoglycemia in rhesus monkeys. However, responsiveness to L-dopa was noted [87].

Schaeffer et al. [66] have compared the content and secretion of insulin and glucagon in human fetal pancreas slices in vitro. Neither hormone was present at 25 days of gestation; however, both were detected after 47 days. There was a progressive increase in concentrations of both hormones with increasing gestational age. Incubation with glucose at 300 mg/100 ml (16.7 mM) medium had no effect on the secretion of either hormone, while arginine (5 mM) produced a significant release of both. Interestingly, after gel filtration chromatography, a fraction containing a molecular weight three times that of glucagon and reacting with specific glucagon antibody was found. The analogy to proinsulin may be significant.

Glucagon, like insulin, does not cross the human placenta [88] so that the fetal plasma glucagon must be of fetal origin. By the sixth week of gestation, exogenous glucagon is able to stimulate the accumulation of cyclic AMP in human fetal liver. It can therefore be inferred that the entire cellular pathway (receptor–G protein–adenylate cyclase [see below]) is present and functional. This establishes the fact that the glucagon receptor and the adenylate cyclase system are responsive at this early stage of development [89,90].

Sperling et al. [91] observed a significant increase in pancreatic glucagon in plasma immediately after birth when blood glucose concentration decreased. Levels were stable from 2–24 hours but rose further from day 1 to day 3 of life. Following formula feeds, a marked rise in glucagonlike immunoreactivity occurred.

Fetal Growth Hormone

In a detailed study, Kaplan et al. [67] measured the content and concentration of immunoreactive growth hormone in 117 human fetal pituitary glands from 68 days of gestation to term. In the fetal pituitary gland, the content of growth hormone rose progressively from mean levels of 0.44 ± 0.2 μg at 10 to 14 weeks of gestation to 675 ± 112 μg at 35 to 40 weeks. The human growth hormone (HGH) content correlated positively with gestational age, crown–rump length, and weight of the pituitary gland. The youngest fetus studied (70 days' gestation) had immunoreactive HGH in plasma at a concentration of 14.5 ng/ml. Maximal plasma concentrations were found at 15 to 24 weeks' gestation, with significantly lower levels in the more mature fetus. It was suggested that the appearance and development of the secretory capacity for HGH by the human fetal pituitary gland coincided with developmental changes in the portal system and hypothalamus (Fig. 1-10).

Human growth hormone does not cross the human placenta [92,93]. Although the normally high levels in the preterm and term infant cannot be suppressed by hyperglycemia [94], increased values occur following hypoglycemia. Fetal growth hormone is not necessary for growth in utero.

The paradoxical release of growth hormone by hyperglycemia in

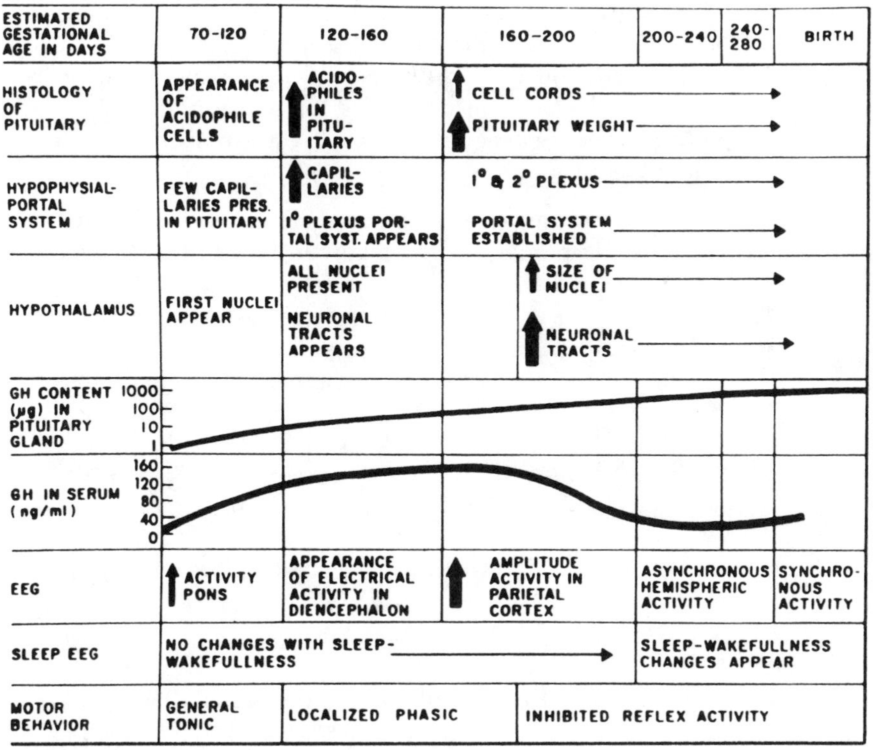

ESTIMATED GESTATIONAL AGE IN DAYS	70-120	120-160	160-200	200-240	240-280	BIRTH
HISTOLOGY OF PITUITARY	APPEARANCE OF ACIDOPHILE CELLS	↑ACIDO-PHILES IN PITU-ITARY	↑ CELL CORDS ———————→ ↑PITUITARY WEIGHT—————→			
HYPOPHYSIAL-PORTAL SYSTEM	FEW CAPIL-LARIES PRES. IN PITUITARY	↑CAPIL-LARIES I° PLEXUS POR-TAL SYST. APPEARS	I° & 2° PLEXUS ——————→ PORTAL SYSTEM ESTABLISHED ——————→			
HYPOTHALAMUS	FIRST NUCLEI APPEAR	ALL NUCLEI PRESENT NEURONAL TRACTS APPEARS	↑SIZE OF NUCLEI —————→ ↑NEURONAL TRACTS —————→			
GH CONTENT (µg) IN PITUITARY GLAND	1000 100 10 1					
GH IN SERUM (ng/ml)	160 120 80 40 0					
EEG	↑ACTIVITY PONS	APPEARANCE OF ELECTRICAL ACTIVITY IN DIENCEPHALON	↑AMPLITUDE ACTIVITY IN PARIETAL CORTEX	ASYNCHRONOUS HEMISPHERIC ACTIVITY	SYNCHRO-NOUS ACTIVITY	
SLEEP EEG	NO CHANGES WITH SLEEP-WAKEFULLNESS ——————————→			SLEEP-WAKEFULLNESS CHANGES APPEAR		
MOTOR BEHAVIOR	GENERAL TONIC	LOCALIZED PHASIC	INHIBITED REFLEX ACTIVITY			

FIGURE 1-10. The ontogeny of HGH secretion by the human fetus as correlated with histologic changes in the pituitary and the development of the portal system and central nervous system. (From Kaplan, Grumbach, and Shepard. Reproduced from the *Journal of Clinical Investigation*, 1972; 51:3080, by copyright permission of the American Society of Clinical Investigation.)

the fetus has been demonstrated following glucose infusion to the pregnant woman by Wolf [95] and to the pregnant monkey by Mintz [96]. Arginine infusion directly into the circulation of the fetal monkey produced no consistent rise in growth hormone [96]. Similarly, arginine had no effect on HGH levels in the human fetus at midterm but resulted in a doubling of plasma HGH in the term fetus.

Grumbach [67,97] hypothesized that neuroendocrine control of growth hormone secretion is related to the development of the release of growth hormone releasing factor (GRF) and growth hormone inhibiting factor as shown (Fig. 1-11):

1. Early in gestation (7 to 10 weeks), there is no circulatory linkage between the median eminence and the adenohypophysis by the portal system, so that the secretion of HGH is either autonomous or only in part regulated by GRF.
2. By midgestation, the portal system develops, and a relatively unrestrained tonic release of GRF results in intense stimulation of HGH secretion by the pituitary acidophils.
3. Late in gestation (30 to 40 weeks), neuroinhibitory influences develop, which are possibly related to the maturation of the hypothalamic monoaminergic neuronal network or to the stimulation of GIF or suppression of GRF.

Autonomic control, alpha adrenergic enhancement, and beta inhibition of HGH release may also be important factors.

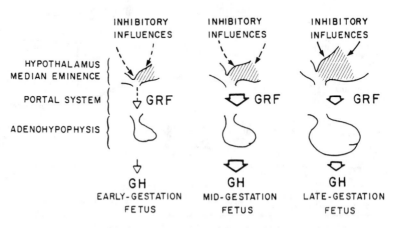

FIGURE 1-11. Graphical representation of the development of regulatory mechanisms for control of HGH secretion in the human fetus. (From Grumbach, Kaplan. In: Gluck L, ed. *Modern Perinatal Medicine.* Chicago: Year Book Medical Publishers, Inc., 1974; 247, with permission.)

Other Fetal Growth Factors

Insulinlike Growth Factors

Formerly known as somatomedins (A and C), these are now identified as insulinlike growth factor I[1] (IGF-I [somatomedin-C]) and insulinlike growth factor II (IGF-II) [98].

Insulinlike growth factor I has been characterized as being an intermediary of growth hormone action on skeletal tissue and as having growth-promoting or insulinlike effects on many other tissues. It is produced in the liver under the influence of growth hormone [99]. Growth rates in normal children correlate with concentrations of IGF-I in plasma. Plasma levels have been low in hypopituitarism and high in acromegaly. In the Laron-type dwarf, HGH values were normal, whereas IGF-I levels were low and did not respond to HGH [100]. Hintz, Seeds, and Johnsonbaugh [101] have evaluated IGF-I levels and growth hormone concentrations in maternal and fetal cord plasma. As noted previously, growth hormone levels were much higher in the fetus than in the mother; however, IGF-I levels were similar in both groups. No significant correlation between IGF-I and growth hormone levels in cord plasma were noted. The low IGF-I levels noted in cord plasma, which were comparable to those in nonpregnant adults, suggested an increased end organ sensitivity in the fetus. During postnatal life, the growth hormone dependency of IGF-I is well documented [102,103]. Thyroxine appears important in the maintenance of serum IGF-I. Nutritional status is another important factor in regulation of the IGFs.

Insulinlike growth factors I and II are important mitogens [98,102]. They may exhibit insulinlike effects, such as increasing glucose transport, oxidation, and lipogenesis in some experimental systems. Because these effects usually have been observed only at high concentrations, they have been considered pharmacologic rather than physiologic actions. These may well be dependent on the target-cell type and developmental stage.

A multitude of specific growth factors from diverse tissues have been identified and chemically characterized. Their role is beyond the scope of this text. The following enumerates a few: transforming growth factors alpha and beta, nerve growth factor, epidermal growth factor, multiplication stimulating factor, platelet derived growth factor, tumor necrosis factor, etc.

Both insulinlike growth factor I and epidermal growth factor have

---

[1]IGF-I is used synonymously with sulfation factor and somatomedin-C in this section.

been found to stimulate glycogen synthesis in fetal rat hepatocytes [103].

Catecholamines

Catecholamines are present in the human fetus in the adrenal medulla and the organs of Zuckerkandl (para-aortic bodies), the latter being the major source of norepinephrine [104]. The catecholamine concentration of these tissues increases during gestation, with maximal levels present at about 20 weeks [105], and with the norepinephrine concentration of liver being comparable to that of the adult. Joelsson and Adamsons [106] and Sandler and associates [107] have demonstrated that catecholamines cross the placenta by midgestation.

Eliot et al. [108] have studied plasma concentrations of the catecholamines (CAT) epinephrine (E) and norepinephrine (NE) during the first 48 hours of life. Umbilical plasma CAT were similarly elevated in term infants delivered by cesarean section or vaginally. Umbilical arterial concentrations of both E and NE exceeded those in umbilical venous samples. NE concentrations exceeded E concentrations throughout the initial 48 hours of life, even though marked decreases occurred in both.

In a study of 12 normoglycemic preterm neonates at 2 hours of age, Pryds et al. [109] observed plasma epinephrine to be 0.24 ng/ml (range 0.01–0.95 ng/ml) while norepinephrine was 0.77 ng/ml (0.25–1.84 ng/ml).

Corticosteroids

The adrenal gland represents the major steroidogenic organ in the human fetus [110]. Diczfalusy emphasized that both the fetus and placenta as the fetoplacental unit are necessary for the overall synthesis of steroid hormones [54,55]. Hence, the fetal adrenals (though not the placenta) synthesize cholesterol, which is then converted to progesterone by the placenta (and to some extent by the fetal adrenal) and finally to corticosteroids by the fetal adrenal. These enzymatic reactions are all functioning at high activity in early gestation in the human. In addition to the complexity of the fetoplacental unit, most neutral steroids readily cross the placenta unaltered (e.g., cortisol), while the conjugated forms are transferred only to a limited extent [111]. Glucocorticoid is important for fetal glycogenesis [90] (see below).

Maternal plasma concentrations of cortisol are several times higher than fetal concentrations. Cord plasma 17-hydroxycorticosteroid is higher in vaginally delivered compared to elective cesarean section delivered infants. Serial plasma cortisol measurements have been reported for normal infants during the first 3 days of life by Gutai et al. [112]. Elevated concentrations decrease from levels of 12–14 µg/dl in cord plasma to 4.3 ± 2.6 (SD) µg/dl after 6 hours of age. Infants responded to intramuscular adrenocorticotropic hormone (ACTH) with a twofold rise in 2 hours. Since a very large proportion of cortisol is bound to transcortin (steroid binding protein), these data do not permit comment on the small amount of free cortisol.

Kenny et al. [113] studied cortisol production rates (CPR) in normal infants, children, and adults. CPR was 18.3 ± 3.6 mg/M²/day in 14 full-term, vaginally delivered infants. These rates were significantly greater than those found in infants over 5 days of age (14.0 ± 2.9 mg/M²/day). The latter were similar to values in older children and adults.

Thyroid Hormones

Fisher et al. [114,115] have extensively studied human maternal-fetal thyroid hormone interrelationships during development, beginning at 11 weeks' gestation. During pregnancy, maternal serum values for T_4 were characteristically elevated and were similar at 11 to 18 weeks, 22 to 34 weeks, and at term. However, free thyroxine levels in maternal serum were significantly higher at 11 to 18 weeks than at term. Maternal thyroid stimulating hormone (TSH) concentrations were similar to those in euthyroid, nonpregnant subjects. In contrast, fetal serum T_4 and free T_4 concentrations were low between 11 and 18 weeks and increased progressively between 22 weeks and term. Thyroxine appeared in serum and amniotic fluid at about the fifteenth week of gestation and increased thereafter. Most of the T_4 was bound to protein in all three compartments (maternal blood, fetal blood, and amniotic fluid). Free T_4 in amniotic fluid did not correlate with either maternal or fetal serum-free T_4. T_3 was unmeasurable in amniotic fluid, although present in cord serum.

Fetal serum TSH concentrations were low between 11 and 18 weeks of pregnancy but seemed to increase abruptly between 18 and 22 weeks to levels similar to those of term infants. TSH in term fetal serum exceeded that in maternal serum.

The placenta appears to be essentially impermeable to thyroid hormones. Using sensitive radioimmunoassay techniques, Sack et al. [116] have found the mean concentrations at term shown in Table 1-3. Abuid et al. [117] have also noted low free T_3 levels at term in cord serum compared to that in maternal serum. These changes during development have been correlated with maturation of the fetal

TABLE 1-3. Mean concentrations of thyroid hormones*

	THYROXINE (μg/100 ml)	FREE THYROXINE (ng 100/ml)	TRIIODOTHYRONINE (ng 100/ml)
Maternal	11.25 ± 0.82†	2.56 ± 0.32	201 ± 16.2
Cord	9.31 ± 0.29	2.67 ± 0.33	55 ± 7.5
Amniotic fluid	0.64 ± 0.07	4.13 ± 0.49	15

*Data was taken from Reference 116.
† Values are given as mean ± standard error of the mean.

hypothalamic-pituitary TSH control system, which appears to mature between 18 and 22 weeks.

• Biochemical Mechanisms of Glucose Regulation

The mechanisms controlling the production of glucose by the mammalian liver involve a variety of control points. Although the metabolism of the adult liver has been studied extensively, this discussion contrasts observations in fetal and neonatal liver with those in the adult. Particular attention should be given to species' differences that occur during development.

The production of glucose by the liver involves two major processes: (1) release of glucose from preformed stores (i.e., glycogen breakdown) and (2) the synthesis de novo from smaller carbon units (i.e., gluconeogenesis). This latter mechanism can be subdivided into (1) the uptake of substrate by the hepatocytes from the blood, (2) the conversion of this substrate into three-carbon fragments from which glucose can be synthesized, (3) the synthesis of glucose from these three-carbon units, and (4) the release of glucose from the liver (Fig. 1-12).

Glycogen Metabolism

The accumulation of glycogen in the mammalian liver during fetal development was first observed by Claude Bernard in 1859 [118]. Since that initial observation, this phenomenon has been described in all mammalian species that have been examined [119,120]. In most species, glycogen only begins to accumulate just before birth (e.g., 3 days before term in the rat); however, in the human, glycogen begins to accumulate in the fetal liver beginning at about the thirteenth week of gestation [121], although it can be detected in liver from much younger fetuses [122]. Glycogen concentrations are approximately 36

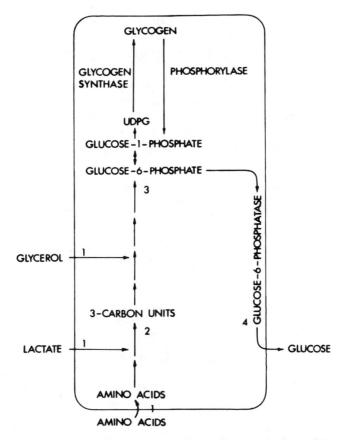

FIGURE 1-12. Pathways for glucose production in the hepatocyte. The numbers refer to each of the major steps in gluconeogenesis (see text): (1) uptake of substrate, (2) conversion to functional 3-carbon units, (3) synthesis of glucose-6-phosphate from these functional units, and (4) release of glucose via glucose-6-phosphatase.

mg/g liver at 20 weeks' gestation. Nonetheless, in all species, the high glycogen concentration is rapidly depleted in the first few hours of life [123]. The concentration of glycogen in the liver of an adult man under fed conditions is approximately 40–60 mg/g, which can be readily mobilized to provide glucose for immediate circulation.

The activation of the enzyme systems for glycogen breakdown and the simultaneous inactivation of the enzyme systems for glycogen synthesis are primarily thought to be responsible for increasing blood glucose concentration. In the adult, phosphorylase (the rate-limiting step of breakdown) is activated, while glycogen synthase (the rate-limiting step of synthesis) is inactivated [124]. The signals most clearly responsible for this mobilization of glycogen are glucagon and cate-cholamines, via cyclic AMP. Hormone-receptor complex in the membrane interact in a yet-to-be-defined manner with the G protein complex. Transformation of G_s:GTP to G_s:GDP results in activation of adenylate cyclase [125]. Although the mechanism has been described most clearly in rabbit muscle, a similar process occurs in mammalian liver (Fig. 1-13). The stimulation of membrane-bound adenylate cyclase leads to an increased synthesis of cyclic AMP. Accumulation within the hepatocyte provides enough of this cyclic nu-

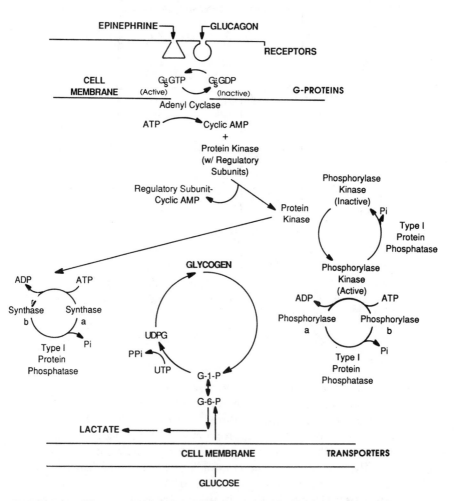

FIGURE 1-13. Hormonal regulation of glycogen metabolism via cyclic AMP. This schema omits release of glucose from the liver, as well as the mechanism(s) for branching and debranching of glycogen. The newly recognized phosphoinositide cascade has also been omitted.

cleotide for binding to the regulatory subunit of protein kinase A (phosphorylase kinase kinase or cyclic AMP-dependent protein kinase) which detaches from the catalytic subunit, thereby rendering it effective and capable of catalyzing the conversion of phosphorylase kinase from a dephosphorylated (inactive) form to an active phosphorylated enzyme in the presence of Mg^{++} and ATP [126]. The phosphorylase kinase then activates phosphorylase by a similar phosphorylation in the presence of Mg^{++} and ATP [127]. The end result of this enzymatic cascade provides active phosphorylase for the breakdown of glycogen.

Simultaneously, the "activation" of protein kinase (presumably the same enzyme involved in phosphorylase activation) acts on a second liver substrate, glycogen synthase a, and inactivates it by a similar phosphorylation reaction, converting it into glycogen synthase b [128]. This reaction provides for a decrease in the synthesis of glycogen.

Another important system for controlling several metabolic processes (including glycogenolysis in liver) is known as the phosphoinositide cascade [129]. Briefly, a specific enzyme, phospholipase C, hydrolyzes phosphatidyl inositol 4,5-bisphosphate into two messengers: inositol 1,4,5-trisphosphate (IP_3) and diacylglycerol. IP_3 mobilizes cytosolic Ca^{++}, which stimulates glycogenolysis. The other messenger, diacylglycerol, enhances this process by activating the enzyme protein kinase C, which in turn inactivates glycogen synthase by phosphorylation.

G protein carries the excitation signal from the activated receptor to phosphoinositidase (phospholipase C). It is apparent then that at least two distinct processes involving G proteins are involved in glycogen synthesis and degradation [125].

Insulin antagonizes the effects of glucagon, epinephrine, and cyclic AMP on hepatic glycogen metabolism in the adult. This hormone has been shown to activate glycogen synthase indirectly [124] and simultaneously inactivate phosphorylase [130]. The mechanism of insulin action in this system involves activation of glycogen-associated type I protein phosphatase [131,132].

Type I protein phosphatase is now recognized as an important controlling enzyme of glycogen metabolism. It dephosphorylates the active form of phosphorylase kinase and phosphorylase a and the inactive form of glycogen synthase [131,132]. The glycogen-bound form of type I protein phosphatase consists of the type I phosphatase catalytic subunit and a glycogen-binding component that is a substrate for protein kinase A [131,132]. Presumably, insulin stimulates glycogen synthesis via phosphatase activation and prevents the breakdown of glycogen. Corticosteroid administration acutely increases hepatic glycogen content [133], a fact that has been attributed to an increase in the conversion of glycogen synthase b to a [134], although some investigators have related this increase to an increase in total glycogen synthase activity [135]. Furthermore, steroids produce a small decrease in phosphorylase activity secondary to an increase in phosphorylase phosphatase activity. DeWulf and Hers have postulated that the induction of phosphorylase phosphatase is the initial steroid-mediated enzymatic alteration [134]. This increased phosphorylase phosphatase activity relieves active phosphorylase inhibition of glycogen synthase b to a conversion, thus promoting glycogen synthase a activity [136]. In summary, corticosteroids promote a rapid accumulation of hepatic glycogen, presumably via an increase in glycogen synthase a activity.

Other factors and their possible roles as intracellular effectors in the regulation of glycogen metabolism in the adult have attracted much attention. Glucose, glucose-6-phosphate, ATP, inorganic phosphate (P_i), and Mg^{++}, as well as a variety of other cellular intermediates have been documented to affect glycogen synthase activity in adult muscle and liver [128,137,138]. Similarly, glucose, ATP, AMP, P_i, and so forth, have profound effects on phosphorylase activity in adult muscle and liver [131,138,139]. In general, these effectors act in concert to promote glycogen accumulation or depletion.

During development in most species, the appearance of glycogen synthase precedes the accumulation of hepatic glycogen stores [140,141], whereas phosphorylase either does not change appreciably during this time or is low in activity. The relative changes in glycogen synthase a and active phosphorylase may be the major controlling factors, since both forms of these two key enzymes are not necessarily important physiologically. During development of the human fetal liver, a large portion of the total phosphorylase is available for activation [89,122]. However, in this same tissue, glycogen synthase a activity is low and constant, while the b form activity increases parallel to the accumulation of glycogen [122]. Furthermore, since the hepatic concentration of glucose-6-phosphate is high (0.4–0.7 mM), the b form of glycogen synthase may be important in the storing of glycogen in fetal liver. In addition, during the initial two-thirds of gestation, the hepatic cellular concentrations of certain metabolic intermediates change, in that the stimulators of glycogen synthase b activity increase and the major inhibitor (inorganic phosphate) decreases [122].

Glycogen stores in human fetal liver are susceptible to hormonal regulation as early as the sixth week of gestation [122]. Glucagon, catecholamines, and cyclic AMP are all capable of promoting a rapid and dramatic depletion of human fetal liver glycogen. In contrast to the adult, a decrease in glycogen synthase activity is associated with no alteration in phosphorylase activity. Insulin, on the other hand, promotes the opposite effects [122]. Corticosteroids have not been examined for effects on human fetal liver glycogen metabolism. However, corticosteroids are required for fetal liver glycogen deposition in animals [140], presumably by effecting an increase in glycogen synthase activity [135,142]. From studies of fetal rat liver, Gruppuso and Brautigan [143] concluded that the late gestational rise in fetal hepatic glycogen content is not dependent on the coincidental increase in fetal insulin concentrations but is best correlated with induction of glycogen synthase. Type I protein phosphatase activities were found in advance of glycogen synthesis and thus are unlikely to be regulatory. On the basis of studies of glycogen regulation in isolated perfused near-term monkey fetal liver, Sparks et al. [144] speculated that galactose may be uniquely important for neonatal glycogen synthesis. The lactose content of milk may be important to the repletion of glycogen in the liver shortly after birth.

Studies of human fetal muscle glycogen metabolism are not available. However, examination of the development of muscle glycogen synthase in the primate fetus indicates a parallel increase in the form b activity and the accumulation of glycogen in the presence of a very low form a activity [145]. Furthermore, epinephrine is capable of depleting glycogen in this tissue in vitro, while insulin produces the opposite effect [146].

Although glycogen synthase and phosphorylase are considered the rate-limiting steps in the synthesis and breakdown of glycogen, other enzymatic steps are necessary to complete either of these processes [147]. Branching enzyme is required for the introduction of new branch points before additional glucose units can be added by glycogen synthase. Similarly, the debrancher complex transfers and removes glucose units so as to expose and eliminate the branch point, thereby allowing phosphorylase to further degrade the molecule. Under normal conditions, the brancher/debrancher system does not appear to limit synthesis or degradation. However, under altered physiologic and pathologic states, these enzyme activities are important in the overall regulation of glycogen metabolism. The traditional view that following a fast and ingestion of carbohydrate, glucose is a major hepatic substrate and serves as a direct precursor for glycogen has been recently reviewed [148]. Evidence has accumulated that gluconeogenic substrates such as fructose, glycerol, or lactate may be preferentially utilized by liver for glycogen synthesis.

Uptake of Substrate

The uptake of glucose, lactate, pyruvate, amino acids, and glycerol by the liver is necessary for glycogenosis and gluconeogenesis. Glucose is taken up so rapidly that the liver is considered freely permeable to it. The rapid stereospecific carrier-mediated transport previously proposed [149] is now attributed to a specific glycoprotein glucose transporter (vide supra) [27]. Conversion to glucose-6-phosphate is under the control of hexokinase and ATP at low plasma glucose concentrations. However, at high glucose concentrations (as after a meal), glucokinase, which has a high Km for glucose, is operative [150]. Although gluconeogenesis from glycerol does take place in the liver, quantitatively it is of small magnitude [151]. Lactate and pyruvate cross the hepatocyte membrane freely, although critical examination of this point is lacking.

Uptake of amino acids for gluconeogenesis is thought to provide a major control point in the regulation of substrate supply to the liver. Studies by Felig and his associates [152] have demonstrated that the primary amino acid released by muscle is alanine. During fasting in an adult man, femoral arteriovenous differences of alanine are more than three times greater than of other amino acids [152] and account for about 30 percent of the total amino acid output from muscle [153]. Furthermore, of the total amino acid uptake by the splanchnic bed of fasting man, alanine accounts for over 50 percent [153]. This figure is corroborated by the studies of Ross, Hems, and Krebs [154], in which the rate of glucose production from alanine was found to be among the highest reported for any amino acid. Thus, alanine appears to be a key amino acid substrate for de novo hepatic glucose synthesis [152]. Adult liver in vitro or in vivo can actively take up amino acids of the alanine group (e.g., α-aminoisobutyrate). This process can be stimulated by glucagon, epinephrine, cyclic AMP, insulin, and corticosteroids [155–158]. The mechanisms responsible for these alterations in amino acid uptake are at present unresolved. The release of alanine and glutamine from muscle may involve multiple mechanisms, including transamination and proteolysis, as well as specific carriers [159,160].

Uptake of substrate by the fetal liver has not been studied in detail. Dancis et al. [161] infused α-aminoisobutyrate into pregnant guinea pigs and demonstrated its accumulation in the placenta and maternal liver but not in the fetal liver. Hill and Young [162] have also surveyed the mechanisms of amino acid transport across the placenta. In general, all these studies have demonstrated that all the essential and nonessential amino acids can be transferred by active transport across the mammalian placenta against a concentration gradient.

In human fetal liver, the accumulation of α-aminoisobutyrate has been observed as early as the sixth week of gestation [163]. This uptake was decreased by alanine and was stimulated by both glucagon and insulin [163].

Three-Carbon Units

In the perfused rat liver, physiologically significant rates of gluconeo-genesis have been reported for only alanine, serine, threonine, and glycine, although other amino acids are potentially gluconeogenic [154]. Conversion of alanine or other substrate into functional three-carbon fragments by the liver is accomplished by specific enzymes, e.g., alanine transaminase. Although definitive studies have not appeared, this enzyme may not be rate-limiting in the overall process.

Compared to the adult, fetal rat liver has very low activities of alanine transaminase, aspartate transaminase, serine dehydratase, tyrosine transaminase, and phenylalanine hydroxylase [164]. These activities may limit the flow of substrate to functional three-carbon units for glucose synthesis. The scant data available for the human fetal liver indicate that patterns for enzyme development generally are not similar to those in other species, especially the rat (e.g., phenyl-alanine hydroxylase [165], tyrosine transaminase [166], and the enzymes for metabolism of sulfur-containing amino acids [167]. Whether any of these activities may be considered rate-limiting is unclear at present.

Gluconeogenesis

Gluconeogenesis from functional three-carbon fragments occurs within the hepatocyte (Fig. 1-14). There are a variety of controls operative at different levels, some of which are mentioned below. Intracellular localization or compartmentalization of the events in gluconeogenesis provides one major area for metabolic control. For example, pyruvate entry into mitochondria is stimulated by catecholamines, glucagon, and steroids [168]. The transmitochondrial passage of α-ketoglutarate and glutamate, as well as other energy-yielding substrates, may provide further control [151].

Enzyme activity, specificity, and localization provide additional control. Phosphoenolpyruvate (PEP) carboxykinase is thought by many to be a major control point, since it is located both in the mitochondrial and cytosolic fractions in human liver [151]. Furthermore, the low activity of this enzyme relative to other gluconeogenic enzymes is suggestive of a rate-limiting step. Increases in this enzyme's activity have been demonstrated, however, after administration of cyclic AMP, glucagon, catecholamines, and steroids [169–172]. Insulin, in contrast, has been shown to suppress PEP carboxykinase activity [172]. Shrago and associates have discussed the control of this enzyme by substrate and amino acids [173].

Many other enzyme activities involved in gluconeogenesis are also

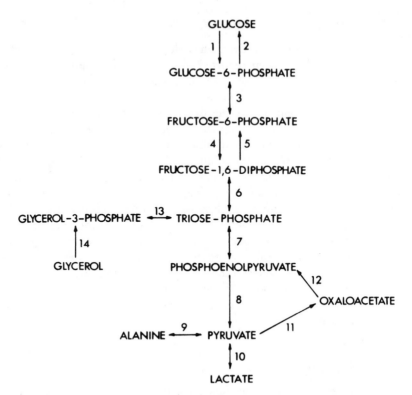

FIGURE 1-14. A simplified view of gluconeogenesis. The numbers refer to the following enzymes: (1) Hexokinase and glucokinase, (2) glucose-6-phosphatase, (3) glucose-6-phosphate isomerase, (4) phosphofructokinase, (5) fructose-1,6-diphosphatase, (6) aldolase, (7) triose phosphate isomerase, phosphoglyceraldehyde dehydrogenase, phosphoglycerate kinase, phosphoglyceromutase, and enolase, (8) pyruvate kinase, (9) alanine transaminase, (10) lactate dehydrogenase, (11) pyruvate carboxylase, (12) phosphoenolpyruvate carboxykinase, (13) glycerophosphate dehydrogenase, and (14) glycerokinase.

specifically regulated. Pyruvate carboxylase is allosterically regulated by acetyl CoA. Pyruvate kinase exists in multiple forms in mammalian liver [174] and is regulated allosterically by fructose-1,6-diphosphate. Fructose-1,6-diphosphatase may be controlled allosterically (e.g., adenine nucleotides) [151], as well as by steroids [175]. Glucose-6-phosphatase regulation is discussed on page 35.

Recently, a new intermediate, fructose-2,6-bisphosphate (F2,6P) has been discovered that can regulate the flow of intermediates involved in hepatic gluconeogenesis and glycolysis at the unidirectional reactions between fructose-6-phosphate and fructose-1,6-biphosphate (Fig. 1-15) [176,177]. This intracellular regulator (F2,6P) is synthesized

BIOCHEMICAL MECHANISMS OF GLUCOSE REGULATION

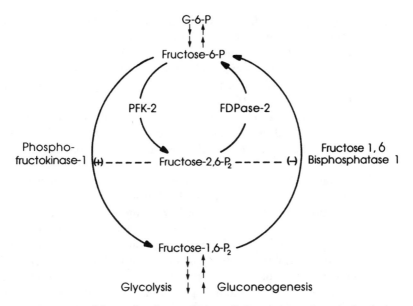

FIGURE 1-15. Schema for the regulation of gluconeogenesis and glycolysis via the intermediate, fructose-2,6-bisphosphate. G-6-P is glucose-6-phosphate; PFK-2 is phosphofructokinase-2; FDPase-2 is fructose diphosphatase-2.

from fructose-6-phosphate under the control of 6-phosphofructo-2-kinase (PFK-2) and fructose bisphosphatase-2 (FDPase-2), activities that reside on the same protein and are regulated by cyclic AMP-dependent protein phosphorylation. In the presence of increased glucose, F2,6P activates phosphofructokinase-1 and inhibits fructose bisphosphate-1, thus inhibiting gluconeogenesis.

These events present a picture of overall gluconeogenic regulation as being stimulated by catecholamines and glucagon via cyclic AMP, decreased by insulin and modulated by corticosteroids [177].

In the fetal rat liver, overall gluconeogenesis from amino acids is virtually absent and develops only some hours after birth [178,179]. In contrast, the midterm fetal sheep liver performs gluconeogenesis at approximately 30 percent of the rate found in the postnatal or adult liver [180].

An important difference for gluconeogenesis among species is the time of appearance of PEP carboxykinase. This enzyme's activity is not detectable in the rat until just prior to birth [178], whereas it is relatively active in fetal dog liver [181]. Another possible control point is that of substrate translocation from the mitochondrion into cytosol and mitochondrial CO_2 fixation [168]. The development of gluconeogenesis has been correlated with the appearance of mitochondrial

CO_2 fixation in the newborn dog [181]. Furthermore, pyruvate carboxylase may be more rate-limiting than PEP carboxykinase in this species [181,182]. This pattern of metabolic maturity is similar to that in the neonatal pig [183–186] but different from that seen in the neonatal rat, in which the development of gluconeogenesis parallels the appearance of PEP carboxykinase activity following birth [187].

Intracellular localization of limiting events has not been explored in human fetal liver, although many of the enzymes of gluconeogenesis have been detected in this tissue: PEP carboxykinase [188,189], pyruvate carboxylase [188], and glucose-6-phosphatase [190,191]. However, development of relative activities of these enzymes has not been clearly established in the human fetal liver.

Studies with fetal rat liver have demonstrated that many of these enzymes are capable of being hormonally regulated either in vivo or in organ culture. Cyclic AMP, glucagon, and epinephrine have been shown to stimulate activity of PEP carboxykinase in utero [178], of glucose-6-phosphatase in utero [192], and of tyrosine transaminase both in utero [193] and in organ culture [194]. Insulin has been shown to decrease PEP carboxykinase [172] and glucose-6-phosphatase [195] and to stimulate tyrosine transaminase activities in fetal liver explants [194].

Studies by Räihä and Schwartz [166] and by Kirby and Hahn [189,196] on human fetal liver explants have suggested that some enzyme activities can be stimulated by cyclic AMP, notably tyrosine transaminase and PEP carboxykinase. The effects of insulin on enzymes in human fetal liver have not been examined.

Human fetal liver appears to be more comparable to that of the dog than to other subprimate mammalian species: (1) PEP carboxykinase is clearly detectable in early human fetal liver [188], and (2) rates of glucose output and gluconeogenesis in human fetal liver [197] are similar to those in the fetal dog [181,182].

Villee first demonstrated gluconeogenesis in slices of midterm human fetal liver [198]. Subsequently, Adam et al. [199] quantified gluconeogenesis in the isolated perfused human fetal liver at 12 to 16 weeks. In human fetal liver explants, Schwartz and Rall [200] demonstrated basal gluconeogenesis from 5 mM alanine of approximately 4 nmoles glucose/g/min, which was stimulated up to tenfold by glucagon, cyclic AMP, or corticosteroids. Insulin, on the other hand, decreased both basal and hormone-stimulated gluconeogenesis in these tissues.

Frazer et al. [201] have studied conversion of $[2,3-^{13}C_2]$ alanine to glucose in newborn human infants at 4–8 hours of age. Both appropriate-for-gestational-age (AGA) and small-for-gestational-age (SGA) infants had functional gluconeogenetic pathways of similar net magnitude.

Glucose-6-Phosphatase and Glucose Release

Even though the release of glucose from the liver occurs so rapidly that the tissue appears freely permeable, a rapid carrier-mediated system has been described [28,149]. Furthermore, as glucose-6-phosphatase is a membrane-bound enzyme [202] and alterations in its activity have often closely correlated with glucose release by the liver, it should be emphasized that the activity of this enzyme may play a key role as the "gatekeeper" of hepatic glucose output.

Since the initial studies demonstrated that adult rat liver glucose-6-phosphatase activity could be increased by steroid administration, starvation, or diabetes [195,203], many investigators have examined the ability of various hormones to regulate this activity. Insulin administered to adult rats was not only capable of decreasing the elevated glucose-6-phosphatase activity associated with diabetes, but was also capable of reducing the glucose-6-phosphatase activity in normal rats in vivo [202,204]. Similar effects have been produced by chronic hyperinsulinemia in third-trimester rhesus fetuses [205,206]. Glucagon, however, was ineffective in altering hepatic glucose-6-phosphatase activity in the dog in vivo [207]. Much attention has focused on the mechanisms involved in the regulation of this activity by steroid hormones and insulin [195].

The release of glucose from human fetal liver has not been studied, but it is assumed to take place as it does in the adult. The development of glucose-6-phosphatase activity in mammalian liver has been documented for a wide variety of species, including the rat [208,209], mouse [120], pig [210], guinea pig [211,212], rabbit [120], and lamb [180,209]. In all these species, the hepatic glucose-6-phosphatase activity is undetectable until just prior to birth, followed by a dramatic increase in activity in the initial postnatal period, surpassing that found in the adult animal [120,212]. This postnatal increase has been attributed to the synthesis of protein de novo [213]. In addition, Greengard and her associates have suggested that the glucagon-cyclic AMP system is the primary physiologic trigger mechanism, since administration of these agents to rat fetuses in utero causes a premature increase in glucose-6-phosphatase activity [192,214,215]. Insulin administration to the newborn rat retarded the normal postnatal increase in activity [214], although insulin administration to fetuses in utero did not alter the glucose-6-phosphatase activity [215]. Prolonged maternal starvation in the rat is associated with fetal hypoglycemia, hypoinsulinemia, and an increase in hepatic glucose-6-phosphatase activity [216].

In contrast to those species described above, the human fetal liver contains considerable glucose-6-phosphatase activity by midgestation [190,191,198] which is already 25 to 30 percent of the level of activity in adult liver. The only other species to exhibit significant glucose-6-phosphatase activity in fetal liver is the rhesus monkey [120,205, 206]. In human fetal liver explants, glucose-6-phosphatase activity is markedly stimulated by cyclic AMP and is suppressed by insulin [217].

• Substrate Transfer across the Placenta

Glucose Transfer

Earlier studies of respiratory quotients before birth and of the blood glucose concentration in fetal blood suggested that carbohydrate is a major source of fetal energy and that glucose freely diffuses across the placenta.

Widdas favored facilitated diffusion as the mechanism for glucose transfer across the placenta [218], noting that a concentration gradient from mother to fetus is always present for glucose, unless glucose has been infused experimentally into the fetal circulation. Chinard and associates [219] infused glucose into women and monkeys prior to and at cesarean section. They observed parallel responses in the blood sugar of the fetus and of the mother in the third month of intrauterine life as well as at term. A significant maternal-fetal gradient of glucose was observed. Battaglia et al. [220] reexamined glucose concentration gradients across the monkey placenta at known periods of gestation. They analyzed maternal arterial and maternal uterine venous and fetal umbilical artery blood for glucose concentrations. The plasma arteriovenous differences for glucose across the uterus (from the maternal surface of placenta) averaged 14.9 mg/100 ml (0.83 mM), while the concentration gradient across the whole placenta averaged 26.6 mg/100 ml (1.48 mM). These investigators reviewed the complexity of the system in which amniotic and fetal pools are superimposed on maternal pools during pregnancy. They emphasized the importance of simultaneous analysis of fetal and maternal arterial and venous (umbilical and uterine) concentrations to assess net transfer of substrates.

Fructose Transfer

In the pregnant human female, fructose is undetectable in the fasting state but rises to a discernible level after the ingestion of sucrose- or fructose-containing foods. The infusion of fructose in a variety of pregnant species, including guinea pigs [221], monkeys, and man [219], has resulted in high maternal fructose levels with very large maternal-fetal or transplacental gradients. Sustained infusions of fructose to the mother result in a slow transfer and a gradually rising level of fructose in the fetus. This behavior of fructose is in marked contrast to the rapid transfer of glucose. In studies by McCann and associates [222], fructose infusions to normal women during labor resulted in large maternal-fetal concentration differences at the time of delivery: maternal levels of 60 to 80 mg/100 ml (3.33–4.44 mM) versus 10 to 15 mg/100 ml (0.55–0.83 mM) in blood from the umbilical vein. Levels in blood from the umbilical artery were always slightly lower than those from the vein. Although detailed studies of fructose injections into fetal monkey or man have not been made to evaluate the reverse transfer across the placenta [223], the studies in situ with the isolated guinea pig placenta indicate a very slow transfer rate of fructose compared to glucose [221]. It is likely that these results are due to specificity of the glucose transporter, as discussed above.

Other Substrates

Amino Acids

Amino acid concentrations in fetal plasma are higher than those in maternal plasma. Amino acids, the sole source of fetal nitrogen, are critical to anabolic processes. Young and Hill [224] have summarized their observations on free amino acid transfer across the placental membrane. In particular, they studied the effect of a fall in maternal blood flow in the pregnant guinea pig and noted that transfer of α-amino nitrogen decreased as placental flow fell. No reduction below 50 percent of the control level occurred even at very low maternal arterial pressures. They speculated on the possibility of a reserve in placental amino acids that may be protective to the fetus. They also noted that maternal plasma concentrations of free amino acids may be relatively unimportant for transfer across the placenta. The placenta is capable of transferring amino acids from maternal to fetal circulation against a large concentration gradient. This may be important early in gestation before the enzymes capable of synthesizing amino acids are developed.

This high fetal-to-maternal plasma amino acid gradient is not unique to the human since ratios as high as 3.8 have been observed in the rat [225]. Virtually all amino acids participate in this enhanced placental transfer. Economides et al. [226] have recently reported on normal preterm human fetuses studied by cordocentesis. They observed a high correlation between fetal and maternal levels for individual amino acids. The fetal concentrations were higher than the maternal. Cretin et al. [227] noted similar correlations between fetal and maternal concentrations of most amino acids at midgestation and at term.

Free Fatty Acids, Triglycerides, Ketones

The role of free fatty acids (FFA) as substrate for the fetus has been reviewed by Hull [228]. Contrary to earlier studies in the human [229] that were interpreted to indicate minimal placental transfer of nonessential fatty acids, studies with labeled fatty acid in several species, but not man in vivo, have indicated rapid transfer. Dancis et al. [230], however, have observed insufficient long chain free fatty acid transfer in the perfused human placenta to account for fetal adipose tissue deposition. The quantitative significance of these observations remains unclear. Hull [228] suggests that fetal tissues, including the brain, may metabolize both fatty acids and ketones for energy.

The presence of essential fatty acids in third trimester fetal adipose tissue is indirect evidence of placental transfer. Direct evidence based on maternal artery-fetal umbilical vein concentration differences of FFA have been inconclusive. The reasons for this have been reviewed and discussed by Battaglia and Meschia [231], who commented on the rapid turnover of these large molecular weight compounds.

In contrast, plasma triglyceride concentrations evaluated by cordocentesis in normal fetuses decrease exponentially with gestational age [232]. Furthermore, there is no relation between fetal and maternal triglyceride levels. This has been interpreted as evidence of minimal net placental (i.e., maternal to fetal) transfer, if any. These fetal levels may reflect fetal triglyceride synthesis and metabolism and result in fetal deposition of fat in the third trimester.

There appears to be rapid transfer of ketones from maternal to fetal circulation, since there is a direct relationship between the concentration of ketones in maternal and fetal plasma [233].

• Blood Glucose Concentrations in the Fetus

While the process of delivery produces an alteration in the continuum of development, the adjustments of the newborn, and of the young infant in particular, must be considered in the light of previous experiences in utero. Fetal biochemical processes important to metabolism that develop in utero have been considered above. The physiologic effects of substrates (metabolic fuels) and hormones on plasma glucose concentration in the fetus follow.

While there have been a number of studies of glucose concentration in the fetal circulation during labor and at the moment of delivery, only recently has information about glucose concentration in fetal blood prior to labor in man or other primates appeared. Holmberg and associates [234] obtained umbilical cord vein samples from the human fetus at vaginal hysterotomy prior to a therapeutic interruption of pregnancy. They found blood glucose values as low as 20 mg/ 100 ml (1.11 mM) in a 22-week-old fetus. Infusions of glucose or fructose to the mother resulted in transfer to the fetus, with higher transfer rates for glucose compared to fructose.

In studies of maternofetal substrate and hormones in early second trimester pregnancy, one of us (Robert Schwartz) observed fetal umbilical vein glucose concentrations of 56 ± 3.4 mg/100 ml (3.11 ± 0.19 mM), compared to maternal levels of 71 ± 3.3 mg/100 ml (3.94 ± 0.18 mM) in 29 pairs after an overnight fast and induction anesthesia (Table 1-2).

More recently, Susa and associates [235] have reported on third trimester rhesus fetuses with ketamine anesthesia to the mothers. In 7 control fetuses (Fig. 1-16), peripheral venous plasma glucose concentration at 113–126 weeks' gestation (term 166 days) was comparable to umbilical vein (UV) plasma glucose (45 ± 13 mg/dl [2.5 ± 0.73 mM]) at delivery at 140 ± 2 days, while umbilical artery values were lower to 0.89 of UV. Maternal peripheral venous (MV) plasma (60 ± 10.1 mg/dl [3.4 ± 0.56 mM]) was highest with the UV to MV ratio at 0.75.

Glucose is considered the major substrate for fetal energy since little is derived from maternal fatty acids. Amino acids are considered primarily as sources for protein synthesis and other nitrogen-containing synthetic processes. Indirect determinations of the respiratory quotient (RQ) in fetal animals were approximately unity and may be interpreted to indicate the major role for glucose.

The Human Fetus

The recent advent of the technique of in utero fetal blood sampling with only local maternal anesthesia has confirmed observations made earlier at elective cesarean section. In addition, correlations with gestational age are now possible. Umbilical venous blood glucose concentration has now been reported in 97 AGA fetuses, ages 17 to 38 weeks, to be 68 ± 13.7 mg/dl (3.8 ± 0.76 mM) compared to a lower level in umbilical artery blood (a ratio of 0.90 of UV) from 25 AGA fetuses. Maternal venous blood was higher by 12 percent ($n = 119$), with a MV-UV difference of 9.0 ± 6.1 mg/dl (0.50 ± 0.34 mM) or UV/MV ratio of 0.89. In another, smaller study (14 fetoscopies 17 to 21 weeks), a significant correlation between maternal arterialized and

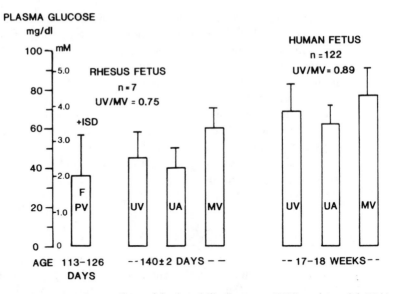

FIGURE 1-16. Comparison of fetal umbilical venous (UV) and arterial (UA) plasma glucose concentrations with simultaneously sampled maternal venous (MV) blood. F-PV refers to peripheral vein sample in the rhesus fetus obtained at hysterotomy and direct exposure of the fetus. The human data was obtained by Economides and Nicolaides. (Data reproduced from Susa JB, Schwartz R. *Diabetes*. 1985; 34 (suppl. 2):36 and from Economides DL, Nicolaides KH. *Am J Obstet Gynecol*. 1989; 160:385, with permission.)

fetal umbilical venous glucose concentrations (mM) was found at midgestation [236]. In addition, maternal hyperglycemia (glucose >80 mg/dl [4.44 mM]) also produced a strong correlation of these two variables (Fig. 1-16).

• Summary

The purpose of this review has been to establish a background in carbohydrate biochemistry and physiology as it relates to the human neonate. The emphasis has therefore been placed on the developing human, although many concepts are derived from studies in animal models.

The biosynthetic mechanisms of the developing fetus have received attention. The maturation of enzymatic processes has been further defined. The complex enzyme systems necessary for glycogen synthesis and metabolism are well-developed in the fetus. Hormonal control, especially by the hypothalamic, pituitary-adrenal, and pancreatic systems, is critical to development. Although tracer techniques have permitted a dynamic analysis in some species, there is insufficient information to correlate adequately the physiologic adjustments of the pregnant woman with the fetus. The development of fluorometric techniques for ultramicroanalysis for substrates and of radioimmunoassay and receptor assays for hormones has expanded the base for understanding the metabolic adjustments in the pregnant woman and her fetus. An emphasis on substrate controls as well as hormonal controls of fetal metabolism has evolved. There is a need for further detailed studies of the maternal-placental-fetal metabolic interactions and their effect on fetal outcome. The newer techniques of nuclear magnetic resonance spectroscopy and cordocentesis should provide further insights.

REFERENCES

1. DEFRONZO RA, ed. *Diabetes/Metabolism Reviews*. New York: John Wiley & Sons, 1987;3:1.
2. STRYER L, ed. *Biochemistry*. 3rd ed. New York: WH Freeman and Co., 1988.
3. MATHEWS CK, VAN HOLDE KE, eds. *Biochemistry*. New York: The Benjamin/Cummings Publ Co., Inc., 1990.
4. JONES CT, ed. *Biochemical Development of the Fetus and Neonate*. Amsterdam: Elsevier, 1982.
5. BELL GI, TAYLOR SI, eds. Diabetes mellitus and molecular biology. In: *Diabetes Care* 1990;13(3):187 and 13(6):547.
6. HERBST JJ, SUNSHINE PP, KRETCHMER N. Intestinal malabsorption in infancy and childhood. *Adv Pediatr.* 1969;16:11.
7. HOLZEL A. Development of intestinal enzyme systems and its relation to diarrhoea. *Pediatr Clin North Am.* 1965;12:635.
8. WISEMAN G. *Absorption from the Intestine*. New York: Academic Press, Inc., 1964.
9. RENOLD AE, THORN GW. Clinical usefulness of fructose. *Am J Med.* 1955;19:163.
10. SOSKIN S, ESSEX HE, HERRICK JF, MANN FC. The mechanism of regulation of blood sugar by the liver. *Am J Physiol.* 1938;124:558.
11. CAHILL GF, OWEN OE. Some observations on carbohydrate metabolism in man. In: Dickens F, Randle PJ, Whelan WJ, eds. *Carbohydrate Metabolism and Its Disorders*. New York: Academic Press, Inc., 1968;497.
12. GUTBERLET RL, SANTOS AQ, DECOELLO S. Altered carbohydrate utilization in sick premature infants. *Pediatr Res.* 1973;7:312.
13. MCILWAIN H, BACHELARD HS, eds. *Biochemistry and the Central Nervous System*. 5th ed. Edinburgh: Churchill Livingstone, 1985.
14. FRIIS-HANSEN B. Body composition during growth—Biochemical data and in vivo measurements. *Pediatrics* 1971;47:261.
15. SHOHL, AT. *Mineral Metabolism*. New York, Reinhold, 1939; 19.
16. BIER DM, LEAKE R, HAYMOND MW, et al. Measurement of "true" glucose production rates in infancy and childhood with 6,6-dideuteroglucose. *Diabetes* 1977;26:1016.

17. BONDY PK, JAMES DF, FARRAR BW. Studies on the role of the liver in human carbohydrate metabolism by the venous catheter technique. I. Normal subjects under fasting conditions and following injection of glucose. *J Clin Invest* 1949;28:238.

18. OWEN OE, MORGAN AP, KEMP HG, SULLIVAN JM, HERRERA MG, CAHILL GF. Brain metabolism during fasting. *J Clin Invest.* 1967;46:1589.

19. SCHWARTZ R, KALHAN SC. Energy sources for neonatal brain metabolism. In: Adamsons K, Fox HC, eds. *Preventability of Perinatal Injury.* New York: Alan R. Liss, Pubs. 1975;187.

20. LEVITSKY LL, FISHER DE, PATON JB, DELANNOY CW. Fasting plasma levels of glucose, acetoacetate, D-betahydroxybutyrate, glycerol and lactate in the baboon infant: Correlation with cerebral uptake of substrates and oxygen. *Pediatr Res.* 1977;11:298.

21. NEHLIG A, DEVASCONCELOS AP, BOYET S. Quantitative autoradiographic measurement of local cerebral glucose utilization in freely moving rats during postnatal development. *J Neurosci.* 1988;8(7):2321.

22. SOKOLOFF L, REIVICH M, KENNEDY C, et al. The [^{14}C]-deoxyglucose method for the measurement of local cerebral glucose utilization: Theory, procedure and normal values in the conscious and anesthetized albino rat. *J Neurochem.* 1977;28:897.

23. DEVASCONCELOS AP, SCHROEDER H, NEHLIG A. Effects of early chronic phenobarbital treatment on the maturation of energy metabolism in the developing rat brain. II. Incorporation of B-hydroxybutyrate into amino acids. *Dev Brain Res.* 1987;36:219.

24. CHUGANI HT, PHELPS ME, MAZZIOTTA JC. Positron emission tomography study of human brain functional development. *Ann Neurol.* 1987; 22:487.

25. KIPNIS DM, HELMREICH E, CORI CF. Studies of tissue permeability. IV. Distribution of glucose between plasma and muscle. *J Biol Chem.* 1959;234:165.

26. PARK CR, MORGAN HE, HENDERSON MJ, REGEN DM, CADENAS E, POST RL. Regulation of glucose uptake in muscle as studied in perfused rat heart. *Recent Progr Horm Res.* 1961;17:493.

27. MUECKLER M, CARUSO C, BALDWIN S, et al. Sequence and structure of a human glucose transporter. *Science* 1985;229:941.

28. FLIER JS, MATSOUKA P. Insulin action and the glucose transporter gene. In: Draznin B, Melmed S, LeRoith D, eds. *Molecular and Cellular Biology of Diabetes Mellitus. Vol III: Insulin Action.* New York: Alan R. Liss, Inc, 1989;175.

29. GOULD GW, BELL GI. Facilitative glucose transporters: an expanding family. *Trends in Biomedical Science* 1990;15:18.

30. FUKUMOTO H, KAYANO T, BUSE JB, et al. Cloning and characterization of the major insulin-responsive glucose transporter expressed in human skeletal muscle and other insulin-responsive tissues. *J Biol Chem.* 1989;264(14):7776.

31. MCLEAN P, BROWN J, GREENBAUM AL. Hormonal regulation of carbohydrate metabolism in adipose tissue. In: Dickens F, Randle PJ, Whelan WJ, eds. *Carbohydrate Metabolism and Its Disorders.* New York: Academic Press, Inc., 1968;397.

32. CROFFORD OB, RENOLD AE. Glucose uptake by incubated rat epididymal adipose tissue. *J Biol Chem.* 1965;240:3237.

33. KATZ J, LANDAU BR, BARTSCH GE. The pentose cycle, triose phosphate

isomerization and lipogenesis in rat adipose tissue. *J Biol Chem.* 1966;241:727.

34. GOLDFINE ID, CARO JF. Molecular and cellular biology of the insulin receptor in diabetes mellitus. In: Draznin B, Melmed S, LeRoith D, eds. *Molecular and Cellular Biology of Diabetes Mellitus. Vol II: Insulin Action.* New York: Alan R. Liss, Inc., 1989;11.

35. EBERT R, CREUTZFELDT W. Gastrointestinal peptides and insulin secretion. *Diabetes/Metabolism Reviews* 1987;3(1):1.

36. UNGER RH, EISENTRAUT AH. Entero-insular axis. *Arch Intern Med.* 1969;123:261.

37. MARLISS EB, AOKI TT, UNGER RH, SOELDNER JS, CAHILL GF. Glucagon levels and metabolic effects in fasting man. *J Clin Invest.* 1970; 49:2256.

38. PAGE MA, WILLIAMSON DH. Enzymes of ketone-body utilization in human brain. *Lancet* 1971;2:66.

39. TILDON JT, CORNBLATH M. Succinyl CoA: 3 Ketoacid CoA transferase deficiency—a cause for ketoacidosis in infancy. *J Clin Invest.* 1972; 51:493.

40. DIERKS-VENTLING C, CONE AL. Ketone body enzymes in mammalian tissues: Effect of high fat diet. *J Biol Chem.* 1971;246:5533.

41. TILDON JT, SEVDALIAN DA. CoA transferase in the brain and other mammalian tissues. *Arch Biochem Biophys.* 1972;148:382.

42. OZAND PT, STEVENSON JH, TILDON JT, CORNBLATH M. The effects of hyperketonemia on glycolytic intermediates in the developing rat brain. *J Neurochem.* 1975;25:61.

43. OZAND PT, STEVENSON JH, TILDON JT, CORNBLATH M. The effects of hyperketonemia on glutamate and glutamine metabolism in developing rat brain. *J Neurochem.* 1975;25:67.

44. BRESSLER R. Physiological chemical aspects of fatty acid oxidation. In: Wakil SJ, ed. *Lipid Metabolism.* New York: Academic Press, Inc., 1970;49.

45. MASORO EJ. *Physiological Chemistry of Lipids in Mammals.* Philadelphia: W. B. Saunders Company, 1968.

46. FRITZ IB, LEE LPK. Fat mobilization and ketogenesis. In: Greep RO, Astwood EB, eds. *Handbook of Physiology,* Section 7, vol. 1. Baltimore: Williams and Wilkins Co., 1974;579.

47. MCGARRY JD, MANNAERTS GP, FOSTER DW. A possible role for malonyl-CoA in the regulation of hepatic fatty acid oxidation and ketogenesis. *J Clin Invest.* 1977;60:265.

48. VAGELOS PR. Regulation of fatty acid biosynthesis. *Curr Top Cell Regul.* 1971;4:119.

49. BORTZ W, LYNEN F. The inhibition of acetyl-CoA-carboxylase by long chain acyl-CoA derivatives. *Biochem Z.* 1963;337:505.

50. WAKIL SJ. Fatty acid metabolism. In: Wakil SJ, ed. *Lipid Metabolism.* New York: Academic Press, Inc., 1970;1.

51. RANDLE PJ, NEWSHOLME EA, GARLAND PB. Regulation of glucose uptake by muscle. *Biochem J.* 1964;93:652.

52. RANDLE PJ, GARLAND PB, HALES CN, NEWSHOLME EA, DENTEN RM, POGSON CI. Interactions of the metabolism and physiological role of insulin. *Recent Progr Hormone Res.* 1966;22:1.

53. SCHONFELD G, KIPNIS DM. Effect of fatty acids on carbohydrate and fatty acid metabolism in rat diaphragm. *Am J Physiol* 1968;215:513.

54. DICZFALUSY E. Recent progress in the fetoplacental metabolism of steroids. In: Vokaer R, DeBock G, eds. *Reproductive Endocrinology.* Oxford: Pergamon Press, 1975;3.

55. DICZFALUSY, E. Endocrine function of the human fetus and placenta. *Am J Obstet Gynecol.* 1974;119:419.

56. GREEP RO, ASTWOOD EB, STEINER DF, FREINKEL N, GEIGER SR, eds. Handbook of Physiology, Section 7: Endocrinology, Vol. 1 Endocrine Pancreas. Washington, DC: American Physiological Society;1972.

57. ROBB P. The development of the islets of Langerhans in the human foetus. *J Exp Physiol.* 1961;46:335.

58. HELLMAN B. The development of the mammalian endocrine pancreas. *Biol Neonate* 1965–1966;9:263.

59. ORCI L, AMHERDT M, MALAISSE-LAGAE F, ROUILLER, RENOLD AE. Insulin release by emiocytosis: Demonstration with freeze-etching technique. *Science* 1973;179:82.

60. VAN ASSCHE FA. *The Fetal Endocrine Pancreas: A Quantitative Morphological Approach.* Belgium: Proefschrift ingediend by de faculteit Geneeskunde der Katholieke Universiteit Lenven. 1970;1–99.

61. VAN ASSCHE FA, GEPTS W. The cytological composition of the foetal endocrine pancreas in normal and pathological conditions. *Diabetologia* 1971;7:434.

62. HELLERSTRÖM C, HELLMAN B. Some aspects of silver impregnation of Langerhans in the rat. *Acta Endocrinol. (Kbh.)* 1960;35:418.

63. PICTET R, RUTTER WJ. Development of the endocrine pancreas. In: Greep RO, Astwood EB, eds. *Handbook of Physiology,* Section 7, vol. 1. Baltimore: Williams & Wilkins Co., 1972;25.

64. ADESANYA T, GRILLO I, SHIMA K. Insulin content and enzyme histochemistry of the human fetal pancreatic islet. *J Endocrinol.* 1966; 36:151.

65. RASTOGI GK, LETARTE J, FRASER TR. Immunoreactive insulin content of 203 pancreases from foetuses of healthy mothers. *Diabetologia* 1970; 6:445.

66. SCHAEFFER LD, WILDER ML, WILLIAMS RH. Secretion and content of insulin and glucagon in human fetal pancreas slices in vitro. *Proc Soc Exper Biol Med.* 1973;143:314.

67. KAPLAN SL, GRUMBACH MM, SHEPARD TH. The ontogenesis of human fetal hormones. I. Growth hormone and insulin. *J Clin Invest.* 1972;51:3080.

68. MILNER RDG, BARSON AJ, ASHWORTH MA. Human foetal pancreatic insulin secretion in response to ionic and other stimuli. *J Endocrinol.* 1971;51:323.

69. SCHWARTZ R. Metabolic fuels in the foetus. Symposium on life before birth. *Proc Roy Soc Med.* 1968;61:1231.

70. ADAM PA, TERAMO K, RÄIHÄ N, GITLIN D, SCHWARTZ R. Human fetal insulin metabolism early in gestation. *Diabetes* 1969;18:409.

71. KALHAN SC, SCHWARTZ R, ADAM PA. Placental barrier to human insulin-I[125] in insulin-dependent diabetic mothers. *J Clin Endocrinol Metab.* 1975;40:139.

72. STEINER DF, KEMMLER W, CLARK JL, OYER PE, RUBENSTEIN AH. The biosynthesis of insulin. In: Greep RO, Astwood EB, eds. *Handbook of Physiology,* Section 7, vol. 1. Baltimore: Williams & Wilkins Co., 1972;175.

73. STEINER DF, CUNNINGHAM DD, SPIGELMAN L, ATEN B. Insulin biosynthesis: Evidence for a precursor. *Science* 1967;157:697.

74. CHEZ RA. The development and function of the human endocrine pancreas. In: Jaffe RB, ed. *The Endocrine Milieu of Pregnancy, Puerperium and Childhood*. Third Ross Conference on Obstetric Research, 1974;43.

75. OBENSHAIN SS, ADAM PA, KING KC, TERAMO K, RAIVIO KO, RÄIHÄ N, SCHWARTZ R. Human fetal insulin response to sustained maternal hyperglycemia. *N Engl J Med*. 1971;283:607.

76. TOBIN JD, ROUX JF, SOELDNER JS. Human fetal insulin response after acute maternal glucose administration during labour. *Pediatrics* 1969; 44:668.

77. BEARD RW, TURNER RC, OAKLEY NW. Fetal response to glucose loading. *Postgrad Med J*. 1971;47:68.

78. MILNER RDG, HALES CN. Effect of intravenous glucose on concentration of insulin in maternal and umbilical cord plasma. *Br Med J*. 1965;1:284.

79. KING KC, BUTT J, RAIVIO K, RÄIHÄ N, ROUX J, TERAMO K, YAMAGUCHI K, SCHWARTZ R. Human maternal and fetal insulin response to arginine. *N Engl J Med*. 1971;285:607.

80. MILNER RDG, ASHWORTH MA, BARSON AJ. Insulin release from human foetal pancreas in response to glucose, leucine and arginine. *J Endocrinol*. 1972;52:497.

81. MILNER RDG. The growth and development of the endocrine pancreas. In: Davis JA, Dobbing J, eds. *Scientific Foundations of Paediatrics*. Philadelphia: W. B. Saunders Company, 1974;507.

82. ECONOMIDES DL, PROUDLER A, NICOLAIDES KH. Plasma insulin in appropriate and small-for-gestational age fetuses. *Am J Obstet Gynecol*. 1989;160:1091.

83. ASSAN R, BOILLOT J. Pancreatic glucagon, and glucagon-like material in tissues and plasmas from human foetuses 6–26 weeks old. In: Jonxis JHP, Visser HKA, Troelstra JA, eds. *Nutricia Symposium Metabolic Processes in the Foetus and Newborn Infant*. Baltimore: Williams & Wilkins Co., 1971;210–219.

84. MILNER RDG, CHOUKSEY SK, MICKLESON KN, ASSAN R. Plasma pancreatic glucagon and insulin: glucagon ratio at birth. *Arch Dis Child*. 1973; 48:241.

85. JOHNSTON DI, BLOOM SR. Plasma glucagon levels in the term human infant and effect of hypoxia. *Arch Dis Child*. 1973;48:451.

86. WISE JK, LYALL SS, HENDLER R, FELIG P. Evidence of stimulation of glucagon secretion by alanine in the human fetus at term. *J Clin Endocrinol Metab*. 1973;37:345.

87. EPSTEIN M, CHEZ RA, OAKES GK, MINTZ DH. Fetal pancreatic glucagon responses in glucose-intolerant nonhuman primate pregnancy. *Am J Obstet Gynecol*. 1977;127(3):268.

88. ADAM PA, KING KC, SCHWARTZ R, TERAMO K. Human placental barrier to I^{125}-glucagon early in gestation. *J Clin Endocrinol Metab*. 1972; 34:772.

89. SCHWARTZ AL, RÄIHÄ NCR, RALL TW. Hormonal regulation of glycogen metabolism in human fetal liver. I. Normal development and effects of dibutyryl cyclic AMP, glucagon and insulin in liver explants. *Diabetes* 1975;24:1101.

90. SCHWARTZ AL, RALL TW. Hormonal regulation of glycogen metabolism in neonatal rat liver. *Biochem J.* 1973;134:985.

91. SPERLING MA, DELAMATER PV, PHELPS D, FISER RH, OH W, FISHER DA. Spontaneous and amino acid-stimulated glucagon secretion in the immediate postnatal period. *J Clin Invest.* 1974;53:1159.

92. GITLIN D, KUMATE J, MORALES C. Metabolism and maternofetal transfer of human growth hormone in pregnant women at term. *J Clin Endocrinol Metab.* 1965;25:1599.

93. KING KC, ADAM PA, SCHWARTZ R, TERAMO T. Human placental transfer of human growth hormone-I[125]. *Pediatrics* 1971;48:534.

94. CORNBLATH M, PARKER ML, REISNER SH, FORBES AE, DAUGHADAY WH. Secretion and metabolism of growth hormone in premature and full term infants. *J Clin Endocrinol Metab.* 1965;25:209.

95. WOLF H, STUBBE P, SABATA V. The influence of maternal glucose infusions on fetal growth hormone levels. *Pediatrics* 1970;45:36.

96. MINTZ DH, CHEZ RA, HORGER EO, III. Fetal insulin and growth hormone metabolism in the subhuman primate. *J Clin Invest.* 1969;48:176.

97. GRUMBACH MM, KAPLAN SL. Fetal pituitary hormones and the maturation of central nervous system regulation of anterior pituitary function. In: Gluck L, ed. *Modern Perinatal Medicine.* Chicago: Year Book Medical Publishers, Inc., 1974;247.

98. HOLLENBERG MD, ATKINSON PR, BALA RM. Regulation of growth factors and their receptors: Implications for the control of normal and abnormal tissue growth. In: Hintz RL, Underwood LE, eds. *Peptide Growth Factors: Relevance to Pediatrics.* Eighty-Ninth Ross Conference. Columbus, Ohio: Ross Laboratories, 1985;2.

99. SPENCER EM. Synthesis by cultured hepatocytes of somatomedin and its binding protein. *FEBS Lett.* 1979;99:157.

100. DAUGHADAY WH, LARON Z, PERTZELAN A, HEINS JN. Defective sulfation factor generation: a possible link to dwarfism. *Trans Assoc Am Physicians.* 1969;82:129.

101. HINTZ RL, SEEDS JM, JOHNSONBAUGH R. Somatomedin and growth hormone in the newborn. *Am J Dis Child.* 1977;131(11):1249.

102. UNDERWOOD LE, D'ERCOLE AJ. Insulin and somatomedins/insulin-like growth factors in fetal and neonatal development. In: Daughaday WH, ed. *Clinics in Endocrinology and Metabolism: Tissue Growth Factors.* 13th ed. United Kingdom: WB Saunders Co., Ltd., 1984;69.

103. FREEMARK M. Epidermal growth factor stimulates glycogen synthesis in fetal rat hepatocytes: Comparison with the glycogenic effects of insulinlike growth factor I and insulin. *Endocrinology.* 1986;119:522.

104. GREENBERG RE, LIND J. Catecholamines in tissues of the human fetus. *Pediatrics.* 1961;27:904.

105. MIRKIN BL. Ontogenesis of the adrenergic nervous system—function and pharmacologic implications. *Fed Proc.* 1972;31:65.

106. JOELSSON I, ADAMSONS K. Effect of pharmacologic agents upon the fetus and newborn. *Am J Obstet Gynecol.* 1966;96:437.

107. SANDLER M, RUTHVEN C, CONTRACTOR S, WOOD C, BOOTH T, PINKERTON JH. Transmission of noradrenaline across the human placenta. *Nature.* 1963;197:598.

108. ELIOT RJ, LAM BS, LEAKE RD, HOBEL CJ, FISHER DA. Plasma catecholamine concentrations in infants at birth and during the first 48 hours of life. *J Pediatr.* 1980;96:311.

109. PRYDS O, CHRISTENSEN NJ, FRIIS-HANSEN B. Increased cerebral blood flow and plasma epinephrine in hypoglycemic, preterm neonates. *Pediatrics.* 1990;85:172.

110. DICZFALUSY E. Steroid metabolism in the fetoplacental unit. *Excerpta Medica Foundation International Congress Series* 1969;183:65.

111. GINSBURG J. Placental drug transfer. *Annu Rev Pharmacol.* 1971;11:387.

112. GUTAI J, GEORGE R, KOEFF S, BACON GE. Adrenal response to physical stress and the effect of adrenocorticotropic hormone in newborn infants. *J Pediatr.* 1972;81:719.

113. KENNY FM, PREEYASOMBAT C, MIGEON CJ with LAWRENCE B, RICHARDS C. Cortisol production rate. II. Normal infants, children and adults. *Pediatrics.* 1966;37:34.

114. FISHER DA, ODELL WD, HOBEL CJ, GARZA R. Thyroid function in the term fetus. *Pediatrics.* 1969;44:526.

115. FISHER DA, HOBEL CJ, GARZA R, PIERCE CA. Thyroid function in the preterm fetus. *Pediatrics.* 1970;46:208.

116. SACK J, FISHER DA, HOBEL CJ, LAM R. Thyroxine in human amniotic fluid. *J Pediatr.* 1975;87:364.

117. ABUID J, STINSON DA, LARSEN PR. Serum triiodothyronine and thyroxine in the neonate and the acute increases in these hormones following delivery. *J Clin Invest.* 1973;52:1195.

118. BERNARD C. De la matière glycogene considéré comme condition de development de certains tissues, chez le foetus, avant l'apparition de la fonction glycogenique du foie. *Comp Rend.* 1859;48:673.

119. SHELLY HJ. Glycogen reserves and their changes at birth. *Br Med Bull.* 1961;17:137.

120. DAWKINS MJR. Biochemical aspects of developmental function in newborn mammalian liver. *Br Med Bull.* 1966;22:27.

121. CAPKOVA A, JIRASEK JE. Glycogen reserves in organs of human fetuses in the first half of pregnancy. *Biol Neonate* 1969;13:129.

122. SCHWARTZ AL. Hormonal regulation of glucose production in human fetal liver. Ph.D. dissertation, Case Western Reserve University, 1974.

123. SHELLY HJ, NELIGAN GA. Neonatal hypoglycemia. *Br Med Bull.* 1966;22:34.

124. BISHOP JS, LARNER J. Rapid activation-inactivation of liver UDPG-glycogen transferase and phosphorylase by insulin and glucagon in vivo. *J Biol Chem.* 1967;242:1354.

125. GILMAN AG. G proteins and regulation of adenylyl cyclase. The Albert Lasker Medical Awards. *J Am Med Assoc.* 1989;262(13):1819.

126. KREBS EG. Role of the cyclic AMP-dependent protein kinase in signal transduction. The Albert Lasker Medical Awards. *J Am Med Assoc.* 1989;262(13):1815.

127. RALL TW, SUTHERLAND E, WOSILAIT W. The relationship of epinephrine and glucagon to liver phosphorylase. *J Biol Chem.* 1956;218:483.

128. LARNER J, VILLAR-PILASI C. Glycogen synthase and its control. *Curr Top Cell Regul.* 1971;3:195.

129. BERRIDGE MJ. Inositol trisphosphate, calcium, lithium, and cell signaling. The Albert Lasker Medical Awards. *J Am Med Assoc.* 1989;262(13):1834.

130. CRAIG J, RALL TW, LARNER J. Influence of insulin and epinephrine on adenosine-3'-5'-phosphate and glycogen transferase in muscle. *Biochim Biophys Acta.* 1969;177:213.

131. STALMANS W, BOLLEN M, MVUMBI L. Control of glycogen synthesis in health and disease. *Diabetes/Metabolism Reviews.* 1987;3(1):127.

132. COHEN P, COHEN PTW. Protein phosphatases come of age. *J Biol Chem.* 1989;264(36):21435.

133. LONG CNH, KATZIN B, FRY EG. The adrenal cortex and carbohydrate metabolism. *Endocrinol.* 1940;26:309.

134. DEWULF H, HERS HG. Roles of glucose, glucagon and glucocorticoids in regulation of liver glycogen synthetase. *Eur J Biochem.* 1968;6:558.

135. EISEN HJ, GOLDFINE ID, GLINSMANN WH. Regulation of hepatic glycogen synthesis during fetal development. Roles of hydrocortisone, insulin and insulin receptor. *Proc Natl Acad Sci USA.* 1973;70:3454.

136. DEWULF H. Control of glycogen metabolism in liver. Ph.D. dissertation, University Catholic de Louvain, 1971.

137. GOLD AH. On the possibility of metabolite control of liver glycogen synthetase activity. *Biochem.* 1970;9:946.

138. VAN DE WERVE G, JEANRENEAUD B. Liver glycogen metabolism: An overview. *Diabetes/Metabolism Reviews.* 1987;3(1):47.

139. SMITH EE, TAYLOR PM, WHELAN WJ. Enzymatic processes in glycogen metabolism. In: Dickens F, Randle PJ, Whelan WJ, eds. *Carbohydrate Metabolism and Its Disorders.* New York: Academic Press, Inc., 1968;89.

140. JACQUOT R, KRETCHMER N. Effects of fetal decapitation on enzymes of glycogen metabolism. *J Biol Chem.* 1964;239:1301.

141. KORNFELD R, BROWN D. The activity of some enzymes of glycogen metabolism in fetal and neonatal guinea pig liver. *J Biol Chem.* 1963;238:1604.

142. JACQUOT R. Some hormonally controlled events of liver differentiation in the perinatal period. In: Hamburgh M, Barrington E, eds. *Hormones in Development.* New York: Appleton-Century-Crofts, 1971; 587.

143. GRUPPUSO PA, BRAUTIGAN DL. Induction of hepatic glycogenesis in the fetal rat. *Am J Physiol (Endocrinol Metab 19).* 1989;256:E49.

144. SPARKS JW, LYNCH A, CHEZ RA, GLINSMANN WH. Glycogen regulation in isolated perfused near term monkey liver. *Pediatr Res.* 1976;10:51.

145. BOCEK RM, BASINGER GM, BEATTY CH. Glycogen synthetase, phosphorylase and glycogen content of developing rhesus muscle. *Pediatr Res.* 1969;3:525.

146. BOCEK RM, YOUNG M, BEATTY CH. Effect of insulin and epinephrine on the carbohydrate metabolism and adenyl cyclase activity of rhesus fetal muscle. *Pediatr Res.* 1973;7:787.

147. HERS H-G, VAN HOOF F, DEBARSY T. Glycogen storage diseases. In: Scriver CR, Beaudet AL, Sly WS, Valle D, eds. *The Metabolic Basis of Inherited Disease.* 6th ed. New York: McGraw-Hill, Inc., 1989;425.

148. KATZ J, MCGARRY JD. Perspectives: the glucose paradox. *J Clin Invest.* 1984;74:1901.

149. WILLIAMS TF, EXTON JH, PARK CR, REGEN DM. Stereospecific transport of glucose in the perfused rat liver. *Am J Physiol.* 1968;215:1200.

150. WEINHOUSE S. Regulation of glucokinase in liver. *Curr Top Cell Regul.* 1976;11:1.

151. EXTON JH. Gluconeogenesis. *Metabolism.* 1973;21:945.

152. FELIG P. Glucose-alanine cycle. *Metabolism.* 1973;22:179.

153. LONDON D, FOLEY T, WEBB C. Evidence for the release of individual amino acids from resting human forearm. *Nature.* 1965;208:588.

154. ROSS D, HEMS R, KREBS HA. The rate of gluconeogenesis from various precursors in the perfused rat liver. *Biochem J.* 1967;102:942.

155. NOALL MW, RIGGS TR, WALKER LM, CHRISTAINSEN HN. Endocrine control of amino acid transport. *Science.* 1957;126:1002.

156. CHAMBERS JW, GEORG RH, BASS AD. Effect of hydrocortisone and insulin on uptake of α-aminoisobutyrate by isolated perfused rat liver. *Mol Pharmacol.* 1965;1:66.

157. CHAMBERS JW, GEORG RH, BASS AD. Effect of catecholamines and glucagon on amino acid transport in liver. *Endocrinol.* 1968;83:1185.

158. CHAMBERS JW, GEORG RH, BASS AD. Effect of glucagon, cyclic 3′,5′-AMP and its dibutyryl derivative on amino acid uptake in the isolated perfused rat liver. *Endocrinol.* 1970;87:366.

159. RUDERMAN NB, BERGER M. The formation of glutamine and alanine in skeletal muscle. *J Biol Chem.* 1974;249:5500.

160. OZAND PT, TILDON JT, WAPNIR R, CORNBLATH M. Alanine formation by rat muscle homogenate. *Biochem Biophys Res Commun.* 1973; 53:251.

161. DANCIS J, MONEY WL, SPRINGER D, LEVITZ M. Transport of amino acids by placenta. *Am J Obstet Gynecol.* 1968;101:820.

162. HILL PM, YOUNG M. Net placental transfer of free amino acids against varying concentrations. *J Physiol.* 1973;235:409.

163. SCHWARTZ AL. Hormonal regulation of amino acid accumulation in human fetal liver explants. Effects of dibutyryl cyclic AMP, glucagon and insulin. *Biochim Biophys Acta.* 1974;362:276.

164. McGEE M, GREENGARD O, KNOX EW. Quantitative determination of phenylalanine hydroxylase in rat tissues. Developmental formation in liver. *Biochem J.* 1972;127:669.

165. RÄIHÄ NCR. Phenylalanine hydroxylase in human liver during development. *Pediatr Res.* 1973;7:1.

166. RÄIHÄ NCR, SCHWARTZ AL. Enzyme induction in human fetal liver in organ culture. *Enzyme.* 1973;15:330.

167. GAULL G, STURMAN JA, RÄIHÄ NCR. Development of mammalian sulfur metabolism. Absence of cystathionase in human fetal tissues. *Pediatr Res.* 1972;6:538.

168. ADAM PA, HAYNES RC JR. Control of hepatic mitochondrial CO_2 fixation by glucagon, epinephrine and cortisol. *J Biol Chem.* 1969; 244:6444.

169. WICKS WD, KENNEY FT, LEE KL. Induction of hepatic enzyme synthesis in vivo by adenosine 3′,5′-monophosphate. *J Biol Chem.* 1969; 244:6008.

170. FOSTER DO, RAY PD, LARDY HA. Studies on the mechanism underlying adaptive changes in rat liver phosphoenolpyruvate carboxykinase. *Biochem.* 1966;5:555.

171. YEUNG D, OLIVER IT. Induction of pyruvate carboxylase in neonatal rat liver by adenosine 3′,5′-cyclic monophosphate. *Biochem.* 1968; 7:3231.

172. BARNETT CA, WICKS WD. Regulation of phosphoenolpyruvate carboxykinase and tyrosine transaminase in hepatoma cell cultures. *J Biol Chem.* 1971;246:7201.

173. SHRAGO E, YOUNG J, LARDY HA. Carbohydrate supply as a regulator of phosphoenolpyruvate carboxykinase activity in rat liver. *Science.* 1967;158:1572.

174. TANAKA T, HARANO U, SUE F, MORIMURA H. Crystalline characterization

and metabolic regulation of two types of pyruvate kinase isolated from rat tissues. *J Biochem.* (Tokyo) 1967;62:71.

175. WEBER G, SINGHAL RL. Role of enzymes in homeostasis. *J Biol Chem.* 1964;239:521.

176. HERS HG, VAN SCHAFTINGEN E. Fructose 2,6-disphosphate 2 years after its discovery. *Biochem J.* 1982;206:1.

177. EXTON JH. Mechanisms of hormonal regulation of hepatic glucose metabolism. *Diabetes/Metabolism Reviews.* 1987;3(1):163.

178. YEUNG D, OLIVER IT. Gluconeogenesis from amino acids in neonatal rat liver. *Biochem J.* 1967;103:744.

179. YEUNG D, OLIVER IT. Development of gluconeogenesis in neonatal rat liver. *Biochem J.* 1967;105:1229.

180. BALLARD FJ, OLIVER IT. Carbohydrate metabolism in liver from fetal and neonatal sheep. *Biochem J.* 1965;95:191.

181. CHLEBOWSKI RT. Autonomic and enzymatic control of glucose production in isolated perfused canine fetal and neonatal liver. Ph.D. dissertation, Case Western Reserve University, 1974.

182. CHLEBOWSKI RT, KALHAN SC, LOWRY M, ADAM PA. Autonomic and enzymatic control of glucose production in the isolated perfused canine fetal and neonatal liver. *Pediatr Res.* 1973;7:381.

183. SWIATEK KR, CHAO KL, CORNBLATH M, TILDON JT. Distribution of phosphopyruvate carboxylase in pig liver. *Biochim Biophys Acta.* 1970; 206:316.

184. SWIATEK KR, CHAO KL, CHAO HL, CORNBLATH M, TILDON JT. Enzymatic adaptation in newborn pig liver. *Biochim Biophys Acta.* 1970; 222:145.

185. TILDON JT, SWIATEK KR, CORNBLATH M. Phosphoenolpyruvate carboxykinase in the developing pig liver. *Biol Neonate.* 1971;17:437.

186. SWIATEK KR, KIPNIS DM, MASON G, CHAO KL, CORNBLATH M. Studies of starvation hypoglycemia in newborn pigs. *Am J Physiol.* 1968; 214:400.

187. BALLARD FJ, HANSON R. Phosphoenolpyruvate carboxykinase and pyruvate carboxylase in developing rat liver. *Biochem J.* 1967;104:866.

188. RÄIHÄ NCR, LINDROOS K. Development of some enzymes involved in gluconeogenesis in human liver. *Ann Med Exp Biol Fenn.* 1969; 47:146.

189. KIRBY L, HAHN P. Enzyme induction in human fetal liver. *Pediatr Res.* 1973;7:75.

190. AURRICHIO S, RIGILLO N. Glucose-6-phosphatase activity in human fetal liver. *Biol Neonate* 1960;2:146.

191. GENNSER G, LUNDQUIST I, NILSSON E. Glycogenolytic activity in the liver of the human fetus. *Biol Neonate* 1971;19:1.

192. GREENGARD O, DEWEY HK. Initiation by glucagon of the premature development of tyrosine transaminase, serine dehydratase and glucose-6-phosphatase in fetal rat liver. *J Biol Chem.* 1967;242:2986.

193. HOLT P, OLIVER IT. Factors affecting the premature induction of tyrosine aminotransferase in fetal rat liver. *Biochem J.* 1968;108:333.

194. WICKS WD. Induction of tyrosine α-ketoglutarate transaminase in fetal rat liver. *J Biol Chem.* 1968;243:900.

195. WEBER G, SINGHAL RL, STRIVASTAVA SK. Action of glucocorticoids as inducer and insulin as suppressor of biosynthesis of hepatic gluconeogenic enzymes. *Adv Enzyme Regul.* 1965;3:43.

196. KIRBY L, HAHN P. Enzyme activities during culture of fetal rat liver. *Can J Biochem.* 1973;51:476.

197. ADAM PA, GLASER G, ROGOFF F, SCHWARTZ AL, RAHIALA E-L, KEKOMÄKI M. Autoregulation and evolution of glucagon control of hepatic glucose production in the human fetus and canine newborn. *Clin Res.* 1972;20:539.

198. VILLEE CA. Regulation of blood glucose in the human fetus. *J Appl Physiol.* 1953;5:437.

199. ADAM PA, KEKOMÄKI M, RAHIALA E-L, SCHWARTZ AL. Autoregulation of glucose production by the isolated perfused human liver. *Pediatr Res.* 1972;6:396.

200. SCHWARTZ AL, RALL TW. Hormonal regulation of incorporation of alanine-U-^{14}C into glucose in human fetal liver explants. Effects of dibutyryl cyclic AMP, glucagon, insulin and triamcinolone. *Diabetes.* 1975;24:650.

201. FRAZER TE, KARL IE, HILLMAN LS, BIER DM. Direct measurement of gluconeogenesis from [2,3-^{13}C$_2$] alanine in the human neonate. *Am J Physiol (Endocrinol Metab 3).* 1981;240:E615.

202. ASHMORE J, HASTINGS AB, NESBETT FB, RENOLD AE. Studies on carbohydrate metabolism in rat liver slices. VI. Hormonal factors influencing glucose-6-phosphatase. *J Biol Chem.* 1955;218:77.

203. LANGDON RG, WEAKLEY DR. Influence of hormonal factors and diet upon hepatic glucose-6-phosphatase activity. *J Biol Chem.* 1955; 214:167.

204. FISHER CJ, STETTEN MR. Parallel changes in vivo in microsomal inorganic pyrophosphatase, pyrophosphate-glucose phosphotransferase and glucose-6-phosphatase activities. *Biochim Biophys Acta.* 1966; 121:102.

205. MCCORMICK KL, SUSA JB, WIDNESS JA, SINGER DB, ADAMSONS K, SCHWARTZ R. Chronic hyperinsulinemia in the fetal rhesus: effects on hepatic enzymes active in lipogenesis and carbohydrate metabolism. *Diabetes* 1979;28:1064.

206. SUSA JB, GRUPPUSO PA, WIDNESS JA, et al. Chronic hyperinsulinemia in the fetal rhesus monkey: effects of physiologic hyperinsulinemia on fetal substrates, hormones and hepatic enzymes. *Am J Obstet Gynecol.* 1984;150:415.

207. CAHILL GF, ZOTTU S, EARLE AS. In vivo effects of glucagon on hepatic glycogen, phosphorylase and glucose-6-phosphatase. *Endocrinol.* 1957; 60:265.

208. WEBER G, CANTERO A. Glucose-6-phosphatase in regenerating, embryonic and newborn rat liver. *Cancer Res.* 1955;15:679.

209. DAWKINS MJR. Changes in glucose-6-phosphatase activity in liver and kidney at birth. *Nature.* 1961;191:72.

210. MERSMANN HJ. Glycolytic and gluconeogenic enzyme levels in pre- and postnatal pigs. *Am J Physiol.* 1971;220:1297.

211. NEMETH A. Glucose-6-phosphatase in the liver of the fetal guinea pig. *J Biol Chem.* 1954;208:773.

212. LEA M, WALKER DG. Metabolism of glucose-6-phosphate in developing mammalian tissues. *Biochem J.* 1964;91:417.

213. DAWKINS MJR. Glycogen synthesis and breakdown in fetal and newborn rat liver. *Ann NY Acad Sci.* 1963;111:203.

214. GIRARD J, CAQUOT D, GUILET I. Control of rat liver phosphorylase,

glucose-6-phosphatase and phosphoenolpyruvate carboxykinase activity by insulin and glucagon during the perinatal period. *Enzyme.* 1973;15:272.

215. GREENGARD O. Enzymic differentiation in mammalian liver. *Science.* 1969;163:891.

216. DOMENECH M, GRUPPUSO PA, SUSA JB, SCHWARTZ R. Induction in utero of hepatic glucose-6-phosphatase by fetal hypoinsulinemia. *Biol Neonate.* 1985;47:92.

217. SCHWARTZ AL, RÄIHÄ NCR, RALL TW. Effect of dibutyryl cyclic AMP on glucose-6-phosphatase activity in human fetal liver explants. *Biochim Biophys Acta.* 1974;343:500.

218. WIDDAS WF. Transport mechanisms in the foetus. *Br Med Bull.* 1961; 17:107.

219. CHINARD FP, DANESINO V, HARTMANN WL, HUGGETT A STG, PAUL W, REYNOLDS SRM. The transmission of hexoses across the placenta in the human and the rhesus monkey *(Macaca mulatta). J Physiol.* 1956;132:289.

220. BATTAGLIA FC, HELLEGERS AE, HELLER CJ, BEHRMAN R. Glucose concentration gradients across the maternal surface, the placenta, and the amnion of the rhesus monkey. *(Macaca mulatta). Am J Obstet Gynecol.* 1964;88:32.

221. FOLKART GR, DANCIS J, MONEY WL. Transfer of carbohydrates across guinea pig placenta. *Am J Obstet Gynecol.* 1960;80:221.

222. McCANN ML, ADAM PA, LIKLY BF, SCHWARTZ R. The prevention of hypoglucosemia by fructose in infants of diabetic mothers. *N Engl J Med.* 1966;275:8.

223. KARVONEN MJ, RÄIHÄ N. Permeability of placenta of the guinea pig to glucose and fructose. *Acta Physiol Scand.* 1954;31:194.

224. YOUNG M, HILL PMM. *Free Amino Acid Transfer Across the Placental Membrane in Foetal and Neonatal Physiology.* London: Cambridge University Press, 1973; 329.

225. DOMENECH M, GRUPPUSO PA, NISHINO VT, SUSA JB, SCHWARTZ R. Preserved fetal plasma amino acid concentrations in the presence of maternal hypoaminoacidemia. *Pediatr Res.* 1986;20:1071.

226. ECONOMIDES DL, NICOLAIDES KH, GAHL W, BERNARDIN I, EVANS M. Plasma amino acids in appropriate and small for gestational age fetuses. *Am J Obstet Gynecol.* 1989;161:1219.

227. CRETIN I, CORBETTA C, SERENI LP, et al. Umbilical amino acid concentrations in normal and growth retarded fetuses sampled in utero by cordocentesis. *Am J Obstet Gynecol.* 1990;162:253.

228. HULL D. Storage and supply of fatty acids before and after birth. Perinatal research. *Br Med Bull.* 1975;31:32.

229. KING KK, ADAM PA, LASKOWSKI DE, SCHWARTZ R. Sources of fatty acids in the newborn. *Pediatrics.* 1971;47:192.

230. DANCIS J, JANSEN V, KAYDEN HJ, BJORNSON L, LEVITZ M. Transfer across perfused human placenta. III. Effect of chain length on transfer of free fatty acids. *Pediat Res.* 1974;8:796.

231. BATTAGLIA FC, MESCHIA G, eds. *An Introduction to Fetal Physiology.* New York: Academic Press, Inc., 1986;123.

232. ECONOMIDES DL, CROOK D, NICOLAIDES KH. Hypertriglyceridaemia and hypoxaemia in small for gestational age fetuses. *Am J Obstet Gynecol.* 1990;162:382.

233. SABATA V. *Carbohydrate and Lipid Metabolism of the Human Fetus.* Praha I: Publishing House of the Czechoslovak Academy of Sciences, 1973.

234. HOLMBERG NG, KAPLAN B, KARVONEN MJ, LIND J, MALM M. Permeability of human placenta to glucose, fructose and xylose. *Acta Physiol Scand.* 1956;36:291.

235. SUSA JB, BOYLAN JM, SEHGAL P, SCHWARTZ R. Impaired insulin secretion in the neonatal rhesus monkey after chronic hyperinsulinemia in utero. *Proc Soc Exp Biol Med.* 1990;194:209.

236. BOZZETTI P, FERRARI MM, MARCONI AM, et al. The relationship of maternal and fetal glucose concentrations in the human from midgestation until term. *Metabolism* 1988;37(4):358.

FACTORS
INFLUENCING
GLUCOSE IN
THE NEONATE

• Techniques and Methods

Although levels of total reducing substance (TRS), true sugar (TS), and glucose have been measured in the blood of newborns since 1911 [1–3], there is still disagreement in defining the normal range of blood sugar values in the neonate, as well as the precise limits of significantly low or high concentrations. Prior to the 1960s, much of the confusion was a result of differences in techniques for collecting, precipitating, and analyzing the blood for true sugar.

Since the early sixties, blood glucose values were found to be related not only to the maturity of the infants studied, but also to the following variables:

1. Maternal factors such as maternal weight [4,5], maternal carbohydrate tolerance, and parenteral fluids given to the mother during labor and delivery [6–12],
2. Mode of delivery [3,6],
3. The precise age of the infants in hours [3],
4. The duration of fasting before sampling [3],
5. The time of initiation and composition of feeding, i.e., breast versus formula feeds [3,13],
6. Parenteral fluids to the infant after birth, and
7. The effects of a variety of intensive care measures.

In addition, the concept of varying size for gestation (AGA = appropriate for gestational age, SGA = small for gestational age, and LGA = large for gestational age) was incorporated into routine newborn evaluations [14,15]. Studies including this important variable have been done during the first hours of life before the first feed [16–18] in infants of obese mothers [5] as well as in AGA full-term infants [11,12]. No additional studies of blood or plasma glucose values controlling for these variables have been reported to our knowledge.

Societal variables, such as the number of very young primiparous (<15 years) and older primiparous (>35 years) mothers, have changed and were compounded in the 1980s by maternal heroin and cocaine addiction and AIDS. Concurrently, advances in obstetrics have improved prenatal care, diagnosis, and prognosis. Newer modalities of management include ultrasound, antitocolytic drugs for premature labor, betamethasone to prevent respiratory distress syndrome (RDS), and the ability to deliver viable infants from high-risk pregnancies and those early in gestation (25–30 weeks).

Neonatal intensive care has also changed dramatically with sophisticated physiologic monitoring, respiratory support, and controlling acid-base and electrolyte abnormalities. All of these modalities are now considered routine in the very low birth weight infant (VLBW) and have resulted in survival rates exceeding 50 percent in infants less than 750 gm birth weight with gestations as short as 25 weeks. All may affect blood glucose levels in the neonate, and few have been incorporated in the study designs reported [11,12].

Except for careful measurements in the term neonate during the first hours [12] and days [11] of life, no new data have been provided to modify the original observations reviewed in 1976 [3; pp 80–86]. Yet, the original data do not adequately describe the current neonatal population, which reflects the changes in society and advances in obstetrical and neonatal intensive care noted above. Nevertheless, all of the data indicate that the blood sugar values in full-term healthy infants decrease during the first hours of life [11,12,19,20] and reach levels within the range of the normal adult (60–90 mg/dl [3.8–5.0 mM]) by 2 [11] to 10 [1,3,20] days of age (Fig. 2-1). The blood glucose levels tend to be even lower in infants of low birth weight [21,22], infants of obese mothers [4,5] and of diabetic mothers [23–25] (Fig. 4-7, Chapter 4). However, the absolute values reported vary, depending upon the multiple variables noted above. In addition, the recent use of reagent strip blood screening techniques, read either by eye or by a meter, to define normal as well as hypoglycemic and hyperglycemic values of blood glucose concentrations in the neonate has further confused the issue [26–29].

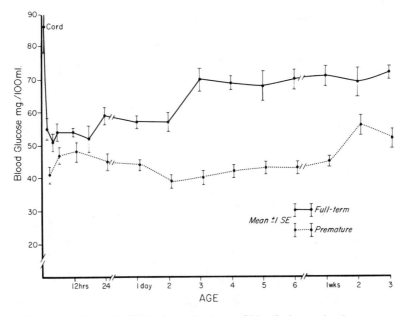

FIGURE 2-1. A total of 206 determinations of blood glucose levels were obtained in 170 full-sized infants (>2.5 kg) and a total of 442 determinations in 104 low birthweight infants (<2.5 kg) throughout the neonatal period. (From Cornblath and Reisner. Reproduced, by permission of *The New England Journal of Medicine*, 273:378, 1965.)

The lack of data has not prevented new definitions for normal, low, or high plasma glucose values based on arbitrary "physiologic" considerations [17,18,30] rather than on data correlating plasma glucose values with brain function [31,32] or neuropsychological outcome. Even more importantly, additional studies are necessary to measure the relationship between blood glucose concentration, blood flow, cerebral glucose transport, counterregulatory hormonal responses, and normal brain metabolism and function as reported by Pryds et al. in preterm infants [32]. Techniques such as PET scanning and magnetic resonance imaging (MRI) can be utilized in such studies in the neonate now.

Currently, the multiple variables (supravide), the lack of basic knowledge of neonatal brain metabolism, and even of statistical data for expected outcome relative to plasma glucose values make the basis for modifying the definitions for normoglycemia, hypoglycemia, and hyperglycemia highly speculative (see Chapter 3, Hypoglycemia in the Neonate).

• Physiologic Influences

At birth, the blood glucose concentration in the infant is proportional to that in the mother, a relative relationship that appears to exist throughout most of fetal life [3; pp 53–54] (see Chapter 1). Thereafter, glucose values fluctuate over a wide range during the first 6–24 hours of life, depending upon the infant's care and treatment, time of first feeding [18,33,34], ambient temperature, degree of handling, prenatal stress, and parenteral calories [35]. Therefore, the age of the infant in hours during the first 48 hours after birth and then in days must be known in order to evaluate and understand the glucose concentrations obtained.

No correlation was found between changes in blood glucose concentrations and the fall in rectal temperature during the *first* hour of life in 13 healthy, vaginally delivered term infants kept at 25°C in the nude [36]. If the temperature is not carefully controlled, this initial chilling may be associated with a significant fall in blood glucose values at 4–6 hours of age [3; p 74] but not at ½, 1, or 24 hours of age. In contrast, Soltesz et al. [37] found no difference in blood glucose values and the rate of disappearance of intravenous glucose in hypothermic versus normothermic newborn infants.

In the term infant, the duration of fasting, the time of initiating the first feeding, as well as its composition and source [13] are also important [11,12]. After a postnatal fast of up to 8 hours' duration, plasma glucose concentrations fell below 40 mg/dl [2.2 mM] in approximately 18 percent of AGA term ($n = 24$) and preterm ($n = 9$) infants and in approximately 75 percent of SGA term ($n = 6$) and preterm ($n = 5$) infants [17]. The lower glucose values were not associated with elevations in plasma ketone concentrations, although increased concentrations of plasma alanine, lactate, and free fatty acids were found [17]. Early adequate dextrose feeds (7.8 gm/kg/day or 30 Kcal/kg/day; 5.4 mg/kg/min) in the first 24 hours of life resulted in increased concentrations of blood glucose in SGA infants of 34–41 weeks gestation, born to either normotensive or preeclamptic mothers [18].

These observations emphasize the need to maintain and record body temperature, age in hours, and time of feedings when evaluating glucose values in full-sized or SGA infants.

In the low birth weight infant (1,250–2,000 gm or 30–34 weeks' gestation) and especially in the very low birth weight (600–1,250 gm/ 24–30 weeks' gestation) infant, careful attention is now routinely given to maintaining temperature, oxygen, parenteral support of glucose, and electrolyte balance. This is achieved by frequent monitoring of oxygenation, glucose values, and metabolic homeostasis (pH, electrolytes, base excess, etc.). These appropriate interventions have obscured any changes in glucose homeostasis that might have occurred as a result of a variety of physiologic factors in this high-risk and abnormal population. This is apparent in the very low birth weight infant (<1000 gm) in whom maintaining the balance between avoiding hypoglycemia and producing hyperglycemia with glucosuria is difficult [38–41].

Even in the larger premature infant between 1,250 and 2,200 gm birth weight, irregular and unpredictable variations in plasma glucose concentrations have been reported after a 4–5 hour fast once feedings have been introduced [21,42].

Within the past decade, many new endocrine factors, especially polypeptide hormones, have been identified and measured at birth and after the first feed. Their role in carbohydrate and glucose homeostasis is being elucidated. Table 2-1 (adapted from Aynsley-Green

TABLE 2-1. Peptides and hormones involved in the utilization of food

Gut motility	Motilin Cholecystokinin Neurotensin Enteroglucagon
Mucosal growth	Gastrin Enteroglucagon
Digestive secretion	Gastrin Secretin Vasoactive inhibitory peptide (VIP) Somatostatin Pancreatic polypeptide
Blood flow	VIP
Absorption	Somatostatin
Enteroinsular axis	Gastric inhibitory peptide (GIP), insulin
Metabolic homeostasis	Insulin Glucagon Growth hormone Cortisol

(From Aynsley-Green. *Annales Nestle Special Edition, Nutrition in Early Life*, 1984, with permission.)

[43]) lists the peptides and hormones that influence glucose concentrations as the newborn adjusts to extrauterine life.

At 18–21 weeks' gestation, mean fetal glucose values were approximately 85 percent of those in maternal blood, whereas concentrations of fetal amino acids were significantly higher than maternal. Insulin, glucagon, gastrin, and pancreatic polypeptide values are higher in maternal venous plasma than in fetal plasma or amniotic fluid, and enteroglucagon and gastric inhibitory peptide are lower [44].

The responsiveness of these substrates and hormones to the first feeding after birth is diminished in preterm infants with a mean gestation of 33.5 weeks and birth weight of 1,950 gm. Over the first 24 days of life, preterm infants (28–33 weeks gestation) given initial bolus feedings of milk show a marked cyclical increase in responsiveness of gastrointestinal hormones following feeding. In contrast, preterm infants maintained on parenteral fluids or receiving milk continuously do not show these surges in hormonal secretions [13,43].

The term infant responds to the first milk feeding with an appropriate increase in concentrations of blood glucose, plasma insulin, gastrin, growth hormone, and enteroglucagon. Plasma pancreatic glucagon concentrations remain unchanged. All of the plasma concentrations of the gastrointestinal hormones increase to values exceeding those in the adult over the first 6–16 days of life in the term infant. Some differences in responsiveness depend upon whether the infant is fed breast milk or formula, but type of milk does not appear to affect blood glucose values.

• Methodologic Effects

Collecting and Handling the Blood Specimen

The source of the blood to be analyzed for glucose is important in interpreting the results. When dextrose is infused via an umbilical artery or central line catheter, the site of the blood sampling may affect the results obtained. If the umbilical artery catheter is low, capillary samples from the lower extremities may be artificially high and not representative of systemic glucose concentrations [45]. This was previously evident from the data of Stur [46]. Equally critical is the error of withdrawing blood without adequate flushing of the dextrose-infused line or sampling proximal or distal to an infusion site.

Care must be exercised in handling the blood sample [47]. The increased rate of in vitro glycolysis in the red blood cells of the newborn infant has been demonstrated by a number of authors [21,48–50] (Fig. 2-2). Twenty-eight blood samples randomly obtained from

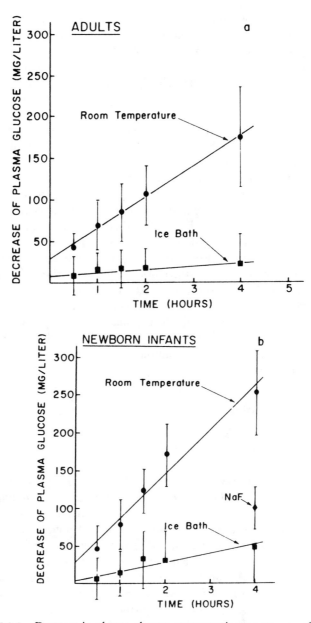

FIGURE 2-2. Decrease in plasma glucose concentration on storage of whole blood from adults (top) and newborns (bottom). Bars are one standard deviation. Rates of decrease (slope, in mg/liter per hour) are adults: room temperature, 36, ice, 3.9; newborns: room temperature, 60, ice, 11. In blood from newborn infants stored with NaF, the decrease at 4 hours was intermediate between that of cooled blood and blood stored at room temperature without preservatives. (From Lin et al. *Clin Chem.* 1976; 22:2031, with permission.)

low birth weight infants less than 3 days of age were found to have a mean (± 1 SD) glucose level of 57 ± 12.5 mg/dl (3.17 mM) [3]. After standing at room temperature for 3 hours, 13 samples had glucose values of <20 mg/dl (<1.1 mM), and 7 had no detectable glucose at all (0.0 mM). Thus, if whole blood from young infants is permitted to stand at room temperature, erroneously low glucose values may be obtained.

Glycolysis can be prevented in shed blood most effectively [50] by keeping the sample on ice as is done with samples for blood gas analysis, or by precipitating the blood at once. Alternatively, the cells can be separated immediately and the plasma analyzed for glucose. Adding sodium fluoride (NaF) (2 mg/ml of blood) to the anticoagulant and keeping the sample refrigerated is also effective in minimizing glycolysis. Sodium fluoride, at this concentration, may affect the accuracy of some methods that use glucose oxidase for analyzing glucose [21] and also interferes with the determinations of sodium, calcium, and urea [50]. Fluoride does not affect the glucose oxidase test if the blood is precipitated with barium or sodium hydroxide and zinc sulfate [3] and the filtrate is used for analysis.

Specific small-volume capillary tubes (e.g., Microtainer Becton Dickenson, USA) containing NaF, EDTA, and thymol have been useful in collecting 50 µl samples. This allows for duplicate analysis in the laboratory [51].

Methodology

Bedside Rapid Techniques

Glucose Oxidase Analyzers. Analyzers (Beckman, YSI) utilizing a glucose oxidase-impregnated membrane and micro whole blood samples (10–25 µl) at the bedside provide accurate results within minutes, especially for values below 40 mg/dl (2.2 mM) and up to 400 mg/dl (22 mM) [26,27]. Several substances in high concentrations may interfere with the glucose oxidase analyzer determination (see Appendix I), but these are unusual in the neonate. Careful, frequent standardization with a known concentration of glucose is required to assure accuracy. These measuring devices can be used effectively and accurately by nursing personnel, albeit after a short period of training and with ongoing surveillance and maintenance [26,52].

Reagent Strip Techniques. These screening methods were developed primarily for estimating blood glucose control in adult patients with diabetes mellitus. Recently, their use has been extended to include diabetic children. This same objective applies to the newer glucose screening reagents and techniques, including the most recent glucose reflectance meters. Their use was never intended to monitor blood glucose values in the neonate. In fact, one manufacturer has recommended that their reagent strips not be used to screen for hypoglycemia in the neonate (Ames revised package insert 1985 for Dextrostix). Nevertheless, neonates have been monitored for both hypoglycemia and hyperglycemia with these screening techniques. Unfortunately, recently the diagnosis of hypoglycemia has been based solely upon such screening results [28], without requiring a confirmatory, reliable laboratory blood glucose determination.

Published reports [26,27,29,53–59] have evaluated a number of screening reagent strips, read either by eye or by a variety of instruments, that estimate blood glucose values at the bedside on small volumes of blood within a short period of time. Essentially all of the reagent strips consist of a dry preparation containing glucose oxidase enzyme, a color reagent with a permanent or fading end point and the necessary cofactors to drive the reaction, contained under a semipermeable membrane through which glucose diffuses from the blood. The screening methods have been tested for precision, accuracy, and reliability over a range of blood glucose values. These reports include blood specimens obtained from neonates, children, and adults at the bedside or artificially reconstructed specimens of blood, plasma, or clear solutions measured at a later time away from the patient. All of these reports compare results with reliable standard glucose analytical techniques.

Sources of error with these rapid reagent strip methods, which result from poor individual operator technique, can include improperly preparing the skin (isopropyl alcohol [60]), placing an inadequate drop of blood on the active portion of the strip, timing the reaction incorrectly, washing or wiping away the blood, and reading the color either against a standard or in a reflectance meter [26,27,61]. In addition, polycythemia or anemia, which are common in the neonate [61–64] can affect the results obtained. Reagent strips must be dated when opened because their accuracy is compromised if exposed to the air for prolonged periods of time.

To summarize:

- No reagent strips have been developed to accurately and reliably diagnose hypoglycemia in the neonate.

- Reagent strips frequently tend to overestimate the numbers of low values for glucose (e.g., <40–50 mg/dl [<2.2–2.8 mM]) (overdiagnosed hypoglycemia).

- Less often, false negatives occur (missed hypoglycemia).

The American medical community [26,27,29,52] and their colleagues abroad [52,61,62,64] agree that, while screening with reagent strips may be useful, it is essential that a plasma glucose determination be done by a reliable laboratory method in order to establish a diagnosis of hypoglycemia or hyperglycemia.

The glucose oxidase analyzer can be used to establish this diagnosis. This method has been demonstrated to be reliable, effective, and efficient in the special care nursery [26,27,52] and should replace reagent strip screening techniques. There is still no substitute for a properly collected and handled specimen of blood analyzed in an accredited laboratory to establish a diagnosis of hypoglycemia or hyperglycemia in the neonate.

Laboratory Glucose Analysis

The proteins in blood interfere with the accurate analysis of glucose in all chemical methods and must be removed either by dialysis as in the automated techniques or by precipitation [65,66]. The precipitating reagents used include perchloric acid (Boehringer) and the alkaline salts of zinc [67]. The latter precipitate glycolytic intermediates, glutathione, sodium fluoride, and nonsugar reducing substances, as well as protein. The analysis of the Somogyi protein-free filtrates with proper chemical techniques indicates true sugar values [68] or glucose if a specific glucose oxidase or hexokinase is used. The ortho-toluidine method as described by Hultman [69] and modified by Hyvarinen and Nikkila [70] has been found to be as specific and reliable as the glucose-oxidase method in the newborn [71]. True sugar values include glucose, fructose, and galactose [72,73], although the latter has a reducing power four-fifths of glucose.

If a specific enzymatic method is used to analyze the perchloric acid filtrate or dialysate of blood from a newborn, the high bilirubin concentration and the reduced glutathione present in high concentration in the red blood cells may inhibit the color development in the glucose-oxidase system, resulting in erroneously low concentrations of glucose [66,67,74]. Peroxides not originating from the oxidation of glucose, as well as other oxidants present in blood, may cause nonspecific oxidation of the chromagen, resulting in falsely high values [71]. These errors may be avoided by the use of barium hydroxide $(Ba(OH)_2)$ and zinc sulfate $(ZnSO_4)$ [75] as the precipitating reagents. Glucose is stable in all of the protein-free filtrates of blood for at least 48 hours with refrigeration.

In addition to specificity, the reliability and reproducibility of the method used for blood glucose determination must be known. Errors in pipetting small samples of blood (0.01–0.2 ml) must be determined by analyzing repeated aliquots of the same blood. The variability of the glucose analysis may be as little as ±2.0 mg/dl (0.11 mM), using 0.5 ml blood and the Somogyi true sugar method (<5 percent) or as great as ±6–10 mg/dl (0.33–0.56 mM; 10–40 percent) with smaller blood samples obtained by inexperienced personnel. The values for true sugars and glucose, as measured by specific methods, are comparable in blood samples from both preterm and term infants during the first days of life.

Since glucose is distributed equally throughout the plasma and intracellular water [76], the concentration of glucose in plasma is somewhat higher than that in whole blood and is not influenced by the hematocrit [77]. Capillary blood, being a variable mixture of arterial and venous blood, may have levels of glucose greater than that in peripheral venous blood [64,78]. This is particularly important in infants with hematocrits of 60 percent or higher. An apparent reduction in whole blood glucose of 10 to 20 percent may occur, depending upon the hematocrit, even with a reliable laboratory technique. On the other hand, the results with screening methods utilizing reagent strips may result in even greater apparent reductions of 30 to 40 percent, with hematocrits exceeding 50 to 60 percent [63].

Only diffusible glucose is available to glucose-dependent tissues such as the brain. Plasma glucose concentrations closely reflect this value and should be used to define hypoglycemia, normoglycemia, and hyperglycemia.

In summary, glucose concentrations measured in the neonate may be influenced by any or all of the following:

- Collecting and handling the blood
    Source of blood
    Accuracy in collecting sample
    Prevention of glycolysis
- Method of analysis
    Bedside rapid methods
        Glucose oxidase analyzer
        Reagent strip screening
    Laboratory
        Precipitating proteins and other interfering substances
        Specificity of methods
        Reproducibility

- Other factors

    Hematocrits in whole blood versus plasma values

    Interfering substances with reagent strips as well as glucose oxidase analyzers

• Glucose Concentrations in the Neonate

Term Infants

The First Hours of Life

At birth, the glucose concentration in the blood from the umbilical vein is related to that in the mother (approximately 85 percent of her level) and is usually higher than that from the umbilical artery. The absolute values vary, depending upon the time of the last meal, the duration and nature of the delivery, and the parenteral administration of dextrose [6–10]. Thus, the blood glucose values in the umbilical vein can vary between 40 and 90 mg/dl (2.2 and 5.0 mM) after a normal vaginal delivery during which the mother was given no intravenous dextrose. On the other hand, concentrations as high as 160 to 200 mg/dl (8.9 to 11.1 mM) have been reported in umbilical vein blood if the mother has been given parenteral dextrose prior to and during delivery (see Table 2-2).

Following birth, there is usually a fall in the infant's concentration of blood glucose, the rate being dependent on the starting values, with stabilization at mean blood glucose values of 45 to 60 mg/dl (2.5 to 3.3 mM) between 4 and 6 hours of age (see Fig. 2-3) [11,12,19,20,79]. Table 2-3 and Figure 2-3 summarize observations made between 1961 and 1987 of blood glucose concentrations prior to the first feed in term infants. These values are remarkably similar considering the changes in obstetric and pediatric management that have occurred over that time period.

In infants fasted for long periods of time (6 to 24 hours), the blood glucose values usually stabilized after the first 2 hours of life. It is noteworthy that blood glucose values that are low at birth can actually increase rather than fall (see Fig. 2-3, Group IV).

Effect of Feedings

Once feedings are begun during the first hours of life, the mean plasma glucose concentrations tend to rise (Fig. 2-4), but wide fluctuations in individual values persist. The range was found to be from 40 to 120 mg/dl (2.2 to 6.67 mM) in infants between 1 and 28 days of age

TABLE 2-2. Levels of blood (plasma) sugar (mg/dl) in normal full-term infants after initiation of feedings

	HOURS FASTING	AGE (days)								
		1	2	3	4	5	6	7–13	14–20	21–27
I* (N = 51)	4									
Mean		55	57	62	68	67				
Range				15–120						
II† (N = 10–35)	4½									
Mean		57	57	70	69	68	70	71	69	72
Range		21–85	46–77	49–88	58–61	36–90	55–82	58–88	46–88	62–104
III‡ (N = 26–69)	3–4									
Mean		65	71	73	83		80			
Range		17–119	48–98	50–114	56–116		54–102			
IV§ (N = 92–113)	3–4									
Mean		56	61	64						
Range		33–74	46–81	48–79						

*Group I were analyzed by the Somogyi method (true blood sugar) and reported by Norval et al. [1].
†Group II were analyzed by glucose oxidase (blood glucose) and reported by Cornblath and Reisner [80].
‡Group III were analyzed by a Beckman glucose analyzer (plasma glucose) and reported by Srinivasan et al. [11].
§Group IV were analyzed by glucose oxidase (serum glucose) and reported by Heck and Erenberg [12].

TABLE 2-3. Levels of sugar (mg/dl) in whole blood in low birth weight infants

	AT BIRTH CORD	AGE (hours)								
		0–3	4–6	12	18	24	30	36	42	48
I*										
Mean	71	47 {0–6}		45	43	43	44	41	46	50
Range	24–140	26–72 {0–6}		18–107	15–62	16–60	18–90	25–60	18–78	19–80
N	21	20 {0–6}		23	23	14	15	10	14	14
II†										
Mean		41	47	48	45 {18–24}			44 {36–48}		
Range		24–72	21–70	25–89	23–84 {18–24}			18–73 {36–48}		
N		20	26	22	37 {18–24}			49 {36–48}		

	AGE (days)													
	0	1	2	3	4	5	6	7	8	9	10	11	12	13
III‡														
Mean	45	53	55	60	60	58	63	63	66	65	71	65	63	64
Range	. . . . 15 to 115 mg/dl													
N	33							28 (7–13 days)		24 (14–20)		23 (21–27)		22 (28–55)
IV§														
Mean	44	44	39	40	42	43	43	45 (7–13 days)		56 (14–20)		52 (21–27)		48 (28–55)
Range	18–73	15–73	20–64	21–79	18–78	22–83	22–83	28–61		23–98		18–77		22–83
N	49	45	45	43	32	33	33	40		33		26		43

*Group I: True blood sugar determined by the Somogyi method [81].
†Group II: Blood glucose determined by glucose oxidase method [21].
‡Group III: True blood sugar determined by the Somogyi method after 2–3 hour fast [2].
§Group IV: Blood glucose analyzed by glucose oxidase method after 3½–4 hour fast [21].

MEAN CONTROL BLOOD SUGAR CURVES

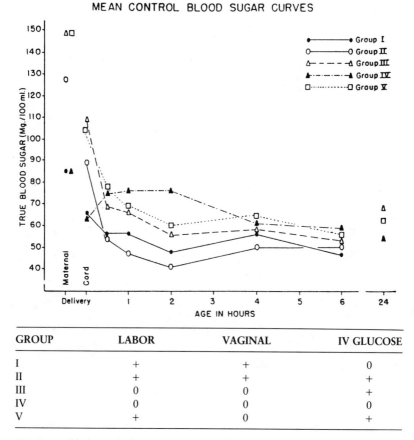

(From Cornblath et al. Reproduced by permission of *Pediatrics* 27:378, copyright 1961.)

FIGURE 2-3. Blood sugar determinations were obtained on 50 full-sized infants between birth and 24 hours of age.

[80]. After 24 hours of age, fewer low concentrations of blood glucose were found. In one study, mean concentrations of plasma glucose attained values similar to those of the older infant after 24 hours of age [11], whereas in another, comparable values occurred within 48 hours of life [12]. These findings contrast with the results from earlier studies in which mean adult values were not observed until after 72 hours of age.

Variables that can affect blood glucose concentrations within the first days of life include initial age, source and volume of feedings, and the sampling time related to feeding. The interpretation of these values depends upon an adequate size of an appropriate reference population and the statistical analysis of the results [52].

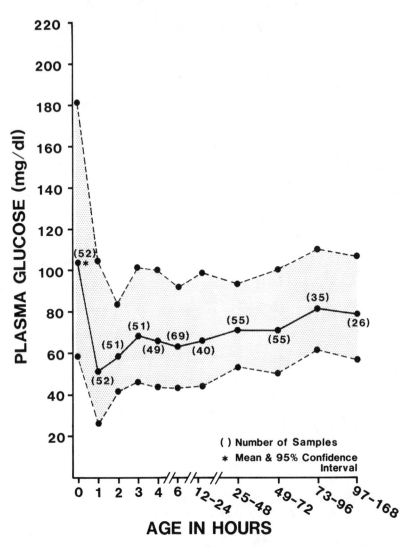

FIGURE 2-4. Predicted plasma glucose values during first week of life in healthy term neonates appropriate for gestational age. (From Srinivasan. *J Pediatr.* 1986; 109:905, with permission.)

Low Birth Weight

The First Hours of Life

In contrast with the body of knowledge about blood glucose concentrations in full-term infants in the first hours of life, there is inadequate information about low birth weight infants, especially with current management and with the survival of very low birth weight (VLBW) infants.

Current care of low birth weight preterm infants has changed dramatically in the past 15 years. Almost all preterm infants are given nutritional support soon after birth, while only a few larger infants may still be fasted briefly. In contrast, earlier studies of low birth weight infants [21,34,81,82] did provide data on fasting up to 48 and even 72 hours [34]. This information was valid under the conditions existing at that time, but is no longer applicable to current low birth weight or VLBW nursery populations.

Studies prior to 1970, in infants ranging in weight from 735 to 2,190 gm and of indeterminate gestation, reported blood true sugar and glucose concentrations within the first 48 hours of postnatal life prior to formula feedings [21,81,82] (Fig. 2-1). Cord blood glucose concentrations were similar to those in term infants. Thereafter, mean blood glucose values were distinctly lower than those reported in term infants (Fig. 2-1) and remained around 45 mg/dl (2.5 mM) (range of means 41–55 mg/dl [2.28–3.06 mM]) for the next 48 hours. While 15 to 20 percent of individual determinations were less than 30 mg/dl (1.67 mM), few (1.2 percent) were less than 20 mg/dl (1.11 mM). Prolonged (48–72 hours) fasting significantly increased the frequency of low blood glucose values [34].

Fasting values are not relevant to the care of preterm low birth weight or VLBW neonates who are given parenteral support if early feedings (prior to 2 to 4 hours of age) are not deemed feasible. Their importance lies in recognizing the wide fluctuations in blood glucose concentrations that were observed previously over hours and even days without any overt clinical correlations.

These early studies show mean glucose values obtained 3 to 4 hours after feedings, which by today's standard would be considered nutritionally inadequate, that were consistently lower than those in fed term infants (Fig. 2-1). Their mean values did not reach those considered within the accepted range for older infants and children throughout the period of observation.

No studies within the past 15 years have addressed the question of expected preprandial plasma glucose concentrations to be found in infants being cared for in neonatal intensive care units (NICU) today.

Glucose Concentrations in Cerebrospinal Fluid

Abnormal values have been defined for both the absolute concentration of glucose in the cerebrospinal fluid (CSF) as well as the CSF/blood glucose ratio. Concentrations of CSF glucose below 50 mg/dl

(2.78 mM) are considered significantly low at all ages [83]. CSF glucose/blood (plasma) glucose ratios below 0.4 are also abnormally low. Normal ratios average between 0.74 and 0.81 in the neonate [84,85], between 0.4 to 0.6 in older infants and children [86], and between 0.8 to 1.0 in adults [83,84,87].

A number of studies of CSF and blood total reducing substances have been done in both the full-term and low birth weight neonate [88–90] prior to 1950. In young infants, CSF sugar concentrations higher than those in blood were reported in 8 to 50 percent of infants. Unfortunately, it is impossible to determine from these studies the reliability of the values for blood total reducing substances measured without precautions to prevent glycolysis.

Using a specific method to measure glucose in samples within 30 minutes of sampling, the ratio of CSF glucose/blood (plasma) glucose was 0.81 (range 0.44 to 2.5) in 87 AGA term and 0.74 (range 0.55 to 1.0) in 30 preterm infants. All infants were considered normal, with no evidence of any infection or intracranial hemorrhage [85].

Low CSF glucose concentrations or hypoglycorrhachia have been associated with bacterial, tuberculous, fungal and viral meningitis, syphilis, sarcoidosis, subarachnoid hemorrhage, and hypoglycemia. The CSF/blood (plasma) glucose ratio varies, depending upon the etiology of the low CSF glucose values. The ratio may be less than 0.5 in the presence of intracranial hemorrhage and significantly lower than that (<0.1–0.3) with bacterial meningitis [85]. However, in 16 pediatric patients with low plasma glucose values and CSF glucose concentrations <50 mg/dl (2.78 mM), only one had a CSF/blood (plasma) ratio <0.5, the others were >0.6. This relationship between the CSF and blood glucose was observed when the blood glucose was obtained between 1 and 114 minutes, usually less than 30 minutes, prior to the lumbar puncture.

In the presence of a low CSF glucose concentration, a plasma and CSF determination are both necessary to diagnose hypoglycemia. Hypoglycorrhachia can occur hours to days following a significant cerebral or subarachnoid bleed in the neonate and persist for days to weeks (as long as 57 days) [91]. The relationships among glucose, electrolytes (e.g., potassium), and central nervous system (CNS) bleeds, cerebral infarcts, and CNS abnormalities are just beginning to be elucidated [92].

While the CSF glucose can fall quickly in the presence of acute hypoglycemia, the rise in CSF glucose following oral or parenteral glucose appears to take from 30 minutes to 4 hours. Thus, a CSF glucose value may not reflect the current blood value. It is recommended that a blood be obtained for a plasma glucose determination (*not* reagent strip screen) within 30 minutes prior to a lumbar puncture in order to determine a valid CSF/blood (plasma) glucose ratio [86].

• Normoglycemia, Hypoglycemia, and Hyperglycemia in the Neonate

Since 1908, blood sugar concentrations have been measured in newborn infants, yet the definitions of significantly high and low blood glucose values remain controversial. Initially, the new technology was used to measure values in term infants [93, 94].

Clinical interest in blood sugar determinations increased with the availability of insulin for the treatment of diabetes mellitus in 1922. The recognition of iatrogenic brain damage from exogenous insulin and the diagnosis of clinical hypoglycemic syndromes that produced illness, neurologic sequelae, and death were responsible.

In 1929, Van Creveld [95] was the first to recognize that the blood sugar values in premature infants (defined by birth weight alone) between 1,500 and 2,500 gm were lower than those in term infants reported previously. Although the low values persisted during the first weeks of life, he attributed this to immaturity of hepatic regulation. He did not attribute any symptoms or significance to these lower concentrations.

By 1937, Hartmann and Jaudon [96] also noted the lower blood sugar concentrations in term infants and infants of diabetic mothers (IDMs) during the first days of life but also attributed no significance to them. They did report on 286 cases of significant hypoglycemia studied over a 15-year period. They carefully distinguished between serum "apparent," whole and capillary blood, and "true" sugar values and assigned a different significance to the glucose values obtained by each technique. Only newborns, infants, and children with severe manifestations or recurrent or persistent clinical hypoglycemia were described as significant. This report included a classification of hypoglycemia, diagnostic tests, and reports of microscopic sections of the pancreas that distinguished between hyperplasia and hypertrophy of the islets and isolated islet cell tumors.

Other reports of that era (1938–1954) were related to specific syndromes, e.g., glycogen storage disease [97], or isolated tumors of the islet cells or adenomatosis, often discovered at autopsy [98].

In 1953, McQuarrie [99] presented his extensive experience with idiopathic hypoglycemia of infancy. He excluded "normal newly born infants with transient hypoglycemia" of which he had seen "many patients . . . but have made no special study of (this) type of case." He then described 25 patients with recurrent severe hypoglycemia with onset between 1 day and 5 years of age (21 of 25 with an onset under 2 years). He suggested that early recognition and effective treatment with ACTH might prevent brain damage.

At the same time, Komrower [100] and Farquhar [22, 25] reported infants of diabetic mothers and normal infants with very low blood sugar levels (some even zero) and concluded these low values were "physiologic" in the neonate and of no clinical significance. These low concentrations occurred most often in infants of diabetic mothers fasted up to 5 days of age [101], an accepted medical practice of that decade for both term and premature infants to avoid aspiration and respiratory problems.

Concurrently, the 1950s and 1960s also saw the beginning of interest in careful physiologic and biochemical measurements of high-risk infants in order to more fully define those factors that put them at risk and might be remediated [102–106]. These included measurements of neutral temperature, ambient oxygen concentration, electrolytes, blood gases, substrates, and carefully controlled clinical trials of different antibiotics, sulfonamides, and other therapeutic modalities.

The observation that transient symptomatic hypoglycemia occurred in eight infants of toxemic mothers was contrary to the prevalent opinion that low blood glucose concentrations were of little significance in the neonate [107]. In order to establish that, in fact, the symptomatic infants had blood glucose values significantly lower than unaffected neonates, it was necessary to determine a statistical definition of hypoglycemia and hyperglycemia. Furthermore, in asymptomatic infants, these definitions might provide a basis for prevention, diagnosis, and intervention.

A statistical approach is dependent upon reliable assays, careful definitions of the populations studied, their care and outcome, and sufficient numbers of subjects to allow a proper statistical analysis. Such a survey was done in the 1960s in full-term, normal-sized infants, low birth weight infants, and twins. When combined with Whipple's triad, i.e., (1) clinical manifestations, (2) a significantly low blood glucose measurement, and (3) clearing of symptoms with restoration of blood glucose concentration to normal, these results, based on two values exceeding two standard deviations below the mean, have provided a convincing definition for significant, symptomatic hypoglycemia since the 1960s [21, 80].

These criteria were widely accepted and provided a basis for screening and evaluating a number of neonates with previously unexplained clinical manifestations. As a result, a number of new entities were found to have hypoglycemia as a major contributing factor, e.g., Beckwith-Weidemann syndrome (see p. 206), congenital hypopituitarism (see p. 187), congenital optic nerve hypotrophy (see p. 183), complication of exchange transfusions for Rh disease [108], and early recognition of hyperinsulinemia (see p. 193), glycogen storage diseases (see p. 249), and newer metabolic disorders (see p. 361).

In addition to a statistical definition, another way to identify significant hypoglycemia is to correlate acute, subacute, and chronic neurophysiologic and/or biochemical changes that occur in response to specific blood glucose concentrations. Acute changes may result in adrenomedullary responses [32], abnormal patterns in auditory [31] or visual [32] evoked potentials, generalized electroencephalographic alterations, abnormal positron emission tomography scans, magnetic resonance imaging, and early clinical manifestations of neuroglycopenia [107]. Hypoglycemia may affect the cardiovascular as well as the central nervous system acutely. Subacute and chronic effects may be manifest as abnormal behavior, neuropsychiatric aberrations, and mental retardation. There may be chronic seizures and neuromuscular abnormalities as well. Ultimately, interpretation of these observations will depend upon accurately measuring and correlating plasma glucose concentrations with cerebral blood flow, intracerebral glucose uptake, and brain energy metabolism and function [32].

In the 1970s, based on "physiologic" considerations in the mature individual, it was suggested that any blood glucose value less than 40 mg/dl warranted the diagnosis of hypoglycemia [17, 30]. Although no evidence was provided to support this hypothesis, proponents did utilize this new value as the one criterion for all neonates at all ages. However, based on the original definition for neonatal hypoglycemia, prospective follow-up studies of hypoglycemic and normoglycemic controls did not indicate significant neurologic handicaps in either group of high-risk premature and SGA infants [109]. The hypoglycemic group did have less of an improvement in IQ between 4 and 6 years of age compared to that in controls. To our knowledge, no other outcome data relating blood glucose values in neonates with abnormalities in CNS function were reported during that decade.

In the 1980s, with the survival of VLBW premies, the development of PET and MRI scanning and correlations between blood glucose concentrations and neurologic function such as evoked potentials [31,32] and electroencephalogram (EEG) changes, objective data began to accumulate in some animal models. These were often complex experiments involving hypoxia, changes in blood flow and glucose uptake, as well as hypoglycemia. In contrast, uncomplicated fetal hyperinsulinemia has been produced in the third trimester rhesus monkey [110]. Hypoglycemia developed postnatally and persisted for 6 to 10 hours untreated. Although there was some delay in adaptation to the test situation in the experimental group, long-term (up to 5 years) behavioral and neurologic follow-up could not discriminate between control and hypoglycemic animals [110].

Data in adults and preliminary results in neonates suggested that changes in auditory evoked potentials occurred when serum glucose values fell below 70 mg/dl (3.9 mM) in the normal adult [111] and 47 mg/dl (2.6 mM) in 1 of 5 hypoglycemic neonates [31]. These acute electrophysiologic changes may persist for hours but are transient and have not been correlated with long-term adverse outcome. More recently, a prospective controlled feeding study in 661 infants under 1,850 gm birth weight was completed. A retrospective analysis was made of over 6,000 blood glucose determinations obtained in conjunction with this feeding study. Lucas et al. [112] utilized only the first blood glucose concentration obtained on any given day between birth and 2 + months of age for their analysis. Multiple regression analyses was used to control for confounding factors. They concluded that 5 or more days (not necessarily consecutive) of a blood glucose value less than 47 mg/dl (2.6 mM) correlated positively with an increased risk of neurodevelopmental abnormalities at 18 months of age [52]. They emphasized the long duration involved and the fact that a single blood glucose value less than 47 mg/dl (2.6 mM) does not indicate CNS damage in itself. In fact, the data suggest that the normal plasma glucose concentration exceeds 47 mg/dl (2.6 mM) rather than provides a cutoff for hypoglycemia [52].

With current techniques available, data are required to correlate both acute consequences of various concentrations of blood glucose with objective neurologic malfunctions and their long-term consequence. The latter is difficult and requires a prospective controlled study with both hypoglycemic and normoglycemic controls, as well as long-term follow-up. Without such a study, the recently revised specific definitions of hypoglycemia have little to support their acceptance or use.

Definitions of Normoglycemia, Hypoglycemia, and Hyperglycemia

Any single blood glucose value reflects a balance between glucose utilization and glucose production (endogenous from liver, exogenous from digestion of carbohydrate) as modulated by hormonal interactions. Hormones both stimulate (insulin) and inhibit glucose uptake and utilization (glucagon, epinephrine, growth hormone, corticosteroids). In addition, events preceding the measurement such as fasting, feeding, or abrupt cessation of parenteral glucose, as well as those occurring subsequently, affect the interpretation. Biologic variability, homeostatic adaptability, as well as compensatory mechanisms of individual human infants preclude assigning an absolute or single value as the dividing line between normality and abnormality for any measurement made to define neonatal homeostasis. All of these variables, compounded by the problems of collecting and analyzing the sample, clearly indicate that assigning a characteristic or a prognostic significance to any one specific glucose determination is unwarranted.

This variability presents a dilemma of interpretation and management for the individual physician caring for a specific newborn infant. In the absence of information relating specific ranges of blood glucose concentrations to either significant acute neurophysiologic changes or permanent neurodevelopment outcome, the available statistical data in normal term infants can serve as a basis for clinical management of the neonate.

Term Infant

All relevant data from studies with reliable glucose determinations in normal term infants through 1987 have been analyzed even though these included a variety of feeding regimens, modes of delivery, and management of the mother's labor and delivery (e.g., parenteral glucose versus no fluid) [3,11,12,28,80]. This analysis serves as the basis for normal, intermediate, and abnormal ranges presented to aid in managing glucose homeostasis in the term neonate.

With the initial cord blood glucose values ranging between 80–150 mg/dl (4.4–8.3 mM), newborn infants stabilize their mean plasma concentrations around 50 to 60 mg/dl (2.8 to 3.3 mM) by 4 to 6 hours of age. Individual values may range between 30 to 100 mg/dl (1.7 to 5.6 mM) and a significant number (15–20 percent) may have had one or even two glucose concentrations between 15 and 30 mg/dl (0.83 and 1.67 mM) during those initial hours. These are most common between 2 and 4 hours of age. At approximately 24 hours of age, these mean concentrations are 60 to 65 mg/dl (3.33 to 3.61 mM) (range 40–90 mg/dl [2.22–5.0 mM]). Thereafter, mean glucose values of 65 to 75 mg/dl (3.61 to 4.17 mM) are not uncommon, but may increase to 80 mg/dl (4.44 mM) [11], depending upon the feeding regimen. The normal range of plasma glucose concentrations after 48 hours of age is between 50 to 100 mg/dl (2.78 to 5.56 mM).

Symptomatic hypoglycemia as a result of hyperinsulinism, congenital hypopituitarism, or maternal diabetes mellitus has been documented in the first hours of life in term infants, based upon reliable laboratory blood glucose determinations and a prompt response to parenteral glucose. The glucose concentrations were almost always less than 20 mg/dl (1.11 mM), and the clinical manifestations cleared promptly following adequate therapy. These plasma glucose concentrations (<20–25 mg/dl [1.11–1.39 mM]) are clearly abnormally low and warrant the diagnosis of significant hypoglycemia. The significance of glucose values between 25 and 40 mg/dl (1.39 and 2.22 mM) still requires clarification and depends upon duration and clinical manifestations. This range can be considered as intermediate and an indication to raise the blood glucose to the normoglycemic levels.

To date, there is no clinical or physiologic evidence to support the significance of the statistical definition of hyperglycemia derived some 25 years ago as 125 mg/dl (6.9 mM) for both term and low birth weight infants. There are two important consequences of increased blood glucose concentrations: (1) producing hyperosmolality in the brain and other organs and (2) exceeding the renal maximal tubular reabsorption, inducing an osmotic diuresis. The plasma glucose concentrations in transient diabetes mellitus (see Chapter 6) far exceed these statistical definitions of the upper range of normal. This again illustrates that a progressive range of severity exists as a result of biologic variability and individual adaptation (Table 2.4).

Preterm Infant

In the fetus, the blood glucose concentration is approximately 85 percent of that in the mother, whose blood glucose values can fluctuate between 60 and 120 mg/dl (3.3 and 6.7 mM). These variations depend upon the period of gestation, duration of fasting, and maternal diet. Thus, the fetus may have experienced a range of glucose concentrations between 50 and 100 mg/dl (2.78 and 5.56 mM) throughout gestation.

The VLBW premature newborn represents a stage in adaptation between the fetus and the mature term baby. However, prematures differ from the term infant in body composition (e.g., less fat, relatively larger brain), hepatic glycogen stores, and maturity of enzymatic processes and hormonal controls. In addition, circulatory and respiratory adjustments, including those that affect the brain, influence glucose utilization. All of these variable factors contribute to the labile blood glucose concentrations found in the VLBW [113] and the lower values in the larger premature infants [48,80]. In fact, it is remarkable that so many of these high-risk infants sustained their blood glucose concentrations at levels found in normal term infants during a period when parenteral support was uncommon and oral intake minimal to moderate [21].

TABLE 2-4. Plasma glucose concentrations in normal term infants

AGE (hrs)	HYPOGLYCEMIA	Intermediate	NORMOGLYCEMIA	Intermediate	HYPERGLYCEMIA
		(mg/dl)			
0–6	0–25	25–40	40–100	100–125	>125
6–24	0–30	30–45	45–100	100–125	>125
>24	0–40	40–50	50–100	100–125	>125
		(mM)			
0–6	0–1.4	1.4–2.2	2.2–5.6	5.6–6.9	>6.9
6–24	0–1.7	1.7–2.5	2.5–5.6	5.6–6.9	>6.9
>24	0–2.2	2.2–2.8	2.8–5.6	5.6–6.9	>6.9

There is no current data, either of a statistical nature or relating glucose concentrations to prognosis, available upon which to base an adequate definition for normoglycemia, hypo-, or hyperglycemia in these VLBW and premature infants. An arbitrary recommendation may be based on any or all of the following: (1) the range of values found in the fetus, (2) the statistical data from the 1960s, and/or (3) the data used for the term infant (supra vide).

In view of the complexity of care provided preterm low birth weight infants, it is no longer relevant to apply previously derived statistical standards to current premature populations.

Utilizing the last option, severe hypoglycemia is defined as a plasma value less than 25 mg/dl (1.39 mM). The values noted for the term infant above can also be used for diagnosis and management of the premature and VLBW infant, recognizing that these are only estimates.

The clinical significance of hyperglycemia depends upon the maturity, age, and status of the infant. The definition of values for hyperglycemia requires individual monitoring for glucosuria and hyperosmolality, which should be considered when the glucose concentration exceeds 125 mg/dl (6.94 mM). In these high-risk premature infants, the goal for sustaining normoglycemia should be to maintain a range of plasma glucose concentrations between 40 and 100 mg/dl (2.22 and 5.56 mM). Prospective controlled follow-up studies correlating reliable plasma glucose concentrations, maturity, and documented clinical observations with neurologic function and neurodevelopmental outcomes are necessary before more definitive recommendations for the ranges of normality and abnormality can be made for all neonates.

• Summary

Current knowledge would not support a precise "cutoff" definition of hypoglycemia, normoglycemia, or hyperglycemia in the neonate, either term or preterm. Recent data in term infants indicate that plasma glucose concentrations stabilize in 24–48 hours after a variable transient period (hours) of lower values.

Studies since 1929 have consistently reported lower blood glucose values in preterm or low birth weight infants for a period of weeks. Current management is directed toward maintaining plasma glucose concentrations in these high-risk infants in the normoglycemia range found in mature full-term neonates, infants, and children.

Thus, one can offer reasonable ranges of plasma glucose values for approximate definitions, recognizing that the intermediate ranges between normal and abnormal can be used for guidelines and, on occasion, even therapy, but not for diagnosis.

REFERENCES

1. NORVAL MA, KENNEDY RLJ, BERKSON J. Blood sugar in newborn infants. *J Pediatr.* 1949;34:342.
2. NORVAL MA. Blood sugar values in premature infants. *J Pediatr.* 1950;36:177.
3. CORNBLATH M, SCHWARTZ R, eds. *Disorders of Carbohydrate Metabolism in Infancy, 2nd ed.* Philadelphia: WB Saunders Co., 1976;74–86.
4. KLIEGMAN RM, GROSS T. Perinatal problems of the obese mother and her infant. *Obstet Gynecol.* 1985;66:299.
5. KLIEGMAN R, GROSS T, MORTON S, DUNNINGTON R. Intrauterine growth and postnatal fasting metabolism in infants of obese mothers. *J Pediatr.* 1984;104:601.
6. LIGHT IJ, KEENAN WJ, SUTHERLAND JM. Maternal intravenous glucose administration as a cause of hypoglycemia in the infant of the diabetic mother. *Am J Obstet Gynecol.* 1972;113:345.
7. KENEEP NB, KUMAR S, SHELLEY WC, STANLEY CA, GABBE SG, GUTSCHE BB. Fetal and neonatal hazards of maternal hydration with 5% dextrose before caesarean section. *Lancet.* 1982;1:1150.
8. MENDIOLA J, GRYLACK LJ, SCANLON JW. Effects of intrapartum maternal glucose infusion on the normal fetus and newborn. *Anesth Analg.* 1982;61:32.
9. CARMEN S. Neonatal hypoglycemia in response to maternal glucose infusion before delivery. *J Obstet Gynecol Neonatal Nurs.* 1986; 15:319.
10. SINGHI S. Effect of maternal intrapartum glucose therapy on neonatal blood glucose levels and neurobehavioral status of hypoglycemic term newborn infants. *J Perinat Med.* 1988;16:217.
11. SRINIVASAN G, PILDES RS, CATTAMANCHI G, VOORA S, LILLEN LD. Plasma glucose values in normal neonates. A new look. *J Pediatr.* 1986; 109:114.
12. HECK LJ, ERENBERG A. Serum glucose levels in term neonates during the first 48 hours of life. *J Pediatr.* 1987;110:119.
13. AYNSLEY-GREEN A. The control of the adaptation to postnatal nutrition. *Monogr Paediatr.* 1982;16:59.
14. LUBCHENCO L, HANSMAN C, DRESSLER M, BOYD E. Intrauterine growth as estimated from liveborn birth weight data at 24 to 42 weeks of gestation. *Pediatrics.* 1963;32:793.
15. BALLARD J, KAZMIER K, DRIVER MA. A simplified assessment of gestational age. *Pediatr Res.* 1977;11:374.
16. LUBCHENCO LO, BARD H. Incidence of hypoglycemia in newborn infants classified by birth weight and gestational age. *Pediatrics.* 1971;47:831.
17. STANLEY CA, ANDAY EK, BAKER L, DELIVORIA-PAPADOPOLOUS M. Metabolic fuel and hormone responses to fasting in newborn infants. *Pediatrics.* 1979;64:613.
18. WRIGHT LL, STANLEY CA, ANDAY EK, BAKER L. The effect of early feeding on plasma glucose levels in SGA infants. *Pediatrics.* 1983;22:539.
19. CREERY RDG, PARKINSON TJ. Blood glucose changes in the newborn. I. The blood glucose pattern of normal infants in the first 12 hours of life. *Arch Dis Child.* 1953;28:134.

20. CORNBLATH M, GANZON AF, NICOLOPOULOUS D, BAENS GS, HOLLANDER RJ, GORDON MH, GORDON HH. Studies of carbohydrate metabolism in the newborn infant. III. Some factors influencing the capillary blood sugar and the response to glucagon during the first hours of life. *Pediatrics.* 1961;27:378.

21. BAENS GS, LUNDEEN E, CORNBLATH M. Studies of carbohydrate metabolism in the newborn infant. VI. Levels of glucose in blood in premature infants. *Pediatrics.* 1963;31:580.

22. FARQUHAR JW. Control of the blood sugar level in the neonatal period. *Arch Dis Child.* 1954;29:519.

23. REIS RA, DECOSTA EJ, ALLWEISS MD. The management of the pregnant diabetic woman and her newborn infant. *Am J Obstet Gynecol.* 1950;60:1023.

24. PENNOYER MM, HARTMANN AF SR. Management of infants born of diabetic mothers. *Postgrad Med.* 1955;18:199.

25. FARQUHAR JW. The significance of hypoglycaemia in the newborn infant of the diabetic woman. *Arch Dis Child.* 1956;31:203.

26. CONRAD PD, SPARKS JW, OSBERG I, ABRAMS L, HAY WW JR. Clinical application of a new glucose analyzer in the neonatal intensive care unit: comparison with other methods. *J Pediatr.* 1989;114:281.

27. LIN HC, MAGUIRE C, OH W, COWETT R. Accuracy and reliability of glucose reflectance meters in the high-risk neonate. *J Pediatr.* 1989; 115:998.

28. SEXSON WR. Incidence of neonatal hypoglycemia: a matter of definition. *J Pediatr.* 1984;105:149.

29. KEENER PA, TIDEMAN A, MAIJALA D, LEMONS JA. Reliability of the Glucometer reflectance photometer in assessing hypoglycemia in the neonate. *J Perinatol.* 1986;6:51.

30. PAGLIARA AS, KARL IE, HAYMOND M, KIPNIS DM. Hypoglycemia in infancy and childhood. *J Pediatr.* 1973;82:365 (I), 558 (II).

31. KOH THHG, AYNSLEY-GREEN A, TARBIT M, EYRE JA. Neural dysfunction during hypoglycaemia. *Arch Dis Child.* 1988;63:1353.

32. PRYDS O, CHIRSTENSEN NJ, FRIIS-HANSEN B. Increased cerebral blood flow and plasma epinephrine in hypoglycemic preterm neonates. *Pediatrics.* 1990;85:172.

33. DITCHBURN RK, WILKINSON RH, DAVIES PA, AINSWORTH P. Plasma glucose levels in infants weighing 2,500 g and less fed immediately after birth with breast milk. *Biol Neonate.* 1967;11:29.

34. BEARD AG, PANOS TC, MARASIGAN BV, EMINIANS J, KENNEDY HF, LAMB J. Perinatal stress and the premature neonate. II. Effect of fluid and calorie deprivation on blood glucose. *J Pediatr.* 1966;68:329.

35. RUBECZ I, MESTYAN J. Energy metabolism and intravenous nutrition of premature infants. *Biol Neonate* 1973;23:45.

36. JAMES LS. Personal communication.

37. SOLTESZ G, MESTYAN J, JARAI I, FEKETE M, SCHULTZ K. Glucose utilization and the changes in plasma nutrients after intravenously injected glucose in premature infants kept at and below the neutral temperature. I. The disappearance rate of glucose. *Biol Neonate* 1971; 19:241.

38. DWECK HS, CASSADY G. Glucose intolerance in infants of very low birth weight. I. Incidence of hyperglycemia in infants of birth weights 1,100 grams or less. *Pediatrics.* 1974;53:189.

39. CSER A, MILNER RDG. Glucose tolerance and insulin secretion in very small babies. *Acta Paediatr Scand.* 1975;64:457.

40. DWECK HS, MIRANDA LEY. Perinatal glucose homeostasis: the unique character of hyperglycemia and hypoglycemia in infants of very low birth weight. *Clin Perinatol.* 1977;4:351.

41. PILDES RS. Current literature and clinical issues: neonatal hyperglycemia. *J Pediatr.* 1986;109:905.

42. CORNBLATH M, WYBREGT SH, BAENS GS. Studies of carbohydrate metabolism in the newborn infant. VII. Tests of carbohydrate tolerance in premature infants. *Pediatrics.* 1963;32:1007.

43. AYNSLEY-GREEN A. Metabolic and endocrine interrelations during the adaptation to postnatal nutrition in the human neonate. *Annales Nestle Special Edition Nutrition in Early Life,* 1984;29.

44. AYNSLEY-GREEN A, SOLTESZ G, eds. *Hypoglycaemia in Infancy and Childhood.* Edinburgh: Churchill Livingstone, 1985.

45. JACOB J, DAVIS RF. Differences in serum glucose determinations in infants with umbilical artery catheters. *J Perinatol.* 1988;8:40.

46. STUR O. Studies on the physiologic hypoglycemia of newborns. *Biol Neonate.* 1963;6:38.

47. CORNBLATH M, JOASSIN G, WEISSKOPF B, SWIATEK KR. Hypoglycemia in the newborn. *Pediatr Clin North Am.* 1966;13:905.

48. VAN CREVELD S. Carbohydrate metabolism of premature infants; blood sugar during fasting. *Am J Dis Child.* 1929;38:912.

49. ZINKHAM W II. An *in vitro* abnormality of glutathione metabolism in erythrocytes from normal newborns. *Pediatrics.* 1959;23:18.

50. LIN YL, SMITH CH, DIETZLER DN. Stabilization of blood glucose by cooling with ice: an effective procedure for preservation of samples from adults and newborns. *Clin Chem.* 1976;22:2031.

51. BLAIR SC, SCHIER GM, GAN IET, MOSES RG. Improved method for capillary blood glucose collection. *Diabetes Care.* 1987;10:785.

52. CORNBLATH M, SCHWARTZ R, AYNSLEY-GREEN A, LLOYD JK. Hypoglycemia in infancy: the need for a rational definition. *Pediatrics.* 1990; 85:834.

53. HAWORTH JC, DILLING LA, VAN WOERT M. Blood glucose determinations in infants and children, the reflectance meter/enzyme test strip system. *Am J Dis Child.* 1972;123:469.

54. FRANZ ID, MEDINA G, TAEUSCH HW. Correlation of Dextrostix values with true glucose in the range less than 50 mg/dl. *J Pediatr.* 1975; 87:417.

55. PEARLMAN RH, GUTCHER GR, ENGLE MJ, MacDONALD MJ. Comparative analysis of four methods for rapid glucose determination in neonates. *Am J Dis Child.* 1982;136:1051.

56. SHERWOOD MJ, WARCHAL ME, CHEN S-T. A new reagent strip (Visodex) for determination of glucose in whole blood. *Clin Chem.* 1983; 29:438.

57. HAY WW JR, OSBERG IM. The "Eyetone" blood glucose reflectance colorimeter evaluated for in vitro and in vivo accuracy and clinical efficacy. *Clin Chem.* 1983;29:558.

58. HURRERA MD, HSING YH. Comparison of various methods of blood sugar screening in newborn infants. *J Pediatr.* 1983;102:769.

59. BROOKS KE, RAWAL N, HENDERSON AR. Laboratory assessment of three

new monitors of blood glucose: Accu-Chek II, Glucometer II, and Glucoscan 2000. *Clin Chem.* 1986;32:2195.

60. GRAZAITIS DM, SEXSON WR. Erroneously high Dextrostix values caused by isopropyl alcohol. *Pediatrics.* 1980;66:221.

61. TOGARI H, ODA M, WADA Y. Mechanism of erroneous Dextrostix readings. *Arch Dis Child.* 1987;62:408.

62. BARREAU PB, BUTTERY JE. The effect of haematocrit values on determination of glucose levels by reagent strip. *Med J Aust.* 1987; 147:286.

63. GIBBONEY W, COHEN S, KEENER PA, LEMONS JA. Effect of hematocrit on blood glucose measurements. *J Perinatol.* 1986;6:54.

64. KAPLAN M, BLONHEIM O, ALON I, EYLATH U, TRESTIAN S, EIDELMAN AI. Screening for hypoglycemia with plasma in neonatal blood of high hematocrit. *Crit Care Med.* 1989;17:279.

65. SUNDERMAN WF, COPELAND BE, MacFATE RP, MARTENS VE, NAUMAN HN, STEVENSON GF. Manual of American Society of Clinical Pathologists Workshop on Glucose. *Am J Clin Path.* 1956;26:1355.

66. FOX RE, REDSTONE D. Sources of error in glucose determinations in neonatal blood by glucose oxidase methods, including dextrostix. *Am J Clin Pathol.* 1976;66:658.

67. SOMOGYI M. Determination of blood sugar. *J Biol Chem.* 1945;160:69.

68. FALES FW, RUSSELL JA, FAIN JN. Some applications and limitations of the enzymic, reducing (Somogyi), and anthrone methods for estimating sugar. *Clin Chem.* 1961;7:389.

69. HULTMAN E. Rapid specific method for determination of aldosesaccharides in body fluids. *Nature.* 1959;183:108.

70. HYVARINEN A, NIKKILA EA. Specific determination of blood glucose with O-toluidine. *Clin Chem Acta.* 1962;7:140.

71. EK J, DAAE LN. Whole blood glucose determination in newborn infants, comparison and evaluation of five different methods. *Acta Paediatr Scand.* 1967;56:461.

72. HARTMANN AF, GRUNWALDT E, JAMES DH. Blood galactose in infants and children. *J Pediatr.* 1953;43:1.

73. HAWORTH JC, FORD JD. Blood-sugar in infants after lactose feedings. *Lancet.* 1960;2:794.

74. RELANDER A, RÄIHÄ CE. Differences between the enzymatic and O-toluidine methods of blood glucose determinations. *Scand J Clin Lab Invest.* 1963;15:221.

75. SOMOGYI M. Notes on sugar determinations. *J Biol Chem.* 1952;195:19.

76. MACKAY EM. The distribution of glucose in human blood. *J Biol Chem.* 1932;97:685.

77. HAWORTH JC, DILLING L, YOUNOSZAI MK. Relation of blood glucose to haematocrit, birthweight, and other body measurements in normal and growth-retarded newborn infants. *Lancet.* 1967;2:901.

78. CORNBLATH M, LEVIN EY, GORDON HH. Studies of carbohydrate metabolism in the newborn. I. Capillary-venous differences in blood sugar in normal newborn infants. *Pediatrics.* 1956;18:167.

79. KETTERINGHAM RC, AUSTIN BR. Blood sugar during labor, at delivery and postpartum, with observations on newborns. *Am J Med Sci.* 1938;195:318.

80. CORNBLATH M, REISNER SH. Blood glucose in the neonate, clinical significance. *N Engl J Med.* 1965;273:378.

81. WARD OC. Blood sugar studies on premature babies. *Arch Dis Child.* 1953;28:194.
82. MAMUNES P, BADEN M, BASS JW, NELSON J. Early intravenous feeding of the low birth weight neonate. *Pediatrics.* 1969;43:241.
83. MARKS V, ROSE FC, eds. *Hypoglycaemia, 2nd ed.* Oxford: Blackwell Scientific Publ. 1981;417.
84. VOLPE JJ, ed. *Neurology of the newborn, 2nd ed.* Philadelphia: WB Saunders, 1987.
85. SARFF LD, PLATT LH, MCCRACKEN GH. Cerebrospinal fluid evaluation in neonates: comparison of high-risk infants with and without meningitis. *J Pediatr.* 1976;88:473.
86. SILVER TS, TODD JK. Hypoglycorrhachia in pediatric patients. *Pediatrics.* 1976;58:67.
87. MARKS V. True glucose content of lumbar and ventricular fluid. *J Clin Pathol.* 1960;13:82.
88. OTILA E. Studies on the cerebrospinal fluid in premature infants. *Acta Paediatr.* 1948;35(suppl. 8):3 (see p. 65).
89. LIEBE S. Zur Diagnose und Prognose geburtstraumatischer intrakranieller Blutungen. *Mschr Kinderheilk.* 1940;83:1.
90. WAITZ R. Le liquide cephalorachidien due Nouveau-ne. *Rev Franc Pediatr.* 1928;4:1.
91. MATHEW OP, BLAND HE, PICKENS JM, JAMES EJ. Hypoglycorrhachia in the survivors of neonatal intracranial hemorrhage. *Pediatrics.* 1979; 63:851.
92. STUTCHFIELD PR, COOKE RWI. Electrolytes and glucose in cerebrospinal fluid of premature infants with intraventricular haemorrhage: role of potassium in cerebral infarction. *Arch Dis Child.* 1989;64:470.
93. COBLINER. *Ztschr f Kinderh.* 1911;1:207. (Cited by Van Creveld.)
94. GOETZKY. *Ztschr f Kinderh.* 1921;27:195. (Cited by Van Creveld.)
95. VAN CREVELD S. Carbohydrate metabolism of premature infants. I. The blood sugar during fasting. *Am J Dis Child.* 1929;38:912.
96. HARTMANN AF, JAUDON JD. Hypoglycemia. *J Pediatr.* 1937;11:1.
97. SCHULMAN JL, SATUREN P. Glycogen storage disease of the liver. I. Clinical studies during the early neonatal period. *Pediatrics.* 1954;14:632.
98. SHERMAN H. Islet-cell tumor of pancreas in a newborn infant (nesidioblastoma). *Am J Dis Child.* 1947;74:58.
99. MCQUARRIE I. Idiopathic spontaneously occurring hypoglycemia in infants. *Am J Dis Child.* 1954;87:399.
100. KOMROWER GM. Blood sugar levels in babies born of diabetic mothers. *Arch Dis Child.* 1954;29:28.
101. GELLIS SS, HSIA DY-Y. The infant of the diabetic mother. *Am J Dis Child.* 1959;97:1.
102. BHAKOO ON, SCOPES JW. Minimal rates of oxygen consumption in small-for-dates babies during the first week of life. *Arch Dis Child.* 1974;49:583.
103. SCOPES JW, AHMED I. Minimal rates of oxygen consumption in sick and premature newborn infants. *Arch Dis Child.* 1966;41:407.
104. GANDY GM, ADAMSONS K JR, CUNNINGHAM N, SILVERMAN WA, JAMES LS. Thermal environment and acid-base homeostasis in human infants during the first few hours of life. *J Clin Invest.* 1964;43:751.
105. SINCLAIR JC, SILVERMAN WA. Relative hypermetabolism in undergrown, human neonates. *Lancet.* 1964;2:49. (Letter to the Editor.)

106. JONXIS JH, VAN DER VLUGT JJ, DEGROOT CJ, BOERSMA ER, MEIJERS EDK. The metabolic rate in praemature, dysmature, and sick infants in relation to environmental temperature. In Jonxis JH, Visser HKA, Troelstra JA, eds. *Nutricia Symposium on Aspects of Praematurity and Dysmaturity*. Springfield, Ill.; Charles C Thomas, Pubs., 1968; 201–209.

107. CORNBLATH M, ODELL GB, LEVIN EY. Symptomatic neonatal hypoglycemia associated with toxemia of pregnancy. *J Pediatr*. 1959;55:545.

108. MILNER RDG, FEKETE M, ASSAN R. Glucagon, insulin and growth hormone response to exchange transfusion in premature and term infants. *Arch Dis Child*. 1972;47:186.

109. PILDES RS, CORNBLATH M, WARREN I, et al. A prospective controlled study of neonatal hypoglycemia. *Pediatrics*. 1974;54:5.

110. SCHRIER AM, WILHELM PB, CHURCH RM, et al. Neonatal hypoglycemia in the rhesus monkey: Effect on development and behavior. *Infant Behavior & Development*. 1990;13:189.

111. DEFEO P, GALLAI V, MAZZOTTA G, et al. Modest decrements in plasma glucose concentration cause early impairment in cognitive function and later activation of glucose counterregulation in the absence of hypoglycemic symptoms in normal man. *J Clin Invest*. 1988;82:436.

112. LUCAS A, MORLEY R, COLE JJ. Adverse neurodevelopmental outcome of moderate neonatal hypoglycaemia. *Br Med J*. 1988;297:304.

113. WU S, SRINIVASAN G, PILDES RS, PATEL MK. Plasma glucose values during the first month of life in infants <1000 gm. *Pediatr Res*. 1990; 27:231A.

HYPOGLYCEMIA IN THE NEONATE

In 1937, Hartmann and Jaudon [1] were the first to report on a series of 286 neonates and infants with hypoglycemia that they had studied over a 15-year period. Only newborn infants with severe manifestations and recurrent or persistent clinical low "true" blood sugar values were considered to have significant hypoglycemia. These authors carefully distinguished between "apparent" blood sugar values or total reducing substances and "true" blood sugar. "True blood sugar" would be somewhat greater than the blood glucose values measured today. In addition, they distinguished between degrees of severity of hypoglycemia. This approach emphasizes the concept that all deviations from biologic norms represent a continuum of abnormality from mild to severe. Thus, "mild hypoglycemia" was arbitrarily defined between 40 and 50 mg/dl (2.2 and 2.78 mM), "moderate" between 20 and 40 mg/dl (1.1 and 2.2 mM) and "extreme" less than 20 mg/dl (1.1 mM) based on their extensive clinical experience.

Between 1938 and 1959, only isolated patients were reported with specific syndromes of prolonged or severe hypoglycemia (islet cell tumor or adenomatosis [2], idiopathic [3–5]) or inborn metabolic deficiencies (e.g., glycogen storage disease [6]).

Multiple studies (see Chapter 2) between 1929 and 1955 confirmed that blood sugar values, however measured and regardless of source, were lower in premature (low birth weight) infants and infants of diabetic mothers than in term neonates. Blood sugar values in term newborns were less than those seen in older infants and children. However, no clinical significance was attributed to these low values.

In 1959, the initial description of the clinical syndrome of transient symptomatic neonatal hypoglycemia in eight infants changed the concept and significance of hypoglycemia in both preterm and full-term neonates [7]. The initial skepticism as to whether or not the entity existed was dispelled as verification was reported from nurseries around the world [7–24].

The frequency of symptomatic neonatal hypoglycemia was estimated to occur at a rate of 2–3 per 1,000 live births [13,20,25–31].

The infants at risk were predominantly males who were small for gestational age [12,32–34], the smaller of twins (Fig. 3-1) [35], and often born to toxemic mothers [7–9]. Associated problems included pre- or coexisting central nervous system damage [18,36], hypocalcemia, polycythemia [18–21,23,27–29,37,38] and cardiac enlargement [39,40].

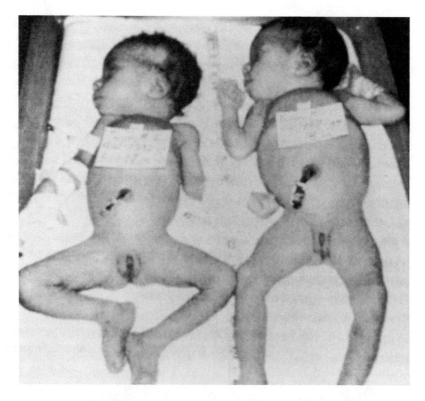

FIGURE 3-1. Discordant twins, 1332 gm and 1871 gm birth weight. The smaller twin had symptomatic hypoglycemia on the second day of life.

Clinical manifestations, including apnea, tremors, apathy, cyanosis, convulsions, tachypnea, limpness, and/or irritability, usually occurred before 72 hours of age in the majority of affected infants [7–24,30,41].

The clearing of clinical manifestations following restoration of the blood glucose concentration to normal is essential to establish the diagnosis [7,30,41].

If untreated for prolonged periods of time, this hypoglycemia may have profound consequences, including death [42,43] or a variety of neurologic handicaps [16,21,23,37,44–50].

Thus, the initial definition of neonatal hypoglycemia included clinical manifestations that were associated with a low plasma glucose value (<25 mg/dl [<1.39 mM]) and cleared following therapy that restored the blood glucose concentration to normoglycemia (>40 mg/dl [2.22 mM]) [7,27,51].

The recognition of asymptomatic neonatal hypoglycemia [20,21, 23,27,28,37,51–60] required a statistical definition of significant hypoglycemia. One such definition is based on blood glucose values more than two standard deviations below the mean in apparently normal infants (see Chapter 2). These values, which varied with gestation, birth weight, and age in hours and days, were based on populations of well full-term and low birth weight infants in the 1960s [61,62]. Recently, these values for normal full-term infants have been reevaluated during the first days of life, resulting in a modest increase in the concentrations defining both normoglycemia and hypoglycemia [63,64] (see p. 70, Fig. 2-4).

Along with the recognition of the frequency and significance of hypoglycemia in the neonate, a number of new and old syndromes associated with low levels of blood glucose were described or rediscovered.

Some were characterized by *transient hypoglycemia,* as in moderate to severe erythroblastosis [18,65–72], cold injury [73–75], adrenal hemorrhage [51,76], and infection [77,78].

Other syndromes presented with life-threatening, *severe persistent or recurrent* hypoglycemic episodes (see Chapter 5, p. 177), as in the Beckwith-Wiedemann syndrome, "infant giants," islet cell adenomas, hyperinsulinism [79], congenital hypopituitarism with or without congenital optic nerve hypoplasia, and other congenital or familial disturbances in carbohydrate, amino acid, organic acid, or lipid metabolism. Although uncommon, these infants are particularly at serious risk and require early recognition, diagnosis, and therapy.

In recent years, there have been dramatic improvements in prenatal care with earlier monitoring and intervention. This has resulted in the survival of high-risk infants, especially those who are asphyxiated at birth or have a high morbidity and mortality because of extreme prematurity and very low birth weight. In fact, fetal hypoglycemia has been documented [80], and low blood glucose values soon after birth are being reported more frequently [31,72,81,82] than ever before. A large number of infants may have significantly low values for blood or plasma glucose during the first 6 hours of life and particularly before the initiation of feedings either orally or parenterally [83].

In view of the complexity of and changes in care provided preterm high-risk infants, it may no longer be relevant to apply previously derived statistical standards to current premature populations [85–87]. New definitions [88], other than statistical norms, will be required to determine what concentrations of plasma glucose represent abnormal values for the very low birth weight and low birth weight premature infant [89].

As a result, a different approach to the concept of hypoglycemia is necessary. There is a continuum of low blood glucose values of varied duration and severity. The impact of the low plasma glucose concentration in any one infant depends on other risk factors, such as hypoxia, asphyxia, sepsis, age, maturity, and ability to compensate by metabolic and endocrine adjustments.

Previously, studies in both animals and man supported the concept that the immature brain was more tolerant to a number of stresses, including hypoglycemia [90] and anoxia than the mature brain (see recent reviews [91,92]). Recently, this has been questioned, without sufficient evidence [89]. While no definitive answers are available, it appears prudent to maintain similar plasma glucose concentrations for all neonates, regardless of gestation. This range has not been shown to be associated with any deviations from normal metabolic, physiologic, or neurologic function. Furthermore, current concepts would not support a specific hypoglycemic value that segregates normal (above a specific concentration) from abnormal (below that concentration), resulting in acute or chronic neurologic damage.

Whatever the basis for definition, almost everyone agrees that, regardless of its origin or the presence or absence of clinical manifestations, hypoglycemia should be treated promptly once the diagnosis has been reliably established in order to restore the blood glucose concentrations to a normal physiologic range [20,23,27,28,30,37,41, 55,59,89,93–95].

• Definition of Hypoglycemia

Hypoglycemia can be defined in terms of a spectrum of clinical consequences (acute, intermediate, long-term, or delayed), physiologic-metabolic effects (counterregulatory hormone and substrate responses), and/or neurologic dysfunction (acute, transient, permanent, and/or long term) (see Table 3-1). To date, none of these approaches have provided sufficient specific data for defining ranges of plasma glucose that could be defined as mild, moderate, or severe neonatal hypoglycemia, as proposed by Hartmann and Jaudon [1].

The definitions here are based on a review of our own experience and clinical reports of persistent or pathological causes of symptomatic hypoglycemia (hyperinsulinism, congenital optic nerve hypoplasia and panhypopituitarism, etc.), patients with clinical manifestations that respond to glucose therapy, and all of the statistical data reviewed in both term and preterm infants.

Hypoglycemia in the term neonate during the first 24 hours of age is defined as a plasma glucose concentration less than 40 mg/dl (2.22 mM). This definition provides an indication to raise the plasma glucose level to sustain a concentration between 50 and 100 mg/dl (2.78 and 5.56 mM). This represents a reasonable definition of normoglycemia and does *not* imply that the lower plasma glucose concentration, alone, produces neurodevelopmental abnormalities.

Beyond 24 hours of age, this plasma value may be increased to 40 to 50 mg/dl (2.22 to 2.78 mM). Values below this range, again, are an indication to raise plasma glucose levels and do not imply neuroglucopenia or neurologic damage (Table 3-2).

At all ages and gestations, plasma glucose values less than 20–25 mg/dl (1.11–1.39 mM) should be treated by parenteral glucose and monitored at regular intervals to assure that these low values do not persist or recur (see Chapter 5, p. 179) (Table 3-2).

These glucose concentrations are based on laboratory analysis of plasma glucose obtained in a manner to avoid the increased glycolysis known to occur in newborn red blood cells. The blood should be handled expeditiously in a manner similar to samples analyzed for blood gas analyses (see Chapter 2, p. 62).

It should be emphasized that glucose oxidase reagent strip techniques are not reliable when screening for hypoglycemia and *cannot*

TABLE 3-1. Definitions of hypoglycemia

1. Clinical manifestations: response to glucose
2. Statistical surveys: normal populations
3. Functional correlations: acute ⟶ chronic
    a. Physiologic, Metabolic
    b. Neurologic
4. Outcomes
    a. Neurologic
    b. Behavioral
    c. Intellectual

TABLE 3-2. Current definition of hypoglycemia (all neonates)

AGE	PLASMA GLUCOSE
First 24 hours	<40 mg/dl (2.2 mM)
After 24 hours	<40–50 mg/dl (2.2–2.8 mM)

- Indication to raise the plasma glucose level to 50–100 mg/dl (2.7–5.6 mM).
- Lower plasma concentrations alone have not been shown to produce neurodevelopmental abnormalities.

All ages	<20–25 mg/dl (1.1–1.4 mM)

- Treat with parenteral glucose.
- Monitor at regular intervals.

be used as the basis for the diagnosis of hypoglycemia [30,41,76,89]. Several reasons for this include:

1. The result obtained depends upon the hematocrit,
2. The precision required for performance and timing is rarely achieved,
3. There is a wide variance of ± 5 to 15 mg/dl (0.28 to 0.83 mM) when compared to laboratory determinations, and
4. There is a striking lack of reproducibility.

This is true especially at blood glucose values less than 40–50 mg/dl (2.22–2.78 mM) whether the strips are read by eye or by meters [96,97]. In contrast, screening at the bedside with a laboratory-quality glucose oxidase analyzer (Yellow Springs Instrument, Beckman) can produce reliable results on single specimens of blood with an acceptable variance of ± 1.5 mg/dl (0.8 mM) when done by a trained person, e.g., a neonatal nurse or technician.

We still recommend that at least two successive values that are significantly low be obtained, if possible, before making the definitive diagnosis of hypoglycemia in the neonate [76]. A blood sample for laboratory analysis should be obtained before parenteral therapy is initiated. This sample alone in the grossly symptomatic infant may suffice for the diagnosis. Repetitive blood glucose values are unambiguously low, almost always below 25 mg/dl (1.39 mM), in those infants with organic causes of hypoglycemia [31], i.e., hyperinsulinism or hypopituitarism (see Chapter 5, p. 196).

Frequency

The frequency of neonatal hypoglycemia depends upon the criteria for diagnosis [76,98] and the population surveyed, as well as the method for blood collection and glucose analysis. The impact of early intervention in high-risk and very low birth weight infants at birth will further modify occurrence figures [72,99]. Over the past three decades, with dramatic changes in neonatal and obstetrical care and monitoring of normal, abnormal, term, and low birth weight infants, the frequency of hypoglycemia has varied.

Initially, in the 1960s, the rate was estimated to be 2–3/1,000 live births using laboratory blood glucose determinations as the basis for diagnosis. However, during the first hours after birth, the frequency varied anywhere from 14 percent in normal term infants to 18 to 67 percent of SGA preterm neonates [82,83]. When based on all admissions to an intensive care nursery, the rates were generally between 5–20 percent, depending upon the populations included, e.g., high risk, SGA, IDM [76, pp. 158–159]. In contrast, Pildes et al. reported an incidence of 5.7 percent from a survey of all low birth weight infants who had daily blood glucose measurements for the first 5 days of life (1963–1964) [29].

Raivio and Hallman [18] in 1968 emphasized the infant at risk rather than total nursery populations as an important consideration in monitoring for hypoglycemia. Thus, hypoglycemia occurred in 20 percent of their SGA infants, in 16 percent of their IDMs, in 15 percent of terminally ill infants, and in 18 percent of severe erythroblastotic infants (cord hemoglobin less than 10 mg/dl). Currently, the at-risk population to be monitored has expanded significantly (see following section on clinical management). With more intensive monitoring and interventions in the 1970s, the overall rate was estimated at 4.4/1,000 live births. A frequency of 16 percent was reported among all low birth weight infants [51] and of 18 percent among SGA infants whose deficiency in weight (>30 percent) exceeded that in length (<15 percent) [82].

In 6,665 deliveries resulting in 6,627 live births between January 1982 and December 1984, Sutton and Kingdom [31] found 43 infants with blood glucose concentrations less than 18 mg/dl (1.0 mM), a frequency of 6.5/1,000 live births. Thereafter, few population studies have been reported.

In studies of full-term, normal infants born between 1981 and 1983, Srinivasan et al. [63] reported 3 of 344 were symptomatic hypoglycemic infants (1 percent). In contrast, Heck and Erenberg [64] found that 33 (29 percent) of 114 infants born in 1982–1983 had at least one serum glucose level less than 40 mg/dl (2.2 mM). All of the latter were asymptomatic. The reasons for these differences are not apparent, but again emphasize the difficulty of obtaining and analyzing frequency data.

In a prospective controlled feeding study done between 1981 and

1983 [100], Lucas et al. [93] also included a protocol for measuring blood glucose values in a group of 661 infants with birth weights less than 1,850 gm. A total of 6,808 samples were taken on separate days for glucose analysis. They reported an overall frequency of 66 percent, with a single blood sugar value of less than 47 mg/dl (2.6 mM) as the criterion for hypoglycemia. In this group, 28 percent had blood glucose values less than 29 mg/dl (1.7 mM), 10 percent less than 11 mg/dl (0.61 mM), and 37 percent between 29 and 47 mg/dl (1.7 and 2.6 mM). Values less than 47 mg/dl (2.6 mM) were recorded on 3 or more days, not necessarily consecutive, in 104 infants (16 percent). In contrast to these high estimates, both Pildes and Raivio reported at a Ciba Discussion Meeting in London in October, 1989 [89] that current standards of care, with the almost immediate introduction of parenteral glucose in such low birth weight infants, had resulted in a significant decrease in the frequency of hypoglycemia, but an increase in the incidence of hyperglycemia. In fact, among 38 infants with a mean birth weight of 802 gm and mean gestational age of 27 weeks who survived and were given maintenance parenteral glucose and monitored during the first 28 days of life, only 0.4 percent (3) of 848 plasma glucose determinations were <25 mg/dl (1.4 mM) and 2.4 percent (20) <40 mg/dl (2.2 mM). The latter were found on at least two occasions in seven infants. In contrast, 22.6 percent (192) plasma glucose values were >125 mg/dl (6.9 mM) and 12.3 percent (104) were >150 mg/dl (8.3 mM) [99].

• Clinical Manifestations

Clinical presentation of hypoglycemia is never specific, especially in the neonate, and may include a wide range of local or generalized manifestations that are common in the sick infant.

Episodes of twitching, cyanosis, seizures, apnea, irregular respirations, irritability, apathy, limpness, hypothermia, difficulty in feeding, exaggerated Moro reflex [18], high-pitched cry, and coma have all been attributed to or have resulted from significant hypoglycemia. On occasion, vomiting [55], tachypnea [29,40], bradycardia [60], and "eye-rolling" [8] have also been associated with hypoglycemia.

The clinical manifestations should subside within minutes to hours in response to adequate treatment with intravenous glucose if hypoglycemia alone is responsible. These signs and symptoms are not at all specific and have been associated with a variety of neonatal problems with or without secondary hypoglycemia (see Table 3-3).

Some infants with hypoglycemia are rarely symptomatic for unexplained reasons. These include infants of diabetic mothers, those with transitional hypoglycemia during the first hours of life associated

TABLE 3-3. Differential diagnosis in newborns with episodes of apnea, cyanosis, "jitteriness," limpness, twitching, high-pitched cry, difficulty in feeding, coma, and convulsions

CLINICAL ENTITY

Central Nervous System
Congenital defects
Congenital infections (e.g., toxoplasmosis, cytomegalic inclusion disease)
Acquired infections (e.g., meningitis)
Subdural hematoma
Hemorrhage
Kernicterus

Sepsis
Bacterial
Viral
TORCH

Heart Disease
Congenital (hypoplastic left heart syndrome)
Acquired
Arrhythmia

Asphyxia, Anoxia
Perinatal
Meconium aspiration
Respiratory distress syndrome

Iatrogenic
Cold injury
Overheating
Drugs to mother
Narcotic withdrawal
Sulfonylureas
Propylthiouracil
B tocolytics
Abrupt cessation of hypertonic parenteral glucose
Postoperatively in neonate

Endocrine Deficiency
Adrenal hemorrhage
Hypothyroid

Multiple Congenital Anomalies
Trisomy 18

Metabolic Aberrations
Pyridoxine dependency
Hypocalcemia
Hyponatremia
Hypernatremia
Hypomagnesemia

with perinatal asphyxia or fasting, and older infants with type I glycogen storage disease. While alternate substrates such as lactate, ketones, glycerol, and selected amino acids may support brain metabolism in the neonate, current data are still inadequate to use measurements of these substrates in making clinical decisions for diagnosis or therapy.

• Clinical Management of the Neonate at Risk

Clinical management of neonatal hypoglycemia is based on four basic principles: (1) monitoring infants at highest risk, (2) confirming that the plasma glucose concentration is low and is responsible for the clinical manifestations present, (3) demonstrating that the symptoms have responded following glucose therapy with restoration of the blood glucose to normoglycemic levels, and (4) observing and carefully documenting all of these events.

Infants at the highest risk for requiring routine monitoring [41] of blood glucose and glucose support regardless of their symptoms would include the following:

1. Small for gestational age less than third percentile [12,32–34,101], especially those discordant for weight versus length [82],
2. Smaller of discordant twins [35,102] (weight difference ≥25 percent) (Figs. 3-2 and 3-3),
3. Large for gestational age greater than ninetieth percentile [51,83],
4. Very low birth weight infants (<1250 gm) [99,103],
5. Infants of:
    a. Insulin-dependent diabetic mothers (see p. 125),
    b. Gestational diabetic mothers (see p. 149),
    c. Massively obese mothers [104,105],
    d. Preeclamptic mothers [7–9],
    e. Mothers who were given large amounts of [106,107] or any [108] parenteral glucose during labor and delivery,
    f. Mothers given parenteral glucose too rapidly prior to delivery [107,109],
6. Isolated hepatomegaly
7. Significant hypoxia [20,51],
8. Perinatal distress [21–23, 51,101],
9. Apgar scores <5 at 5 minutes or thereafter [51],
10. Severe erythroblastosis (cord Hb <10 gm/dl) [18,72],
11. Any infant with microphallus or anterior midline defect, especially with hyperbilirubinemia (see Chapter 5, p. 188),
12. Family history of neonate with hypoglycemia or unexplained death in infancy, and

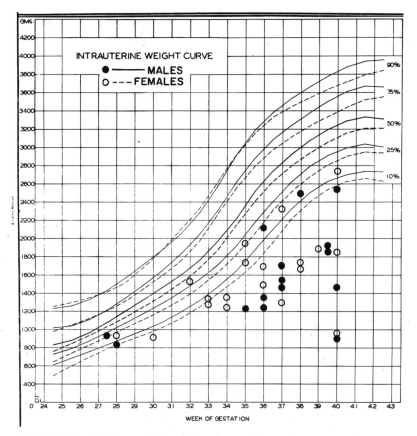

FIGURE 3-2. Weights at birth of 34 infants with transient neonatal symptomatic hypoglycemia plotted against weeks of gestation. (From Lubchenco et al. *Pediatrics*. 1963; 32:793 and Lubchenco et al. *Pediatrics*. 1966; 37:403, with permission)

13. Infant with exomphalos, macroglossia, and/or gigantism (see p. 206).

In these high-risk infants, routine screening should be done at 2, 4, 6, 12, 24, and 48 hours of age or *whenever any of the clinical manifestations noted above occur*. Figure 3-4 provides a graphic flow sheet for screening, confirming, and treating the most common types of hypoglycemia encountered in level 1, 2, and 3 nurseries currently.

Failure to Fully Respond to Therapy

Persistence of the clinical manifestations or failure to respond completely in hours after normalization of the plasma glucose concentration indicates that the hypoglycemia may have been associated with

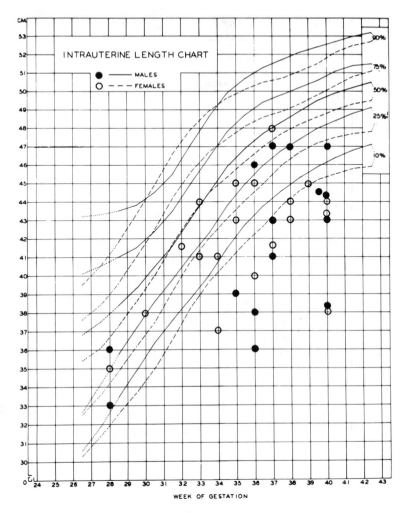

FIGURE 3-3. Lengths for the infants shown in Fig. 3-2.

or secondary to another abnormality [21,23,30,41,76]. A systematic clinical and laboratory diagnostic evaluation to determine the primary disease is important since hypoglycemia may be secondary to a variety of neonatal conditions that in themselves may be life-threatening or debilitating (see Table 3-3).

Monitoring is indicated in infants with:

1. Central nervous system pathology including intrauterine or peri-natal infections, congenital defects, and hemorrhage,
2. Sepsis, especially bacterial, gram negative [78],

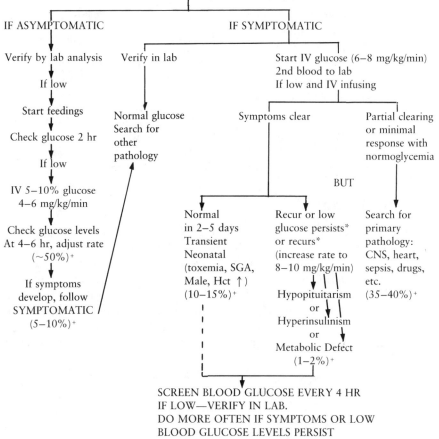

Screen by Chemical Determination in All High Risk Infants
(2, 4, 6, 12, 24, 48 hr of age or when symptomatic)

IF ASYMPTOMATIC   IF SYMPTOMATIC

Verify by lab analysis   Verify in lab   Start IV glucose (6–8 mg/kg/min)
                                                     2nd blood to lab
If low   If low and IV infusing

Start feedings   Normal glucose   Symptoms clear   Partial clearing
                          Search for   or minimal
Check glucose 2 hr   other   response with
                          pathology   normoglycemia
If low

IV 5–10% glucose   BUT
4–6 mg/kg/min
                          Normal   Recur or low   Search for
Check glucose levels   in 2–5 days   glucose persists* primary
At 4–6 hr, adjust rate   Transient   or recurs*   pathology:
(~50%)+   Neonatal   (increase rate to CNS, heart,
                          (toxemia, SGA, 8–10 mg/kg/min) sepsis, drugs,
If symptoms   Male, Hct ↑)   etc.
develop, follow   (10–15%)+   Hypopituitarism   (35–40%)+
SYMPTOMATIC   or
(5–10%)+   Hyperinsulinism
                                         or
                                         Metabolic Defect
                                         (1–2%)+

SCREEN BLOOD GLUCOSE EVERY 4 HR
IF LOW—VERIFY IN LAB.
DO MORE OFTEN IF SYMPTOMS OR LOW
BLOOD GLUCOSE LEVELS PERSIST

* Obtain critical blood sample before and after glucagon followed by diagnostic-therapeutic trial.
+ Frequency among cases of neonatal hypoglycemia.

FIGURE 3-4.   Flow diagram for detection and management of suspected hypoglycemia. (From Cornblath and Poth. In: Kaplan, ed. Philadelphia: WB Saunders, 1982, with permission)

3. Congenital heart disease [110,111],
4. Hypoxia and/or asphyxia, hypoxic ischemic encephalopathy [112],
5. Adrenal hemorrhage,
6. Hypothyroidism,
7. Multiple congenital anomalies [113],
8. Neonatal tetany [76],
9. Postexchange transfusion [69,71,114],

10. Drugs taken by or given to mother [115–117]:
    a. Narcotic withdrawal,
    b. β-sympathomimetic tocolytic drugs to inhibit labor,
    c. Propylthiouracil,
    d. Sulfonylureas in diabetic mothers,
11. Abrupt cessation of hypertonic parenteral glucose [118],
12. Malposition of umbilical artery catheter [119,120], and
13. Postoperative, e.g., pyloric stenosis [121].

Although support of the plasma glucose level is indicated, the primary disease is often the cause of morbidity or mortality in these infants. There is little evidence currently to attribute any untoward outcomes to the associated or resulting hypoglycemia.

• Therapy

Recommended preventive interventions include the early use of oral feedings [52], parenteral fluids, and lipid supplementation [122].

Once the diagnosis of hypoglycemia has been established by reliable determinations of significantly low concentrations of plasma glucose, therapy should be initiated promptly (Table 3-4). In the asymptomatic infant during the first hours after birth, oral glucose may be given and another plasma glucose measurement obtained within 30 to 60 minutes postprandial [41,118]. If still low, parenteral

---

TABLE 3-4. Therapy in neonatal hypoglycemia

Immediate: 0.25 g/kg as 1 ml/kg of 25 percent glucose IV
(rate of 1 ml/min) or as 2.5 ml/kg of 10 percent glucose IV at a rate of 1–2 ml/min.

Continue with: 6–8 mg/kg/min glucose,
58–96 ml/kg/day as 12 to 15 percent dextrose in water,*
85–115 ml/kg/day as 10 percent dextrose in water.

After 12 hours: Add 40 mEq/L NaCl (0.2 N saline).

After 24 hours: Add 1–2 mEq/kg/day KCl.

If symptoms persist or recur or glucose is below 40 mg/100 ml after 4–6 hours:
Increase rate to 10–12 mg/kg/min.
Thereafter add, if necessary,

hydrocortisone 5 mg/kg/day IM every 12 hours or
prednisone 2 mg/kg/day orally.

When the glucose is normal for 24 hours: taper glucose to 5 percent at 6 mg/kg/min, then at 4 mg/kg/min and wean slowly.

---

*See Appendix IV for specific rates and concentrations.

glucose therapy is indicated. In the symptomatic infant, a blood sample should be obtained for a glucose determination at the time that the parenteral administration of glucose is started. If the glucose in this sample is significantly low and the symptoms clear after therapy, the diagnosis of symptomatic hypoglycemia has been established.

The oral glucose feed may be given by nipple or by gavage as a 5 percent dextrose in water solution at 10 ml/kg.

Parenteral glucose therapy is based on the clinical studies and physiologic data of Schwartz et al. [123,124] and Pildes et al. [125,126].

Initially, glucose at 0.25 g/kg as 1 ml/kg of 25 percent or 2.5 ml/kg of 10 percent glucose in water is given intravenously at the rate of 1–2 ml/min.

A continuous infusion of glucose is given immediately following, at the rate of 6–8 mg/kg/min. The concentration of glucose to be used is determined by the total daily fluid requirements, which depend upon the age, weight, and maturity of the infant (Table 3-4 and Appendix IV).

Plasma glucose concentrations should be followed at 1- to 3-hour intervals initially to determine the effectiveness of the therapy. Once stable, plasma glucose may be monitored at 4- to 8-hour intervals preprandial.

If levels of plasma glucose cannot be maintained over 50 mg/dl (2.8 mM) after 4 to 6 hours of parenteral glucose, the rate is progressively increased with monitoring to 10 to 15 mg/kg/min if necessary to achieve normoglycemia.

After 12 hours of fluid therapy, sodium is added at 1–2 mEq/kg/day as a hypotonic sodium chloride solution (40 mEq/liter or "quarter strength saline") to prevent edema [19] or iatrogenic hyponatremia [10,51].

After 24 hours, potassium (1 to 2 mEq/kg/day) should be added to the parenteral fluids. This can be given as KCl or as buffered potassium phosphate.

Oral feedings should be introduced as soon as possible after clinical manifestations subside.

If symptoms recur or persist or if plasma glucose concentrations cannot be maintained over 50 mg/dl (2.8 mM) after 4 to 6 hours of 10–12 mg/kg/min, hydrocortisone (5 mg/kg/day orally or IV every 12 hours), or prednisone (2 mg/kg/day orally daily) should be added to the regimen.

If the rate of glucose infusion exceeds 10–12 mg/kg/min or the hypoglycemia is present after 5–7 days, the infant may have a recurrent or persistent type of hypoglycemia (see Chapter 5, p. 198 for diagnosis and therapy).

It is important to maintain the parenteral glucose and steroids until all clinical manifestations have cleared and the levels of plasma glucose have been stabilized over 50 mg/dl (2.8 mM) for a period of at least 24 hours. It is equally important to carefully document the observations and plasma glucose values to establish the sequence of events.

The concentration of parenteral glucose should then be decreased gradually to 5 percent so the rate of infusion is reduced to 6 mg/kg/min, then to 4 mg/kg/min, and slowly discontinued over 4 to 6 hours, while oral feedings adequate in calories are taken.

If the intravenous glucose infiltrates or is stopped abruptly, a reactive hypoglycemia may ensue as soon as 30 minutes thereafter, and symptoms may recur.

The steroids should be discontinued slowly over several days, using the levels of plasma glucose as a guide.

• Prognosis and Follow-up

The prognosis in newborns with hypoglycemia represents a complex and a multifaceted problem. Of primary importance is the effect on survival. The mortality associated with severe unrecognized hypoglycemia ("nesidioblastosis," islet cell adenoma, congenital hypopituitarism), as well as the neuropathologic changes in the brain associated with untreated "classical" hypoglycemia in the SGA infant [42,43], indicate that a significantly low plasma glucose level persisting over prolonged periods of time can be lethal.

Nevertheless, the effects of hypoglycemia on long-term mental or neurodevelopmental outcome is far from clear [21,23,47,50,93,127–131]. The long-term consequences of significant neonatal hypoglycemia are poorly understood because of the often primary or secondary devastating problems associated with prematurity [132], especially very low birth weight [133,134]. Such problems include hypoxic ischemic encephalopathy [112], congenital anomalies, respiratory distress, multiple metabolic aberrations, asphyxia, cerebral pathology, or sepsis. While a number of dire consequences have been attributed to even brief periods of asymptomatic hypoglycemia (usually in medical litigation), the available data do not support such conclusions.

Animal Data

In adult rats, Siesjö and associates [91,92] have studied the effects of isolated hypoglycemia on the electroencephalogram (EEG), brain energy metabolism, neurophysiology, and neuropathology. In these elegant studies, they developed a model that controlled for hypotension, anoxia, ischemia, and acidosis.

A summary of their extensive experimentation clearly indicated that profound (EEG isoelectric) and prolonged (>30 minutes) hypoglycemia was necessary to demonstrate cell necrosis in the adult rat brain. In control animals, a similar degree of hypoglycemia without the EEG changes was not associated with brain necrosis [135]. These changes were correlated with cerebral blood flow, glucose uptake, oxygen consumption, intracellular energy, and electrolyte changes. Hypoglycemic neuronal damage required that cellular energy states be perturbed, indicating that the mechanisms of cell necrosis were the consequences of energy failure and membrane depolarization. The energy failure was characterized by decreases in concentrations of phosphocreatine and adenosine phosphates, membrane depolarization, by an influx of calcium, an efflux of potassium, with an ensuing acceleration of proteolytic and lipolytic reactions [91,92].

The distribution of the hypoglycemic neuronal necrosis, which was unique and differed from that in ischemia or seizures, suggested the operation of a fluid-borne extracellular toxin [91]. This probably was an excitatory amino acid, such as glutamate or aspartate. These accelerated cell death by causing a dendrosomatic lesion attributed to calcium influx [92].

These techniques and results provide leads for further research into new therapeutic interventions and basic clinical studies.

Vannucci and his collaborators have investigated the effects of hypoglycemia alone or in association with either hypoxemia (8 percent oxygen) or anoxia (100 percent nitrogen) in neonatal rats [136,137] and puppies [138–140]. Petroff et al. [90] and Kliegman [141] have also studied the effects of hypoglycemia alone on brain metabolism in neonatal dogs.

In contrast to the adult rat, newborn animals tolerated as long as 60–120 minutes of blood glucose concentrations under 18 mg/dl (<1.0 mM) without changes in behavior or untoward pathologic or pathophysiologic consequences. If then exposed to anoxia (100 percent nitrogen), hypoglycemic rats died sooner than normoglycemic rats (5 versus 25 minutes). However, if given glucose prior to exposure to anoxia, no differences in survival times were noted [136].

Furthermore, 3–7 day old dogs, after similar periods of hypoglycemia (<18 mg/dl [<1 mM]), showed identical rates of demise and changes in acid-base parameters, pCO_2, heart rate, and blood pressure as normoglycemic controls following asphyxiation. This evidence also indicates the resistance of the neonatal animal to low levels of plasma glucose.

Increases in cerebral blood flow and utilization of alternate substrates [141] have been implicated as the explanation for these differences or resistance to hypoglycemia. Utilizing NMR spectroscopy, Petroff et al. [90] have shown a modulation of excitatory amino acids and a decline in inhibitory neurotransmitters and high-energy phosphates in the neonatal dog as compared to adult animals. However, the data on whole brain versus regional cerebral blood flow and measurements of excitatory amino acids, energy sources, and utilization in these young animals still require further study.

The long-term consequences of prolonged hyperinsulinemic hypoglycemia have been studied in newborn rhesus monkeys by Schrier and colleagues. They utilized an in utero model of hyperinsulinemia [142] to produce neonatal hypoglycemia by the continuous subcutaneous delivery of insulin for up to 4 hours after birth. This resulted in plasma glucose concentrations of 14 ± 4 mg/dl (0.78 mM) for 6.5 ± 1 hours in one group of experimental animals and 16 ± 4 mg/dl (0.89 mM) for 10 ± 1 hours in another. The control group maintained plasma glucose concentrations of 45 ± 10 mg/dl (2.5 mM).

The animals were randomized at birth and then transferred to an experimental psychologist with 30 years' experience in primate behavioral assessment. A cognitive and behavioral testing program was begun under blinded conditions when each animal was 8 months of age. There were no neurologic abnormalities. Testing continued for 22 months, or the equivalent of late childhood in the human. None of the measures of cognitive abilities or behavior distinguished experimental animals with 6.5 hours of hypoglycemia from controls. Ten hours of hypoglycemia resulted in motivational and adaptability problems that made it impossible for some animals to learn even the simplest tasks. However, when provided with additional attention and adequate motivation, these same experimental animals performed as well as controls in all tests designed to measure cognitive abilities [142].

Schrier et al. [142] concluded that neonatal hypoglycemia of 10 hours' duration results in adaptive difficulties in rhesus monkeys, but if special attention is devoted to these animals, there are no enduring cognitive effects or behavioral deficits.

Clinical Data

There have been at least 13 series of cases correlating subsequent neurodevelopmental outcome of neonates with neonatal hypoglycemia, *but without controls* [7,8,19,28,36,44,48,50,60,143–146].[1] The definition of hypoglycemia varied among studies, being less than 20 mg/dl (1.1 mM) in 7, ≤20 mg/dl (1.1 mM) in 3, <25 mg/dl (1.4 mM)

---

[1]The following discussion is based in part on material reviewed by JC Sinclair and PH Steer and presented at a Ciba Foundation Discussion Meeting on Hypoglycemia in Infancy (London, England, October, 1989) [89].

in 2, and unknown in 1. In the majority of reports (9/13), symptomatic hypoglycemia indicated symptoms in association with hypoglycemia but no criteria on whether or not the infant's symptoms responded specifically to glucose therapy. In three reports, the term was used more precisely to designate clinical manifestations that responded to glucose therapy specifically. Most reports did not define the details of measurements of abnormal neurodevelopmental outcome. In summarizing the case series, of the total of 158 symptomatic infants with significantly low blood glucose values, it should be noted that, in 70 percent, no criterion of response of symptoms to glucose therapy was noted; in only 13 percent of infants did the criteria for inclusion describe clearing of symptoms; and in 17 percent, symptoms did not respond to therapy. In this latter group, it was quite likely that the clinical manifestations and outcomes were due to associated or underlying pathology. In addition, the lack of nonhypoglycemic controls, the failure to consider other pathology, and the small numbers of asymptomatic infants followed up raise serious questions about the validity and precision of any inference based on these case series.

Thus, the prognosis and relative risk for neurodevelopmental abnormality in neonatal hypoglycemia cannot be determined by case studies alone. A long-term, prospective controlled study is necessary to resolve these objections and to allow a correlation between neonatal hypoglycemia and outcome.

Such a study would require, at a minimum, the following basic criteria (see footnote 1) [147]:

1. A sound epidemiologic and statistical design to assure adequate numbers in cohorts, avoid sampling bias, provide complete follow-up assessed blindly, and adjust for extraneous prognostic factors,
2. Reliable, accurate plasma glucose determinations and clinical criteria for defining hypoglycemia, both with and without symptoms,
3. A prospective study to include normoglycemic controls, with a follow-up of at least 7–9 years,
4. Either a controlled intervention at predetermined plasma glucose concentrations or a controlled prevention of hypoglycemia, and
5. A specific definition of outcome to include, in addition to precise developmental and mental achievements and neurologic status, metabolic, endocrine, and physical growth criteria as well.

Only in this way will it be possible to establish the prognosis and relative risk of neonatal hypoglycemia as a primary causative factor in abnormal outcome.

No such study exists, and only fragments of this total objective have been reported. Therefore, in infants with neonatal hypogly-cemia, only general conclusions of adverse outcome are possible. Pre-cise estimates cannot be made on the data available.

While seven controlled studies that have evaluated neurodevel-opmental outcomes of both hypoglycemic or nonhypoglycemic con-trols have been reported, none included a randomized trial of intervention for either the treatment or prevention of neonatal hy-poglycemia. Three were follow-ups of infants of diabetic mothers who usually had transient asymptomatic hypoglycemia. None showed an association between neonatal hypoglycemia and outcome in this group.

The other four studies [21,47,93,130] were concerned exclusively or primarily with low birth weight infants in whom hypoglycemia is usually associated with symptoms. Three of these controlled studies [21,47,130] were reported in the 1970s and were based on infants diagnosed in the 1960s. The latest study and the largest was included in a multicenter feeding study [93,100]. While a protocol for obtain-ing plasma glucose samples was included, there was none for assess-ing therapy, and no precautions were taken in handling the blood specimens to prevent glycolysis.

Two of the three early controlled studies reported a risk for sub-sequent neurodevelopmental abnormalities associated with neonatal hypoglycemia (blood glucose values <20 mg/dl [1.1 mM]) in low birth weight infants [21,47]. The risk was substantial with sympto-matic but not asymptomatic hypoglycemia [21]. The third study found no significant association of neonatal hypoglycemia with later cere-bral abnormalities [130]. All three studies, while designed to address specifically the problem of neonatal hypoglycemia, contain serious deficiencies, e.g., sampling bias, small sample size, and incomplete follow-up. These raise serious questions about the validity of their findings concerning the prognosis of neonatal hypoglycemia.

The recent study by Lucas et al. [93] has enlarged the area of uncertainty from neonates with blood sugar values <20 mg/dl (1.1 mM) or at most <30 mg/dl (1.7 mM), and usually symptomatic to a plasma level <47 mg/dl (2.6 mM) regardless of symptoms. In addi-tion, duration of low glucose concentrations in days over the first 9 weeks of life have now been introduced as an independent variable. However, the fact that hypoglycemia was not a primary concern of this prospective controlled feeding study is apparent from the data that indicate some infants were permitted to have plasma glucose values <20 mg/dl (1.1 mM) for as long as 3–7 days. In addition, the glucose values reported and used in their analysis for prognosis were the first ones obtained each day, and the number of days with any specific glucose value were usually not consecutive days. The adjustment for confounding factors and the large sample size were positive aspects of this study. In these high-risk infants under 1,850 gm birth weight, a first glucose value <47 mg/dl (2.6 mM) on 5 or more days correlated positively with abnormal neurologic and developmental outcome at 18 months of age. The significance of this relationship is obscure and requires a prospective controlled intervention study for clarification.

In a recent critical analysis of all reported studies of neonatal hypoglycemia and subsequent neurodevelopment, Sinclair and Steer (Ciba Foundation Discussion Meeting, October 1989) [89,147] concluded:

> . . . the important question of the benefits and risks of striving to maintain blood glucose levels within a prescribed range in low birth weight infants remains unresolved. This is an astounding statement to make in 1989, given the importance attached to the regulation of blood glucose, the volume of research over the past 30 years concerning perinatal changes in glucose supply and the attention given to the monitoring of blood glucose in present-day neonatal intensive care units. Glucose, along with oxygen and warmth, is considered a fundamental need of the newborn. But of the three, it is only contrasting policies in the provision of glucose that have not been put to the test in randomized clinical experiments. . . . The most important contribution of the report of Lucas et al. . . . would be finally to provoke a definitive prospective randomized trial of alternative policies of the provision and/or control of glucose in the care of low birth-weight infants.

The only addition to this conclusion would be that such a trial should include all hypoglycemic infants regardless of birth weight or gestation.

· Pathogenesis and Pathophysiology

"Pathogenetically, idiopathic neonatal hypoglycemia can be regarded as failure to adapt to independent extrauterine life". . . . Raivio (1968) [128]. The multiple physiologic and biochemical changes that occur during the rapid period of adaptation at birth reflect prenatal events, perinatal stresses, and the interaction of multiple hormones and substrates at and after birth. Hypoglycemia essentially represents an imbalance between glucose production or input and glucose utilization or uptake. The regulation and complexity of glucose metabolism throughout fetal development has been detailed in Chapter 1. Only data pertinent to the pathogenesis of the various manifestations of transient neonatal hypoglycemia are summarized here.

Hypoglycemia is the end result of multiple altered regulatory mechanisms. Some may have occurred or begun before birth, such as falling or low estriols or maternal hypoxia, resulting in reduced glucose transport across the placenta and in lower fetal hepatic glycogen. Fetal hypoglycemia early in labor has been associated with growth retardation, preeclampsia, accidental hemorrhage, and maternal hypoglycemia, but not with reduced fetal pO_2 or base excess. Ketones and amino acids, which readily traverse the normal placenta, may be abnormal with maternal toxemia or diabetes. The placental transfer of free fatty acids, ketones, and glycerol, and their metabolism and utilization in sparing glucose can influence extrauterine adaptation.

With all of these variables, plus the dynamic changes in energy requirements for air breathing and temperature maintenance, as well as circulatory changes and increased activities of both digestive and excretory functions, the concepts of excess utilization or uptake of glucose or inadequate intake or production of glucose are, indeed, complex.

Excess utilization or uptake and loss may result from:

1. An absolute or relative hyperinsulinism—IDM, erythroblastosis, LGA, SGA, or islet cell or other endocrine pathology,
2. Neonatal adaptation, stress, and/or incomplete aerobic oxidation with hypoxia, asphyxia, or infection,
3. Relatively excessive amounts of glucose-dependent tissues—brain to liver ratio in SGA,
4. Inadequate glucose-sparing substrates—FFA, ketones, glycerol, amino acids, lactate.

Inadequate production or input may result from:

1. Inadequate or delays in feedings or providing parenteral calories and glucose,
2. Aberrant control mechanisms that regulate effective gluconeogenesis, glycolysis, lipolysis; also hypothalamic, pituitary, and peripheral endocrines,
3. Transient developmental immaturity of critical metabolic pathways reducing endogenous production of glucose and/or other substrates, and
4. Deficient metabolic reserves of precursors or glucose-sparing substrates.

There is evidence for each of these mechanisms in individual or groups of hypoglycemic neonates.

Excess Utilization (Uptake or Loss)

Excessive utilization as defined by the rapid clearance of an intravenously administered bolus of glucose has been reported in neonates with hypoglycemia by a number of investigators [8,60,148–151]. Gentz et al. [60] associated the rapid clearance of glucose with clinical manifestations and reduced values of plasma FFA, which could be reversed by the administration of hydrocortisone or HGH. Yet, HGH values in the neonate are elevated and respond appropriately to hypoglycemia, but are not suppressed by hyperglycemia [152]. Although cortisol production rates are appropriate for surface area, four of eight hypoglycemic infants had low production rates [153]. Epinephrine excretion has also been reported to be decreased in some infants with spontaneous transient hypoglycemia during the first hours of life [154].

Other studies have implicated elevated concentrations of plasma insulin either following glucose administration (12/29 hypoglycemic infants) [150,155] or under basal conditions [101,156]. Both groups, those with and those without an elevated insulin response to parenteral glucose, showed the same hyperglycemic response to glucagon [157]. Relative hyperinsulinism would also occur with adrenal, thyroid, or pituitary pathology (see Chapter 5).

In a group of 15 proven septic infants who had increased disappearance rates for intravenous glucose, none had an increase in plasma insulin concentration. However, five had hypoglycemia following a 3–4 hour fast, and three were symptomatic [78].

While an increased clearance of glucose occurred, the exact disposition of the glucose could not be determined by these studies. Previously, the relatively large brain-to-liver ratio in the SGA infant as compared to the AGA [158] has been implicated as one factor in increasing glucose utilization in these infants [27].

Measurements of glucose-sparing of alternate substrates to support the brain have been reported during the development of hypoglycemia (e.g., during fasting), and have been found to be present in normal concentrations [159]. However, no turnover studies or total body estimates of these alternate substrates have been made to actually assess the amount and availability of these metabolites. Supplementing the diet of preterm neonates of 36 weeks' gestation with medium chain triglycerides reduced the frequency of hypoglycemia significantly from 35 to 7 percent [122].

Furthermore, in SGA infants, oral alanine has increased the levels of glucagon and alanine, but not those of glucose or insulin [160]. Yet, oral alanine produced an increase in glucose, glucagon, insulin, and alanine in the AGA newborn. Glucagon has been given as a continuous infusion in the treatment of transient neonatal hypoglycemia with inconstant effects [161].

Inadequate Production (Input)

The SGA infant with his increased metabolic needs [162–164], oxygen consumption [165] and heat requirements [164] requires adequate total calories as soon as possible after birth. The absolute glucose needs depend upon the availability of glucose-sparing substrates [166,167], as well as glycogen stores [168] and glucose precursors. Thus, the diminished quantities of glycogen [169], fat [170], glycerol [171], and ketone bodies [171] in these infants may be critical. The apparent unavailability of gluconeogenic amino acids [160,172,173] and lactate [173] further increases the fuel requirements and compromises glucose homeostasis in these high-risk babies.

Hyperinsulinemia [101,150,155,174], both absolute and relative, has been found in some of these hypoglycemic infants. This inhibits the endogenous production of glucose by the liver as well as lipolysis, decreasing FFA and ketones, gluconeogenesis, and conversion of lactate and pyruvate to glucose. Thus, both increased utilization and decreased production result from excess insulin [175].

The rapid changes in the ability to clear various monosaccharides [176], in the responses to exogenous and endogenous hormones, substrates and precursors [27] indicate that multiple critical metabolic pathways mature during the first hours to days of life.

In animals, there is a delay between the appearance of rate-limiting enzyme activities and effective gluconeogenesis [177,178]. This is thought to be due to alterations in the redox potential within the cells. Shifts of redox potential as evidenced by altered lactate/pyruvate, β-hydroxybutyrate/acetoacetate, and alpha ketoglutarate/glutamate ratios in the plasma from the high-risk SGA hypoglycemic infant may reflect intracellular changes as well. Thus, anoxia, asphyxia, or intrauterine metabolic modifications resulting from an imbalance of substrates might transiently inhibit the ability of the cell to function or to respond to regulating hormones appropriately [179–181].

Recently, studies of glucose kinetics have been performed in AGA and SGA infants using stable isotopes of glucose for analyses [182–184]. In one study of eight SGA term infants, with a mean birth weight of 2,087 gm and 38 weeks' gestation, $[6,6-^2H_2]$ glucose was measured in infants with a mean basal plasma glucose concentration of 53.7 ± 7.9 mg/dl (3 ± 0.4 mM) compared to eight AGA term infants with a mean of 61.3 ± 10.1 mg/dl (3.4 ± 0.6 mM). There were no differences in plasma insulin levels (mean 5.2 ± 2.9 versus

10.2 ± 5.1 μU/ml [31.2 ± 17.4 versus 61.2 ± 30.6 pM]). The glucose turnover (Ra) was 4.25 ± 0.98 mg/kg/min in the SGA infants compared to 3.53 ± 0.32 mg/kg/min in the AGA infants, a significant difference ($p < 0.05$) [185].

In other studies using uniformly labeled D-[U-^{13}C] glucose, of 23 preterm AGA, 14 term AGA, and 9 SGA infants, parenteral glucose administration (6 mg/kg/min) did not suppress hepatic glucose output uniformly in these infants in contrast to the adult [182,183]. The SGA infants had a more mature response than the AGA infants of similar gestation. There was no correlation between plasma glucose concentrations and glucose production rates in newborns or adults. However, both groups showed an inverse correlation between plasma insulin levels and glucose production rates.

Studies with stable isotope [2,3-^{13}C] alanine incorporation into glucose have also been done in the neonate [185]. The fractional incorporation of alanine into glucose per unit body weight was similar in SGA and AGA newborns. It should be pointed out that there are few studies performed during actual hypoglycemia. All of these data support the concept that multiple mechanisms are involved in transient neonatal hypoglycemia, especially prevalent in SGA infants. Normal full-term newborns in early neonatal life have been studied with L-[1-^{13}C] leucine infusion and respiratory calorimetry [186]. Leucine flux (μM/kg/hr) correlated with body weight and energy expenditure. It was suggested that the relationship between birth weight and protein metabolism is independent of gestational age.

In preliminary studies of hypoglycemia in infants and children, Koh et al. [95] observed abnormalities in auditory and somatic evoked potentials in 10 of 17 patients at glucose levels ranging from 25 to 47 mg/dl (1.4 to 2.6 mM). These changes were also transient, but in three neonates persisted for 1–48 hours after restoration of the blood glucose to normal values. The relationship between these changes and subsequent development has not been determined.

With the recent availability of techniques to measure changes in cerebral function [187], cerebral blood flow [188,189], catecholamine responses [189], and glucose utilization directly in the neonate, data should become available to better define those concentrations of plasma glucose that are correlated with abnormal responses and outcomes.

Pryds et al. [189] compared cerebral blood flow and plasma epinephrine and norepinephrine responses in 13 hypoglycemic infants (mean birth weight = 1,500 gm, mean gestational age = 31.2 weeks) and 12 normoglycemic controls (mean birth weight = 1,310 gm, mean gestational age = 29.5 weeks). Hypoglycemia was defined as a plasma glucose concentration <30 mg/dl (1.7 mM). There was a statistically significant increase in cerebral blood flow in the hypoglycemic group, but not in plasma epinephrine concentrations; norepinephrine levels remained constant throughout the range of blood glucose values. In a comparable study, Pryds et al. [188] reported that cerebral function estimated by electroencephalogram and visual evoked potentials was normal during short periods of low glucose values. They concluded that blood glucose concentrations must be maintained above 30 to 45 mg/dl (1.7 to 2.5 mM) to avoid cerebral hyperperfusion and epinephrine secretion.

Correlating these acute changes in cerebral blood flow, hormone responses, and electroencephalogram findings with long-term neurodevelopmental outcomes will be the challenge of the next decade. More precise direct measurements of cerebral function, metabolic perturbations, blood flow, glucose uptake, and utilization, and correlations with both immediate and long-term outcomes should ultimately resolve some of the current uncertainties.

Case Report (Patient 3.1): Iatrogenic Hypoglycemia

KL was born to a 35-year-old, gravida 2 para 1 mother, whose pregnancy was complicated by a flulike illness in the first trimester, smoking one-half pack of cigarettes per day, and evidence of intrauterine growth retardation (IUGR) at 28 weeks' gestation by ultrasonography. Bed rest did not result in catch-up growth, and pitocin induction was initiated at 37 weeks' gestation. She was born by vaginal delivery after an uneventful labor lasting 3 hours and 40 minutes. Membranes ruptured at the onset of labor. She had Apgar scores of 8 and 9 at 1 and 5 minutes. At 45 minutes after birth, the Dextrostix was <30 mg/dl (1.7 mM). Oral glucose (15 ml 10 percent dextrose/water) was given and a subsequent Dextrostix was 20 mg/dl (1.1 mM). While the intravenous glucose rate was 5 mg/kg/min, the serum glucose was 28 mg/dl (1.6 mM).

At this time, the infant was alert and completely asymptomatic. Temperature was 96.6° and then 98.6°F. Pulse was 152/min, respiration rate (RR) = 52/min, and blood pressure (BP) 47/23. Birth weight was 2,200 gm (<10th percentile), length 48 cm (just below the 50th percentile), and head circumference 33 cm (25–50th percentile). Physical examination was within normal limits without organomegaly.

The hemoglobin was 18 gm/dl, hematocrit 52 percent, and white blood cell count (WBC) 16,800 with normal differential. There were 58 nucleated red blood cells per 100 white blood cells; IgM 8.0 mg/dl. Electrolytes were within normal limits. Calcium was 9.2 mg/dl. Uric acid 1.6 mg/dl; bilirubin increased from 5.7 to 12.6 mg/dl over 6 days. Cholesterol was 82 mg/dl (normal 0–132 mg/dl). TORCH titers were negative.

Intravenous glucose was given first as a 4-ml bolus of 10 percent glucose in water, followed by a rate of 5.6 mg/kg/min. Four hours later, a Chemstix was 20 mg/dl (1.1 mM). The parenteral glucose was increased to 7 mg/kg/min. The goal was to maintain Chemstix in the 60–80 mg/dl range (3.3–4.4 mM). Frequent stick analyses were low (<30–40 mg/dl [1.7–2.2 mM]), yet the infant was always asymptomatic, and laboratory analyses done 2 to 4 times a day were between 55–67 mg/dl (3.1–2.2 mM) during the first 48 hours, and only one was 32 mg/dl (1.8 mM) on day 3. All 10 other values within the first 6 days of life ranged between 45 and 65 mg/dl (2.5 and 3.6 mM).

Using the Chemstix as the guide, the intravenous glucose was discontinued periodically with low values resulting and then restarted and steadily increased to 10, then 13, and finally 20 mg/kg/min by day 4. The infant was edematous, refused feeding, and was vomiting. She was then transferred to a level 3 NICU for further evaluation and an endocrine investigation of the etiology of the "resistant" hypoglycemia.

On admission, aside from the edema from excessive parenteral fluid (300 gm weight gain) and jaundice, the physical examination was entirely within normal limits, as were the routine laboratory studies. A blood sample was analyzed for glucose concentration (33 mg/dl [1.8 mM]), and insulin concentration (4.9 μU/ml [29.4 pM]) and had an insulin/glucose (I/G) ratio of 0.15, well within normal limits.

The parenteral glucose was slowly reduced in volume and concentration from 20 to 15 to 10 to 5 mg/kg/min, with occasional serum glucose values in the 30–40 mg/dl range (1.7–2.2 mM). These were always without symptoms and were within the normal range (45—60 mg/dl [2.5–3.3 mM]) when rechecked several hours later.

A glucagon stimulation test with blood samples taken for glucose, insulin, cortisol, and growth hormone was done 48 hours after transfer. The results were:

TIME (min)	CHEMSTIX (mg/dl)	GLUCOSE		INSULIN		HGH (ng/ml)	CORTISOL (μg/dl)
		(mg/dl)	(mM)	(μU/ml)	(pM)		
0	22	21	1.2	11.0	66	20.0	11.7
10	55	47	2.6	12.5	75		
20	120	60	3.3	11.7	70		
30	96	78	4.3	9.0	54	26.8	14.6

Thyroid function studies at the first hospital were normal: T4 = 15.6 mcg/dl, TSH = 10.8 μU/ml. As the parenteral glucose was discontinued, full formula feedings were established, and the infant was discharged in excellent condition at 11 days of age.

Comment

This SGA, meconium-stained infant had low serum glucose values within an hour after birth. Basing their therapy and relying on Chemstix values for blood glucose, aggressive parenteral glucose administration was initiated. The discrepancies between Chemstix and laboratory glucose concentrations throughout the clinical course and during the glucagon test indicate the fallacy of this approach. Insufficient attention to the laboratory values for glucose and an unrealistic goal of Chemstix values between 60 and 80 mg/dl (3.3 and 4.4 mM) resulted in overtreating this asymptomatic infant. Periodic cessation of parenteral glucose produced the expected reactive hypoglycemia (by Chemstix only, apparently).

The thorough endocrine investigation effectively eliminated congenital hypopituitarism and hyperinsulinemia in this female infant. A slow steady reduction in the concentration and volumes of glucose administered intravenously cured the "hypoglycemia."

This patient illustrates the need to monitor plasma glucose concentrations with glucose oxidase or laboratory methods rather than glucose oxidase screening reagent pads alone. It should be emphasized that it is necessary to repeat or confirm low glucose values before increasing the administration of glucose in concentration and volume. This is especially true in the asymptomatic infant.

• Summary

Low blood glucose values in the neonate are not uncommon and require careful evaluation to determine their significance, persistence, or relevance to the clinical condition of the infant. Thus, plasma glucose concentrations represent an estimate of the metabolic milieu of a particular infant at a specific point in time. While restoration of the plasma glucose concentration to normoglycemic values is desirable, the urgency to do so and the methods to be employed depend upon the entire clinical evaluation of the infant, including the age in hours, the presence of clinical manifestations, and multiple other risk factors.

REFERENCES

1. HARTMANN AF, JAUDON JC. Hypoglycemia. *J Pediatr.* 1937;11:1.
2. SHERMAN H. Islet-cell tumor of pancreas in a newborn infant (nesidioblastoma). *Am J Dis Child.* 1947;74:58.
3. WILKINS L, ed. The diagnosis and treatment of endocrine disorders in childhood and adolescence. Springfield, Ill.: Charles C. Thomas, 1957;464.
4. MCQUARRIE I. Idiopathic spontaneously occurring hypoglycemia in infants. *Am J Dis Child.* 1954;87:399.
5. SCHWARTZ O, GOLDNER MG, ROSENBLUM J, ARVIN J. Neonatal hypoglycemia, report of a case of unusual duration. *Pediatrics.* 1955; 16:658.
6. SCHULMAN JL, SATURN P. Glycogen storage disease of the liver. I. Clinical studies during the early neonatal period. *Pediatrics.* 1954;14:632.
7. CORNBLATH M, ODELL GB, LEVIN EY. Symptomatic neonatal hypoglycemia associated with toxemia of pregnancy. *J Pediatr.* 1959;55:545.
8. CORNBLATH M, WYBREGT SH, BAENS GS, KLEIN RI. Symptomatic neonatal hypoglycemia: Studies of carbohydrate metabolism in the newborn infant. VIII. *Pediatrics.* 1964;33:388.

9. HAWORTH JC, COODIN FJ, FINKEL KC, WEIDMAN ML. Hypoglycemia associated with symptoms in the newborn period. *Can Med Assoc J.* 1963;88:23.

10. BROWN RJ, WALLIS PG. Hypoglycemia in the newborn infant. *Lancet.* 1963;1:1278.

11. HARRIS R, TIZARD JP. The electroencephalogram in neonatal convulsions. *J Pediatr.* 1960;57:501.

12. NELIGAN GA, ROBSON E, WATSON J. Hypoglycaemia in the newborn. A sequel of intrauterine malnutrition. *Lancet.* 1963;1:1282.

13. ZETTERSTRÖM R, [EEG-OLOFSON O, NILSSON L]. Neonatal chemistry. (Discussion workshop.) *Ann NY Acad Sci.* 1963;111:537 and personal communication.

14. TYNAN MJ, HAAS L. Hypoglycaemia in the newborn. *Lancet.* 1963;2:90 (Letter to the Editor.)

15. CREERY RDG. Hypoglycaemia in the newborn. *Lancet.* 1963;1:1423. (Letter to the Editor.)

16. GRAUAUG A. Neonatal hypoglycaemia. *Med J Aust.* 1965;1:455.

17. HAWORTH JC, DILLING L, YOUNOSZAI MK. Relation of blood-glucose to haematocrit, birthweight, and other body measurements in normal and growth-retarded newborn infants. *Lancet.* 1967;2:901.

18. RAIVIO KO, HALLMAN N. Neonatal hypoglycemia. I. Occurrence of hypoglycemia in patients with various neonatal disorders. *Acta Paediatr Scand.* 1968;57:517.

19. RAIVIO KO. Neonatal hypoglycemia. II. A clinical study of 44 idiopathic cases with special reference to corticosteroid treatment. *Acta Paediatr Scand.* 1968;57:540 and personal communication.

20. HAWORTH JC, VIDYASAGAR D. Hypoglycemia in the newborn. *Clin Obstet Gynecol.* 1971;14:821.

21. KOIVISTO M, BLANCO-SEQUEIROS M, KRAUSE U. Neonatal symptomatic and asymptomatic hypoglycaemia: A follow-up study of 151 children. *Dev Med Child Neurol.* 1972;14:603.

22. LACOURT G. Dépistage et prévention de l'hypoglycémie néonate transitoire. *Médecine Sociale et Preventive.* 1974;19:101.

23. FLUGE G. Clinical aspects of neonatal hypoglycaemia. *Acta Paediatr Scand.* 1974;63:826 and personal communication.

24. MACHADE J, EBRAHIM GJ. Hypoglycaemia in the newborn. *East Afr Med J.* 1969;46:67.

25. WYBREGT SH, REISNER SH, PATEL RK, NELLHAUS G, CORNBLATH M. The incidence of neonatal hypoglycemia in a nursery for premature infants. *J Pediatr.* 1964;64:796.

26. NELIGAN GA. Idiopathic hypoglycemia in the newborn. In: Gairdner D, ed. *Recent Advances in Pediatrics.* London: J. & A. Churchill Ltd., 1965, 110.

27. CORNBLATH M, JOASSIN G, WEISSKOPF B, SWIATEK KR. Hypoglycemia in the newborn. *Pediatr Clin North Am.* 1966;13:905.

28. CREERY RDG. Hypoglycaemia in the newborn: Diagnosis, treatment and prognosis. *Dev Med Child Neurol.* 1966;8:746.

29. PILDES R, FORBES AE, O'CONNOR SM, CORNBLATH M. The incidence of neonatal hypoglycemia: A completed survey. *J Pediatr.* 1967;70:76.

30. CORNBLATH M. Hypoglycemia in infancy and childhood. *Pediatr Annals.* 1981;10:356.

31. SUTTON AM, KINGDOM JCP. Neonatal hypoglycaemia: an important early

sign of endocrine disorder. *Br Med J.* 1985;291:1046. (Letter to the Editor.)

32. GRUENWALD P. Chronic fetal distress. *Clin Pediatr.* 1964;3:141.

33. LUBCHENCO L, HANSMAN C, DRESSLER M. Intrauterine growth as estimated from liveborn birth weight data at 24 to 42 weeks of gestation. *Pediatrics.* 1963;32:793.

34. LUBCHENCO LO, HANSMAN C, BOYD E. Intrauterine growth in length and head circumference as estimates from live births at gestational ages from 24 to 42 weeks. *Pediatrics.* 1966;37:403.

35. PILDES RS, FORBES AE, CORNBLATH M. Blood glucose levels and hypoglycemia in twins. *Pediatrics.* 1967;40:69.

36. KNOBLOCH H, SOTOS JF, SHERARD ES JR, HODSON WA, WEHE RA. Prognosis and etiologic factors in hypoglycemia. *J Pediatr.* 1967;70:876.

37. BEARD A, CORNBLATH M, GENTZ J, KELLUM M, PERSSON B, ZETTERSTRÖM R, HAWORTH JC. Neonatal hypoglycemia: A discussion. *J Pediatr.* 1971;79:314.

38. SENIOR B, SADEGHI-NEJAD A. Hypoglycemia: a pathophysiologic approach. *Acta Paediatr Scand.* 1989;(Suppl 352):1.

39. AMATAYAKUL O, CUMMING GR, HAWORTH JC. Association of hypoglycaemia with cardiac enlargement and heart failure in newborn infants. *Arch Dis Child.* 1970;45:717.

40. REID MM, REILLY BJ, MURDOCK AI, SWYER PR. Cardiomegaly in association with neonatal hypoglycaemia. *Acta Paediatr Scand.* 1971; 60:295.

41. CORNBLATH M. Hypoglycemia. In: Nelson NM, ed. *Current therapy in neonatal-perinatal medicine. 2nd ed.* Philadelphia: BC Decker, Inc., 1990;262.

42. ANDERSON, JM, MILNER RDG, STRICH SJ. Effects of neonatal hypoglycaemia on the nervous system: A pathological study. *J Neurol Neurosurg Psychiatry.* 1967;30:295.

43. BANKER BQ. The neuropathological effects of anoxia and hypoglycaemia in the newborn. *Dev Med Child Neurol.* 1967;9:544.

44. HAWORTH JC, MCRAE KN. The neurological and developmental effects of neonatal hypoglycemia: A follow-up of 22 cases. *Can Med Assoc J.* 1965;92:861.

45. HAWORTH JC. Carbohydrate metabolism in the fetus and the newborn. *Pediatr Clin North Am.* 1965;12:573.

46. HAWORTH JC, MCRAE KN. Neonatal hypoglycemia: A six-year experience. *Journal Lancet.* 1967;87:41.

47. PILDES RS, CORNBLATH M, WARREN I, PAGE-EL E, DIMENZA S, MERRITT DM, PEEVA A. A prospective controlled study of neonatal hypoglycemia. *Pediatrics.* 1974;54:5.

48. EEG-OLOFSSON O, GENTZ J, JODAL U, NILSSON LR, ZETTERSTRÖM R. Neonatal symptomatic hypoglycemia. Some results from a follow-up study. *Acta Paediatr Scand.* (Suppl.) 1967;177:85.

49. HAWORTH JC. Neonatal hypoglycemia: How much does it damage the brain? *Pediatrics.* 1974;54:3.

50. FLUGE G. Neurological findings at follow-up in neonatal hypoglycaemia. *Acta Paediatr Scand.* 1975;64:629.

51. GUTBERLET RL, CORNBLATH M. Neonatal hypoglycemia revisited—1975. *Pediatrics.* 1976;58:10.

52. SMALLPEICE V, DAVIES PA. Immediate feeding of premature infants with undiluted breast milk. *Lancet.* 1964:2:1349.

53. BEARD AG, PANOS TC, MARASIGAN BV, EMINIANS J, KENNEDY HF, LAMB J. Perinatal stress and the premature neonate. II. Effect of fluid and calorie deprivation on blood glucose. *J Pediatr.* 1966;68:329.

54. WHARTON BA, BOWER BD. Immediate or later feeding for premature babies? A controlled trial. *Lancet.* 1965;2:969.

55. CAMPBELL MA, FERGUSON IC, HUTCHINSON JH, KERR MM. Diagnosis and treatment of hypoglycaemia in the newborn. *Arch Dis Child.* 1967; 42:353.

56. CHANTLER C, BAUM JD, NORMAN DA. Dextrostix in the diagnosis of neonatal hypoglycaemia. *Lancet.* 1967;2:1395.

57. DITCHBURN RK, WILKINSON RH, DAVIES PA, AINSWORTH P. Plasma glucose levels in infants weighing 2500 g and less fed immediately after birth with breast milk. *Biol Neonate.* 1967;11:29.

58. GRIFFITHS AD. Association of hypoglycaemia with symptoms in the newborn. *Arch Dis Child.* 1968;43:688.

59. RAIVIO KO. Factors affecting the development of symptoms in neonatal hypoglycemia. *Ann Paediatr Fenn.* 1968;14:105.

60. GENTZ JCH, PERSSON B, ZETTERSTRÖM R. On the diagnosis of symptomatic neonatal hypoglycemia. *Acta Paediatr Scand.* 1969;58:449.

61. CORNBLATH M, REISNER SH. Blood glucose in the neonate, clinical significance. *N Engl J Med.* 1965;273:378.

62. BAENS GS, LUNDEEN E, CORNBLATH M. Studies of carbohydrate metabolism in the newborn infant. VI. Levels of glucose in blood in premature infants. *Pediatrics.* 1963;31:580.

63. SRINIVASAN G, PILDES RS, CATTAMANCHI G, VOORA S, LILLEN LD. Plasma glucose values in normal neonates. A new look. *J Pediatr.* 1986; 109:114.

64. HECK LJ, ERENBERG A. Serum glucose levels in term neonates during the first 48 hours of life. *J Pediatr.* 1987;110:119.

65. HAZELTINE FG. Hypoglycemia and Rh erythroblastosis fetalis. *Pediatrics.* 1967;39:696.

66. LUCEY JF, RANDALL JL, MURRAY JJ. Is hypoglycemia an important complication in erythroblastosis fetalis? *Am J Dis Child.* 1967;114:88.

67. BARRETT CT, OLIVER TK JR. Hypoglycemia and hyperinsulinism in erythroblastosis fetalis. *N Engl J Med.* 1968;278:1260.

68. FROM GLA, DRISCOLL SG, STEINKE J. Serum insulin in newborn infants with erythroblastosis fetalis. *Pediatrics.* 1969;44:549.

69. SCHIFF D, ARANDA JV, COLLE E, STERN L. Metabolic effects of exchange transfusion. II. Delayed hypoglycemia following exchange transfusion with citrated blood. *J Pediatr.* 1971;79:589.

70. DRISCOLL SG, STEINKE J. Pancreatic insulin content in severe erythroblastosis fetalis. *Pediatrics.* 1967;39:449.

71. MØLSTED-PEDERSON L, TRAUTNER H, JØRGENSEN KAJ R. Plasma insulin and K values during intravenous glucose tolerance test in newborn infants with erythroblastosis foetalis. *Acta Paediatr Scand.* 1973; 62:11.

72. FANCONI A, BOVET U, TSCHUMI A, LITSCHGI M, BISCHOFBERGER U. Blutglukose beim termingeborenen in der ersten stunde nach der geburt. *Helv Paediatr Acta.* 1982;37:449.

73. MANN TP, ELLIOT RIK. Neonatal cold injury due to accidental exposure to cold. *Lancet.* 1957;1:229.

74. BOWER BD, JONES LF, WEEKS MM. Cold injury in the newborn. *Br Med J.* 1960;1:303.

75. ARNEIL GC, KERR MM. Severe hypothermia in Glasgow infants in winter. *Lancet.* 1963;2:756.
76. CORNBLATH M, SCHWARTZ R, eds. *Disorders of Carbohydrate Metabolism in Infancy.* Philadelphia: WB Saunders Co., 1976;155.
77. YEUNG CY. Hypoglycemia in neonatal sepsis. *J Pediatr.* 1970;77:812.
78. YEUNG CY, LEE VWY, YEUNG CM. Glucose disappearance rate in neonatal infection. *J Pediatr.* 1973;82:486.
79. STANLEY CA, BAKER L. Hyperinsulinism in infants and children. Diagnosis and therapy. *Adv Pediatr.* 1976;23:315.
80. PHILLIPS L, LUMLEY J, PATERSON P, WOOD C. Fetal hypoglycemia. *Am J Obstet Gynecol.* 1968;102:371.
81. HAYMOND MW, KARL IE, PAGLIARA AS. Increased gluconeogenic substrates in the small-for-gestational-age infant. *N Engl J Med.* 1974; 291:322.
82. JARAI I, MESTYAN J, SCHULTZ K, LAZAR A, HALASZ M, KRASSY I. Body size and neonatal hypoglycemia in intrauterine growth retardation. *Early Human Develop.* 1977;1:25.
83. LUBCHENCO LO, BARD H. Incidence of hypoglycemia in newborn infants classified by birth weight and gestational age. *Pediatrics.* 1971; 47:831.
84. AYNSLEY-GREEN A, SOLTESZ G, eds. Hypoglycaemia in infancy and childhood. Edinburgh: Churchill Livingstone, 1985.
85. MILNER RDG. Neonatal hypoglycaemia. *J Perinat Med.* 1979;7:185.
86. MENON RK, SPERLING MA. Carbohydrate metabolism. *Semin Perinatol.* 1988;12:157.
87. HAYMOND MW. Hypoglycemia in infants and children. *Endocrinol Metab Clin North Am.* 1989;18:211.
88. KOH THHG, EYRE JA, AYNSLEY-GREEN A. Neonatal hypoglycaemia - the controversy regarding definition. *Arch Dis Child.* 1988;63:1386.
89. CORNBLATH M, SCHWARTZ R, AYNSLEY-GREEN A, LLOYD JK. Hypoglycemia in infancy: the need for a rational definition. A Ciba Foundation Discussion Meeting. *Pediatrics.* 1990;85:834.
90. PETROFF OA, YOUNG RS, COWAN BE, NOVOTNY EJ JR. 1H nuclear magnetic resonance spectroscopy study of neonatal hypoglycemia. *Pediatr Neurol.* 1988;4:31.
91. AUER RN, SIESJO BK. Biological differences between ischemia, hypoglycemia and epilepsy. *Ann Neurol.* 1988;24:699.
92. SIESJO BK. Hypoglycemia, brain metabolism and brain damage. *Diabetes/Metabolism Rev.* 1988;4:113.
93. LUCAS A, MORLEY R, COLE JJ. Adverse neurodevelopmental outcome of moderate neonatal hypoglycaemia. *Br Med J.* 1988;297:304.
94. PAGLIARA AS, KARL IE, HAYMOND M, KIPNIS DM. Hypoglycemia in infancy and childhood. *J Pediatr.* 1973;82:365(I); 558(II).
95. KOH THHG, AYNSLEY-GREEN A, TARBIT M, EYRE JA. Neural dysfunction during hypoglycaemia. *Arch Dis Child.* 1988;63:1353.
96. CONRAD PD, SPARKS JW, OSBERG I, ABRAMS L, HAY WW JR. Clinical application of a new glucose analyzer in the neonatal intensive care unit: comparison with other methods. *J Pediatr.* 1989;114:281.
97. LIN HC, MAGUIRE C, OH W, COWETT R. Accuracy and reliability of glucose reflectance meters in the high-risk neonate. *J Pediatr.* 1989; 115:998.
98. SEXSON WR. Incidence of neonatal hypoglycemia: a matter of definition. *J Pediatr.* 1984;105:149.

99. WU S, SRINIVASAN G, PILDES RS, PATEL MK. Plasma glucose values during the first month of life in infants <1000 gm. *Pediatr Res.* 1990; 27:231A.

100. LUCAS A, GORE SM, COLE TJ, et al. Multicentre trial on feeding low birth weight infants: effects of diet on early growth. *Arch Dis Child.* 1984;59:722.

101. COLLINS JE, LEONARD JV. Hyperinsulinism in asphyxiated and small-for-dates infants with hypoglycaemia. *Lancet.* 1984;2:311.

102. REISNER SH, FORBES AE, CORNBLATH M. The smaller of twins and hypoglycaemia. *Lancet.* 1965;1:524.

103. DWECK HS, MIRANDA LEY. Perinatal glucose homeostasis: the unique character of hyperglycemia and hypoglycemia in infants of very low birth weight. *Clin Perinatol.* 1977;4:351.

104. KLIEGMAN R, GROSS I, MORTON S, DUNNINGTON R. Intrauterine growth and postnatal fasting metabolism in infants of obese mothers. *J Pediatr.* 1984;104:601.

105. KLIEGMAN RM, GROSS T. Perinatal problems of the obese mother and her infant. *Obstet Gynecol.* 1985;66:299.

106. KENEPP NB, KUMAR S, SHELLEY WC, STANLEY CA, GABBE SG, GUTSCHE BB. Fetal and neonatal hazards of maternal hydration with 5% dextrose before caesarean section. *Lancet.* 1982;1:1150.

107. CARMEN S. Neonatal hypoglycemia in response to maternal glucose infusion before delivery. *J Obstet Gynecol Neonatal Nurs.* 1986; 15:319.

108. SINGHI S. Effect of maternal intrapartum glucose therapy on neonatal blood glucose levels and behavioral status of hypoglycemic term newborn infants. *J Perinat Med.* 1988;16:217.

109. MENDIOLA J, GRYLACK LJ, SCANLON JW. Effects of intrapartum maternal glucose infusion on the normal fetus and newborn. *Anaesth Analg.* 1982;61:32.

110. BENZING F III, SCHUBERT W, HUG G, KAPLAN S. Simultaneous hypoglycemia and acute congestive heart failure. *Circulation.* 1969;40:209.

111. HAYMOND MW, STRAUSS AW, ARNOLD KJ, BIER DM. Glucose homeostatis in children with severe cyanotic congenital heart disease. *J Pediatr.* 1979;95:220.

112. VOLPE JJ. *Neurology of the Newborn, 2nd ed.* Philadelphia: WB Saunders, 1987.

113. ORZALESI M, RENZULLI E, FERRANTE E. Trisomy 18 and neonatal hypoglycaemia. *Lancet.* 1967;2:1211.

114. MILNER RDG, FEKETE M, ASSAN R. Glucagon, insulin, and growth hormone response to exchange transfusion in premature and term infants. *Arch Dis Child.* 1972;47:186.

115. SENIOR B, SLOWE D, SHAPIRO S, MITCHELL AA, HEINONEN OP. Benzothiadiazides and neonatal hypoglycaemia. *Lancet.* 1976;2:377. (Letter.)

116. BRAZY JE, PUPKIN MJ. Effects of maternal isoxsuprine administration on preterm infants. *J Pediatr.* 1979;94:444.

117. EPSTEIN MF, NICHOLLS E, STUBBLEFIELD PG. Neonatal hypoglycemia after beta-sympathomimetic tocolytic therapy. *J Pediatr.* 1979;94:449.

118. CORNBLATH M, POTH M. Hypoglycemia. In: Kaplan S, ed. *Clinical Pediatric and Adolescent Endocrinology.* Philadelphia: WB Saunders, 1982, 157.

119. URBACH J, KAPLAN M, BLONDHEIM O, HIRSCH HJ. Neonatal hypogly-

cemia related to umbilical artery catheter malposition. *J Pediatr.* 1985;106:825.

120. CAREY BE, ZEILINGER TC. Hypoglycemia due to high positioning of umbilical artery catheters. *J Perinatol.* 1989;9:407.

121. HENDERSON BM, SCHUBERT WK, HUG G, MARTIN LW. Hypoglycemia with hepatic glycogen depletion: A postoperative complication of pyloric stenosis. *J Pediatr Surg.* 1968;3:309.

122. SANN L, MOUSSON B, ROUSSON M, MAIRE I, BETHENOD M. Prevention of neonatal hypoglycaemia by oral lipid supplementation in low birth weight infants. *Eur J Pediatr.* 1988;147:158.

123. ADAM PAJ, KING K, SCHWARTZ R. Model for the investigation of intractable hypoglycemia: Insulin-glucose interrelationships during steady-state infusions. *Pediatrics.* 1968;41:91.

124. SCHWARTZ R, ADAM PAJ, KING K, KORNHAUSER D. Glucose control in the newborn infant. In: Jonxis JHP, Visser HKA, Troelstra JA, eds. *Nutricia Symposium. Aspects of Praematurity and Dysmaturity.* Leiden: H. E. Stenfert Kroese N. V., 1968, 210.

125. LILIEN LD, GRAJWER LA, PILDES RS. Treatment of neonatal hypoglycemia with continuous intravenous glucose infusion. *J Pediatr.* 1977; 91:779.

126. LILIEN LD, PILDES RS, SRINIVASAN G, VOORA S, YEH TF. Treatment of neonatal hypoglycemia with minibolus and intravenous glucose infusion. *J Pediatr.* 1980;97:295.

127. HIRABAYASHI S, KITAHARA T, HISHIDA T. Computed tomography in perinatal hypoxic and hypoglycemic encephalopathy with emphasis on follow-up studies. *J Comput Assist Tomogr.* 1980;4:451.

128. RAIVIO KO. Idiopathic hypoglycemia of childhood manifesting in the neonate. *Ann Paediatr Fenn.* 1968;14:110.

129. GRIFFITHS AD, LAURENCE KM. The effect of hypoxia and hypoglycaemia on the brain of the newborn infant. *Dev Med Child Neurol.* 1974; 16:308.

130. GRIFFITHS AD, BRYANT GM. Assessment of effects of neonatal hypoglycemia: A study of 41 cases with matched controls. *Arch Dis Child.* 1971;46:819.

131. EHRLICH RM. Hypoglycaemia in infancy and childhood. *Arch Dis Child.* 1971;46:716.

132. ALLEN MC, JONES MD JR. Medical complications of prematurity. *Obstet Gynecol.* 1986;67:427.

133. BRITTON SB, FITZHARDINGE PM, ASHBY S. Is intensive care justified for infants weighing less than 801 gm at birth? *J Pediatr.* 1981;99:937.

134. KLEIN N, HACK M, GALLAGHER J, FANAROFF AA. Preschool performance of children with normal intelligence who were very low birth weight infants. *Pediatrics.* 1985;75:531.

135. AUER RN, OLSSON Y, SIESJÖ BK. Hypoglycemic brain injury in the rat. Correlation of density of brain damage with the EEG isoelectric time: A quantitative study. *Diabetes.* 1984;33:1090.

136. VANNUCCI RC, VANNUCCI SJ. Cerebral carbohydrate metabolism during hypoglycemia and anoxia in newborn rats. *Ann Neurol.* 1978;4:73.

137. VANNUCCI RC, VASTA F, VANNUCCI SJ. Glucose supplementation does not accentuate hypoxic-ischemic brain damage in immature rats: biochemical mechanisms. *Pediatr Res.* 1985;19:396.

138. VANNUCCI RC, NARDIS EE, VANNUCCI SJ. Cerebral metabolism during

hypoglycemia and asphyxia in newborn dogs. *Biol Neonate.* 1980; 38:276.

139. VANNUCCI RC, NARDIS EE, VANNUCCI SJ, CAMPBELL PA. Cerebral carbohydrate and energy metabolism during hypoglycemia in newborn dogs. *Am J Physiol.* 1981;240:192.

140. ANWAR M, VANNUCCI RC. Autoradiographic determination of regional cerebral blood flow during hypoglycemia in newborn dogs. *Pediatr Res.* 1988;24:41.

141. KLEIGMAN RM. Cerebral metabolic response to neonatal hypoglycemia in growth retarded dogs. *Pediatr Res.* 1988;24:649.

142. SCHRIER AM, WILHELM PB, CHURCH RM, et al. Neonatal hypoglycemia in the rhesus monkey: Effect on development and behavior. *Infant Behavior & Development.* 1990;13:189.

143. CANTAB MB, WALLIS PG. Hypoglycaemia in the newborn infant. *Lancet.* 1963;2:1278.

144. MCKINNA AJ. Neonatal hypoglycemia—some ophthalmic observations. *Can Ophth.* 1966;I:56.

145. CHANCE GW, BOWER BD. Hypoglycaemia and temporary hyperglycaemia in infants of low birth weight for maturity. *Arch Dis Child.* 1966;41:279.

146. COX M, DUNN HG. Idiopathic hypoglycaemia and children of low birth weight. *Develop Med Child Neurol.* 1967;9:430.

147. SINCLAIR JC, STEER PA. Personal communication.

148. MILNER RDG. Neonatal hypoglycaemia: A critical reappraisal. *Arch Dis Child.* 1972;47:679.

149. ZUPPINGER KA. Hypoglycemia in Childhood: Evaluation of Diagnostic Procedures. In: Falkner F, Kretchmer N, Rossi E, eds. *Monographs in Paediatrics.* Basel: S. Karger, 1975.

150. PILDES RS, PATEL DA, NITZAN M. Glucose disappearance rate in symptomatic neonatal hypoglycemia. *Pediatrics.* 1973;52:77.

151. SAULS HS JR, ULSTROM RA. Hypoglycemia. In: Kelley VC, ed. Brenneman's Practice of Pediatrics. vol. 1. Hagerstown: W. F. Prior Co., 1966;Chap. 40.

152. CORNBLATH M, PARKER ML, REISNER SH, FORBES AE, DAUGHADAY WH. Secretion and metabolism of growth hormone in premature and fullterm infants. *J Clin Endocrinol Metab.* 1965;25:209.

153. KENNY FM, PREEYASOMBAT C. Cortisol production rate. VI. Hypoglycemia in the neonatal and postneonatal period, and in association with dwarfism. *J Pediatr.* 1967;70:65.

154. STERN L, SOURKES TL, RAIHA N. The role of the adrenal medulla in the hypoglycemia of fetal malnutrition. *Biol Neonate.* 1967;11:129.

155. LEDUNE MA. Intravenous glucose tolerance and plasma insulin studies in small-for-dates infants. *Arch Dis Child.* 1971;47:111.

156. BHOWMICK SK, LEWANDOWSKI C. Prolonged hyperinsulinism and hypoglycemia in an asphyxiated, small for gestation infant. Case management and literature review. *Clin Pediatr.* 1989;28:575.

157. FEINGOLD DN, STANLEY CA, BAKER L. Glycemic response to glucagon during fasting hypoglycemia: an aid in the diagnosis of hyperinsulinism. *J Pediatr.* 1980;96:257.

158. DAWKINS MJR. Hypoglycaemia in childhood. *Proc Roy Soc Med.* 1964; 57:1063.

159. STANLEY CA, ANDAY EK, BAKER L, DELIVORIA-PAPADOPOLOUS M. Meta-

bolic fuel and hormone responses to fasting in newborn infants. *Pediatrics.* 1979;64:613.

160. WILLIAMS PR, FISER RH JR, SPERLING MA, OH W. Effects of oral alanine feeding on blood glucose, plasma glucagon, and insulin concentrations in small-for-gestational-age infants. *N Engl J Med.* 1975; 292:612.

161. CARTER PE, LLOYD DJ, DUFFY P. Glucagon for hypoglycaemia in infants small for gestational age. *Arch Dis Child.* 1988;63:1264.

162. SINCLAIR JC, SILVERMAN WA. Intrauterine growth in active tissue mass of the human fetus, with particular reference to the undergrown baby. *Pediatrics.* 1966;38:48.

163. SINCLAIR JC, SCOPES JW, SILVERMAN WA. Metabolic reference standards for the neonate. *Pediatrics.* 1967;39:724.

164. MESTYAN J, JARAI I, FEKETE M. The total energy expenditure and its components in premature infants maintained under different nursing and environmental conditions. *Pediatr Res.* 1968;2:161.

165. SCOPES JW, AHMED I. Minimal rates of oxygen consumption in sick and premature newborn infants. *Arch Dis Child.* 1966;41:407.

166. MELICHAR V, DRAHOTA Z, HAHN P. Ketone bodies in the blood of full term newborns, premature and dysmature infants and in infants of diabetic mothers. *Biol Neonate.* 1967;11:23.

167. OWEN OE, MORGAN AP, KEMP HG, SULLIVAN JM, HERRERA MG, CAHILL GF, JR. Brain metabolism during fasting. *J Clin Invest.* 1967;46:1589.

168. SHELLEY JJ, NELIGAN GA. Neonatal hypoglycaemia. *Br Med Bull.* 1966; 22:34.

169. SHELLY HJ. Carbohydrate reserves in the newborn infant. *Br Med J.* 1964;1:273.

170. SHAFRIR E. Adipose tissue and neonatal homeostasis. *Isr J Med Sci.* 1968;4:277.

171. PERSSON B, GENTZ J. The pattern of blood lipids, glycerol and ketone bodies during the neonatal period, infancy and childhood. *Acta Paediatr Scand.* 1966;55:353.

172. MESTYAN J, SCHULTZ K, HORVATH M. Comparative glycemic responses to alanine in normal term and small-for-gestational-age infants. *J Pediatr.* 1974;85:276.

173. DELEEUW R, DEVRIES IJ. Hypoglycemia in small-for-date newborn infants. *Pediatrics.* 1976;58:18.

174. LOWRY C, SCHIFF D. Urinary excretion of insulin in the healthy newborn. *Lancet.* 1968;1:225.

175. COWETT RM. Pathophysiology, diagnosis and management of glucose homeostasis in the neonate. *Curr Prob Pediatr.* 1985;15:1.

176. CORNBLATH M, WYBREGT SH, BAENS GS. Studies of carbohydrate metabolism in the newborn infant. VII. Tests of carbohydrate tolerance in premature infants. *Pediatrics.* 1963;32:1007.

177. PEARCE PH, BUIRCHELL BJ, WEAVER PK, OLIVER IT. The development of phosphopyruvate carboxylase and gluconeogenesis in neonatal rats. *Biol Neonate.* 1974;24:320.

178. BALLARD FJ. The development of gluconeogenesis in rat liver. Controlling factors in the newborn. *Biochem J.* 1971;124:265.

179. OZAND PT, STEVENSON JH, TILDON JT, CORNBLATH M. The effects of hyperketonemia on glycolytic intermediates in developing rat brain. *J Neurochem.* 1975;25:61.

180. OZAND PT, STEVENSON JH, TILDON JT, CORNBLATH M. The effects of hyperketonemia on glutamate and glutamine metabolism in developing rat brain. *J Neurochem.* 1975;25:67.

181. TILDON JT, OZAND PT, CORNBLATH M. The effect of hyperketonemia on neonatal brain metabolism. In: Hommes FA, Vandenberg CJ, eds. The Normal and Pathological Development of Metabolism. New York: Academic Press, 1975, 143.

182. COWETT RM, OH W, SCHWARTZ R. Persistent glucose production during glucose infusion in the neonate. *J Clin Invest.* 1983;71:467.

183. COWETT RM, SUSA JB, OH W, SCHWARTZ R. Glucose kinetics in glucose-infused small for gestational age infants. *Pediatr Res.* 1984;18:74.

184. KALHAN SC, OLIVEN A, KING KC, LUCERO C. Role of glucose in the regulation of endogenous glucose production in the human newborn. *Pediatr Res.* 1986;20:49.

185. FRAZER TE, KARL IE, HILLMAN LS, BIER DM. Direct measurement of gluconeogenesis from [2,3,^{13}C] alanine in the human neonate. *Am J Physiol.* 1981;240:E615.

186. DENNE SC, KALHAN SC. Leucine metabolism in human newborns. *Am J Physiol.* 1987;253:E-608.

187. CHUGANI HT, PHELPS ME. Maturational changes in cerebral function in infants determined by ^{18}FDG positron emission tomography. *Science.* 1986;231:840.

188. PRYDS O, GREISEN G, FRIIS-HANSEN B. Compensatory increase of CBF supports cerebral metabolism in preterm infants during hypoglycemia. *Acta Paediatr Scand.* 1988;77:632.

189. PRYDS O, CHRISTENSEN NJ, FRIIS-HANSEN B. Increased cerebral blood flow and plasma epinephrine in hypoglycemic, preterm neonates. *Pediatrics.* 1990;85:172.

CHAPTER 4

INFANT

OF THE

DIABETIC MOTHER

These infants are remarkable not only because like foetal versions of Shadrach, Meshach and Abednego, they emerge at least alive from within the fiery metabolic furnace of diabetes mellitus, but because they resemble one another so closely that they might well be related. They are plump, sleek, liberally coated with vernix caseosa, full-faced and plethoric. The umbilical cord and the placenta share in the gigantism. During their first 24 or more extrauterine hours they lie on their backs, bloated and flushed, their legs flexed and abducted, their lightly closed hands on each side of the head, the abdomen prominent and their respiration sighing. They convey a distinct impression of having had such a surfeit of both food and fluid pressed upon them by an insistent hostess that they desire only peace so that they may recover from their excesses. And on the second day their resentment of the slightest noise improves the analogy while their trembling anxiety seems to speak of intrauterine indiscretions of which we know nothing [1]

The infant of the diabetic mother (Fig. 4-1), so exquisitely described by Farquhar [1], has survived an unusual genetic and environmental ordeal. This description now applies to fewer and fewer newborn infants of both insulin-dependent and gestational diabetic mothers. Advances in understanding the intrauterine environment, the precise definition of metabolic control, the advantages of pro-

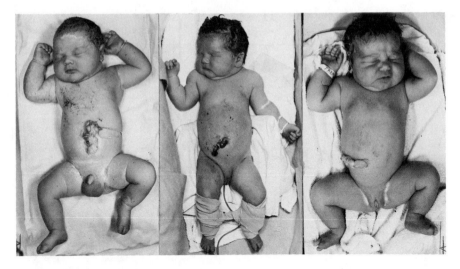

FIGURE 4-1. Unrelated infants of diabetic mothers observed by JW Farquhar. (From *Arch Dis Child*. 1959; 34:76, with the kind permission and cooperation of Dr. Farquhar.)

longed controlled hospitalization, and the recognition and treatment of gestational diabetics have reduced the number of oversized infants, as well as the frequency of perinatal and neonatal mortality and morbidity. The ability to conceive does not apparently differ between diabetic and nondiabetic women. Furthermore, the number of spontaneous abortions in well-controlled diabetic pregnant women does not differ from that in nondiabetic pregnant women [2]. Fetal wastage, neonatal mortality, and morbidity in these babies, although higher than those in nondiabetics, have steadily declined over the past six decades since the introduction of insulin [3–9].

The goals for reproduction in the diabetic are to abolish perinatal mortality and minimize neonatal morbidity. Additionally, normal growth, physical and psychological development, and normal behavioral and psychosocial adjustment should be attained. Ultimately, these aspirations will be fulfilled when sequencing of the human genome identifies the gene responsible for diabetes, so that techniques may be developed to eliminate this disorder. Since this is unlikely to occur in the near future, we must strive to prevent the problems that exist currently.

• The Mother and Her Disease

The analysis of the diverse problems presented by maternal diabetes has been difficult because of the complexity of the metabolic disturbances [10–12]. White [5,13] has suggested a classification based on severity of the disease which would permit comparison of data reported by different clinics.

Table 4-1 presents the classification, modified so as to include less manifest and more subtle forms of the derangement. Class A, which has received emphasis from Miller [14], Carrington [15], O'Sullivan [16], and Coustan [17], appears to represent a heterogenous group which can be subdivided into two groups, gestational diabetes and prior diabetes.

Gestational diabetes is defined as an abnormality of glucose tolerance (oral or intravenous) demonstrable during pregnancy, with reversion to normal within 6 weeks after delivery. This type of diabetes is common in women who are over 25 years of age and obese (over 200 pounds body weight). There is also a genetic predisposition, as evidenced by a strong family history of diabetes, a history of previous overweight infants (>4 kg or 9 lb), and/or of unexplained stillbirths beyond 28 weeks' gestation. O'Sullivan [18] analyzed the natural history of diabetes and noted that 56 percent of prediabetics had an abnormal oral test during the first observed pregnancy. Of 145 patients, 43 percent reverted to normal after delivery. In patients observed in a second pregnancy, the number with glucose intolerance increased. He cautioned, however, that "the individual patient may have nondiagnostic tests at any time in the course of progression to diabetes." Subsequently, the classification has been expanded to identify patients based on (1) the degree of fasting hyperglycemia (> or

---

TABLE 4-1. Revised White classification of diabetes and pregnancy

Gestational diabetes: Abnormal GTT, but euglycemia maintained by diet alone.
Diet alone insufficient, insulin required

Class A: Diet alone, any duration or onset age.
Class B: Onset age 20 years or older and duration less than 10 years.
Class C: Onset age 10–19 years or duration 10–19 years.
Class D: Onset age under 10 years, duration over 20 years, background retinopathy, or hypertension (not preeclampsia).
Class R: Proliferative retinopathy or vitreous hemorrhage.
Class F: Nephropathy with over 500 mg/day proteinuria.
Class RF: Criteria for both classes R and F coexist.
Class H: Arteriosclerotic heart disease clinically evident.
Class T: Prior renal transplantation.

All classes below A require insulin therapy. Classes R, F, RF, H, and T have no onset/duration criteria but usually occur in long-term diabetes. The development of a complication moves the patient to the lower class.

(From References 5–13.)

<110 mg/dl) [19] or (2) the plasma insulin response to glucose (insulinopenia versus hyperinsulinemia) [20]. In contrast, no differences were found in fasting plasma glucagon levels, human chorionic somatomammotropin (HCS), or chorionic gonadotropin concentrations, and in their responses to glucose in gestational diabetic and nondiabetic controls [21,22].

Originally, Priscilla White classified insulin-dependent diabetic pregnancies on the basis of age of onset, duration, severity, and complications. Subsequently, gestational diabetes was included, and more recently patients with renal transplants and ocular complications have been added (Table 4-1).

Pedersen independently classified diabetic pregnancies according to factors that were evident only during pregnancy and carried a poor prognosis (i.e., Prognostic Bad Signs in Pregnancy [PBSP]). Four were of major importance: (1) clinical pyelonephritis, (2) precoma or severe acidosis, (3) toxemia, and (4) "neglectors" (women who have not followed the recommended regimen) [3,22]. He observed that the presence of PBSP was associated with a greater mortality and was of better predictive value if combined with the classification of White. Recent studies have confirmed the earlier reports that the most important factor in assessing fetal outcome is control of maternal diabetes [6, 22–24]. While ketoacidosis and coma have a detrimental effect on the fetus, maternal hypoglycemia apparently does not have an important relationship to survival.

Cousins has summarized the reported studies of obstetric complications from 1965 to 1985 [25]. He has grouped subjects according to (1) gestational diabetes, (2) White's Classes B and C, and (3) White's Classes D, F, and R. The frequency of various problems is presented in Table 4-2. Of note, diabetic ketoacidosis occurred in 7 percent of Classes D, F, and R, but not in the gestational diabetics. In contrast, pregnancy-induced hypertension (toxemia) was found in 16 percent of Classes D, F, and R and in 10 percent of gestational diabetics. The data emphasize again that the gestational diabetic mother must be evaluated and managed separately from the insulin-dependent diabetic.

Importance of Prenatal Care

Control of Maternal Diabetes

Improvement in mortality rate has been attributed to a variety of factors, of which meticulous metabolic control and prenatal care by a medical team appear to be the most significant. Highly motivated pregnant diabetics can usually be managed at home with frequent

TABLE 4-2. Diabetic pregnancy data (1965–1985) analysis for independence of obstetrical complications and diabetic categories

	GESTATION	DIABETIC CATEGORIES				ALL DIABETICS	
		Classes B, C	Classes D, F, R	X^2	P	Number	%
Pregnancy-induced hypertension (%)	10.0	8.0	15.7	15.5	<0.005	2968	11.7
Chronic hypertension	9.9	8.0	16.9	7.7	<0.025	866	9.6
Total hypertension	14.6	14.5	30.9	43.7	<0.005	2205	18.0
Diabetic ketoacidosis	0	8.3	7.1	14.7	<0.005	1508	9.3
Pyelonephritis	4.0	2.2	4.9	3.4	N.S.	991	4.3
Hydramnios	5.3	17.6	18.6	12.9	<0.005	2024	15.7
Preterm labor	0	7.7	4.7	12.2	<0.005	833	9.5
Primary cesarean section	12.4	44.0	56.7	146.0	<0.005	2170	27.1
Repeat cesarean section	—	—	—	—	—	2170	14.3
Total cesarean section	20.4	41.9	58.3	127.0	<0.005	2170	41.5
Maternal mortality	—	—	—	—	—	2614	0.11

Adapted from Cousins. In: Reece, Coustan, eds. *Diabetes Mellitus in Pregnancy.* New York: Churchill Livingstone, 1988, with permission.

home blood glucose monitoring and appropriate diet and insulin therapy to attain normoglycemia. In or out of the hospital, primary attention is directed toward metabolic stability and homeostasis in the mother (and, hence, in the fetus), including good nutrition and the avoidance of ketoacidosis, glycosuria, and irregular or marked fluctuations in the blood glucose concentration. While hypoglycemia has not been directly correlated with fetal morbidity and mortality, its effect on fetal metabolism has not yet been adequately defined in humans. Fetal heart rate irregularities have been recorded in a high percentage of cases in which the mother had hypoglycemia [26]. Boddy and Dawes [27] have noted that in fetal sheep in utero hypoglycemia modifies intrauterine respiratory movement. Until further studies correlating hypoglycemia and its effects on the fetus are available, hypoglycemia should be prevented. In fact, profound hypoglycemia and excessive postprandial hyperglycemia (>130 mg/dl) should both be avoided. For several decades, the evidence has clearly indicated that meticulous diabetic control is associated with improved fetal outcome [9,23,24,28–30].

Gestational diabetes with obesity [31] poses additional dietary problems, since caloric restriction in such patients may result in ketosis secondary to starvation. Four or five small meals equally spaced may be necessary under these circumstances. Supplemental insulin therapy may also be necessary.

Although a few internists persist in recommending them, the use of oral hypoglycemic agents in moderate dosage [32,33] has been reported to result in severe neonatal hypoglycemia in some instances [34]. Seltzer [35] summarized the cases of 11 newborn infants of diabetic mothers who had been treated with oral hypoglycemic agents, resulting in the infants developing life-threatening hypoglycemia within hours of birth. Since these agents traverse the placenta and are metabolized slowly in the fetus and newborn [36], they are contraindicated in the control of diabetes during pregnancy [35].

Fetal Monitoring

Prior to the availability of fetal monitoring techniques, insulin-dependent diabetics (Classes B–F) were often delivered between 35 and 37 weeks' gestation, provided the fetus was of reasonable size. Delivery before 35 weeks was associated with an excessive neonatal mortality, while postponement of delivery until after 37 weeks resulted in a higher stillbirth rate. With the availability of newer monitoring techniques, it has become possible to determine the optimal time for delivery that provides the best chance for infant survival.

Techniques utilized to monitor fetal viability during pregnancy include:

1. Nonstress test,
2. Contraction stress test,
3. Fetal movement,
4. Biophysical profile (using real-time ultrasonography),
5. Hormonal levels in maternal plasma or serum, i.e., placental lactogen (HCS), human chorionic gonadotropin (HCG), and estriol,
6. Maternal urinary hormone excretion rates, i.e., estriol and progesterone, and
7. Maternal serum enzymes, i.e., heat-stable alkaline phosphatase and diamine oxidase.

Techniques now available to assess fetal maturity (especially as related to pulmonary function) include:

1. Examination of amniotic fluid by amniocentesis for
   a. Fat cells,
   b. Lecithin sphingomyelin ratios ("shake" or foam test), phosphatidyl glycerol,
   c. Creatinine, and
   d. Bilirubin, and
2. Ultrasound for fetal and placental size and positions.

Careful maternal fluid and insulin regulation as well as fetal electronic monitoring during labor and delivery are also important. The ideal requirements for monitoring and caring for the high-risk mother, fetus, and neonate demand the establishment of perinatal regional centers with cooperation among the obstetrician, internist, pediatrician, and clinical chemist, all of whom should have a special interest in the diabetic.

Delivery

Prior to the time of delivery (usually determined by the obstetrician, who notifies the internist and pediatrician), the patient may be hospitalized and brought to a stable normal metabolic state. Obstetricians disagree as to the relative advantages of elective cesarean section and vaginal delivery with elective pitocin induction. The timing of delivery is now individualized, based on the consideration of fetal well-being and maturity. Some obstetricians utilize the oxytocin challenge test to evaluate fetal response to the stress of labor. Others utilize physiologic monitoring techniques such as fetal heart rate, fetal size, and uterine contractions, and allow spontaneous labor at term.

In fact, physiologic monitoring of the fetus during labor is now recommended by some obstetricians as an important routine procedure for all diabetic deliveries.

Premature delivery of an immature fetus can be avoided by careful fetal assessment with amniocentesis for lung maturity [37]. Intravenous administration of fluids with glucose and regular insulin should be used to maintain a normoglycemic level and avoid ketosis throughout labor and delivery or during cesarean section. Light et al. [38] have emphasized that both volume and concentration, i.e., amount of glucose per unit of time, must be monitored carefully. Blood glucose and ketone (serum acetone) determinations should be made during this phase. Possible obstetric complications are premature rupture of the membranes, uterine inertia with prolonged labor and shoulder dystocia. Maternal and umbilical vein blood glucose determinations should be obtained at delivery for the future management of the infant. The umbilical blood sample should also be analyzed for hematocrit, bilirubin, calcium, and other electrolytes.

• Congenital Anomalies

As perinatal mortality and neonatal morbidity have improved, attention has focussed on early fetal loss and congenital anomalies. Introducing the measurement of glycosylated hemoglobin in pregnancy [39] directed attention toward glucose control as a factor in etiology. Glycated hemoglobin (the accepted biochemical term) has been measured in clinical laboratories by several techniques: cation resin exchange chromatography, thiobarbituric acid chemical method, isoelectric focussing, electrophoresis, and affinity column chromatography. Only the latter is specific for glucose adducts. Most clinical laboratories use one of the former and require control studies. The literature refers to Hb A_1 which includes all adducts (Hb A_{1a}, A_{1b}, as well as Hb A_{1c}) while Hb A_{1c} refers to the specific glucose adduct. It is not yet possible to establish a precise standard. Comparisons are best made by referring to standard deviation units above the mean. Glycohemoglobin reflects ambient blood glucose concentration over the previous 6–8 weeks and provides a measure of the integrated glucose control.

Leslie and Pyke first reported in 1978 on hemoglobin A_1 in a small sample of 25 pregnant diabetics [40]. Of interest, among the 5 neonates whose maternal Hb A_1 levels exceeded the range of normals, 3 had fatal congenital anomalies. Miller et al., in a retrospective study of 116 pregnant diabetic women whose first Hb A_{1c} was before 14 weeks' gestation, reported that 13 percent of the infants had major congenital anomalies [41], including 3 fatal cardiac defects and 3 fatal brain defects. The frequency of anomalies was 3.4 percent in those whose initial Hb A_{1c} was less than 8.5 percent, and 22.4 percent in those whose Hb A_{1c} was over 8.5 percent (normal Hb A_{1c} = 5.5 ± 0.5 percent). Ylinen et al. [42] found both major and minor fetal malformations in 12 percent of 142 insulin-dependent diabetic pregnancies. Before the sixteenth week of gestation, the mean initial Hb A_{1c} value was significantly higher in pregnancies complicated by fetal malformations compared to those without (9.5 ± 1.8 versus 8.0 ± 1.4 percent) ($p < 0.001$). These retrospective studies indicate that poorly controlled diabetes mellitus in early pregnancy may be associated with an increased risk of malformations and support the recommendation of strict control prior to conception.

Fuhrmann et al. [43,44] reported from East Germany one of the first prospective experiences with strict glucose control prior to conception. Of 57 infants born to 56 well-controlled mothers, only one infant had a fatal cardiac defect. Prepregnancy glucose control in 128 of 420 diabetic pregnant women (292 treated after 8 weeks of gestation) resulted in significant reduction in the rate of birth defects from 7.5 to 0.8 percent. Similar studies from California and Israel have confirmed these observations.

Recently, a multicenter, prospective, controlled, collaborative study (National Institute of Child Health and Human Development Diabetes in Early Pregnancy Study) enrolled 347 diabetic and 389 control women within 21 days of conception [45]. Additionally, 279 diabetic women were entered later. Major malformations were detected in 4.9 percent of the early-entry diabetic women, 2.1 percent of the controls, and 9.0 percent of the late-entry diabetic women. These differences were statistically significant. Contrary to the studies reported above, this study did not identify a correlation between hyperglycemia and glycosylated hemoglobin with malformation. Neither was hypoglycemia (glucose <50 mg/dl [<2.8 mM]) a significant factor. A detailed analysis of this study with Miller's (vide supra) emphasized differences in patient selection (93 percent of the present population fell in Miller's lower-risk group). Mills et al. [43] have emphasized several points: a normal glycosylated hemoglobin should not be taken as a guarantee that diabetes-associated anomalies are absent; conversely, an elevated level does not necessarily indicate an increased risk of anomalies. Neither frequent hyperglycemia nor hypoglycemia was useful in identifying the cause of the excess malformations in the offspring of the diabetic women. Because of the better outcomes seen in the diabetic women who entered early compared to late, they justifiably recommended that women and their physicians strive to attain stable, good diabetic control in the periconceptional period and throughout pregnancy.

The critical period for optimal control depends upon knowledge of embryologic development. Mills and associates found that the significantly more common malformations in infants of diabetic mothers occur before the seventh week of gestation [46]. While virtually every system may be affected during this critical period, there have been reports of the increased frequency of skeletal (sacral agenesis) and cardiac (great vessel) anomalies.

Pathogenesis

The increased incidence of congenital anomalies in infants of diabetic pregnancies has resulted in extensive studies in animals in vivo after spontaneous diabetes or the induction of diabetes with beta cytotropic agents as well as with organ or embryo culture (in vitro). These have been recently reviewed by Pinter and Reece [47], Eriksson [48], and Freinkel [49]. The individual organ systems affected are so diverse that virtually any organ appears to be vulnerable during an appropriately critical stage of development. Pinter and Reece [47] have emphasized that the yolk sac plays an integral role. Freinkel [49] has concluded that the causes of anomalous embryo development in pregnancy of diabetic rodents are multifactorial, including all the aberrant fuels and fuel-mediated components of "the diabetic state" (e.g., high glucose, ketones, somatomedin inhibitor[s], osmolality, etc.). Those tested to date display dysmorphogenic potential ("fuel mediated organ teratogenesis").

Based on animal studies, Freinkel [49] has urged caution in the clinical management of diabetic women pre- and postconception (Fig. 4-2). Because both hypoglycemia and hyperglycemia may be associated with abnormalities in the experimental model, he suggests a goal aimed at avoiding both extremes. Prospective controlled clinical studies of large numbers of subjects will be necessary to resolve this important question.

• Hypoxemia

Hypoxemia has been one of the vexing problems in diabetic pregnancy since it has been implicated in the high rates of unexplained stillbirths, extramedullary hematopoiesis, polycythemia, hyperbilirubinemia, and renal vein thrombosis. In 1959, Gellis and Hsia reported a 7.6 percent stillbirth rate in 768 pregnancies over 28 weeks' gestation [50]. In other series, fetal mortality was as high as 25 percent [28]. The increase in extramedullary hematopoiesis was noted over 40 years ago by Miller [51].

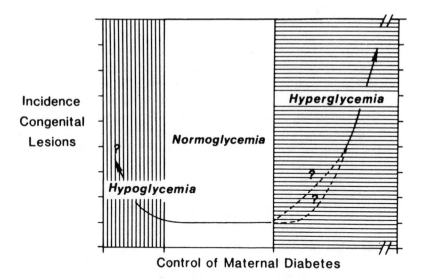

FIGURE 4-2. Therapeutic dilemma in treatment with insulin during early human pregnancy. In the rodent embryo, "hypoglycemia" during the period of glycolytic dependence has been shown to have teratogenic potential. It is not known whether similar vulnerabilities and/or glycolytic dependencies obtained in human embryogenesis during the corresponding developmental interval (i.e., ~ day 16–18 to day 24–25 of gestation). Moreover, in rodents as in humans, the teratogenic thresholds for the multiple dysmorphogenic components of the "diabetic state" (generically designated as "hyperglycemia" here) have not been ascertained. Thus, for the moment, definitive recommendations concerning the intensity of insulin therapy during the first 4–5 weeks of pregnancy cannot be made. However, until more information becomes available, approaches to insulin therapy during the first 4 weeks of pregnancy must be tempered by the recognition that overtreatment as well as undertreatment could be potentially dysmorphogenic at that point in time. (Reproduced from an elegant review by the late Norbert Freinkel who made major contributions to our understanding of the clinicopathological consequences of diabetes in pregnancy. *Horm Metab Res.* 1988; 20:472, with permission.)

In 1965, Naeye noted that overweight infants had liver weights that were 179 percent of controls [52]. Although this was due to an increase in hepatocyte cytoplasm, there was also a threefold increase in hematopoietic tissue compared to controls. Most of these hematopoietic cells were erythroid precursors. Using the quantitative technique of point counting of histologic sections of liver, Singer reported 3 of 4 infants of diabetic mothers (IDMs) over 40 weeks' gestation had clearly increased hematopoiesis [53].

Neonatal polycythemia has been prospectively evaluated by Mimouni et al. [54] in 34 pairs of IDMs and controls carefully matched for 6 variables, including site of sampling, time of sampling, time of cord clamping, gestational age, mode of delivery, and Apgar scores. Polycythemia was defined as a venous hematocrit equal to or greater than 65 percent. The incidence of polycythemia in IDMs was significantly greater than that in controls (29.4 versus 5.9 percent) ($p <$ 0.03). Nucleated red blood cell counts were also significantly elevated in the IDMs. Polycythemia did not correlate with maternal hemoglobin A_{1c} or with increased infant weight percentiles. There was a correlation with neonatal hypoglycemia, but no measurements of fetal insulin secretion were made.

The first definitive experimental studies of fetal hypoxemia induced by chronic hyperinsulinemia were made with serendipity by Carson et al. [55]. Studies of the metabolic effects of infusions of insulin to chronically catheterized fetal sheep resulted in an unexpected outcome: the development of fetal hypoxia in animals infused for 2–4 days but not 2–4 hours. This was associated with a significant decrease in plasma glucose concentration and increase in the molar ratio of glucose to oxygen. These events were reversible, and cessation of insulin infusion resulted in restoration to normal of plasma glucose, glucose-to-oxygen quotient, and blood oxygen content. The mechanisms responsible for these changes were not clarified. Theoretically, these could have been due to limitation of utero-placental-fetal oxygen transfer; alternatively, there could have been enhanced fetal tissue oxygen uptake, or some combination.

Milley et al. [56] confirmed these observations at plasma insulin levels one to two magnitudes lower than those reported by Carson and without changes in plasma glucose concentration. Using microsphere techniques to measure blood flow and cardiac output, they found a decrease in umbilical blood flow as well as in umbilical venous oxygen content. The fall in umbilical blood flow was due to a change in the distribution of cardiac output with a decrease in placental perfusion and an increase to the fetal carcass. Fetal oxygen consumption increased, resulting in fetal arterial hypoxemia. Using a fed sheep model, Milley et al. [57] observed an increased uptake of oxygen, glucose and alpha amino-nitrogen containing substances (amino acids).

In a parallel series of studies, Philipps et al. [58,59] evaluated the effects of continuous hyperglycemia in the chronically catheterized fetal sheep. Plasma glucose levels were elevated twofold. Plasma insulin levels rose; however, responses in individual animals were variable. Whole blood oxygen content of the distal aorta fell consistently by 33 percent of basal values. Since umbilical blood flow and fetal oxygen delivery remained constant, oxygen consumption rose after three days of hyperglycemia. Philipps et al. [60,61] suggested that defined fetal glucose infusions induced stimulation of oxidative metabolism but had little effect upon placental oxygen consumption.

In the human, Widness et al. [62] assessed fetal hypoxemia indirectly by measurement of fetal plasma erythropoietin (Ep) concentration. This hormone is synthesized and released in response to hypoxemia in the kidney in the adult and in both liver and kidney in the fetus. The only known stimulus is hypoxemia. The hormone is not stored, and approximately 4–6 hours of stimulation are necessary before elevations of the plasma level occur. The half-life of plasma erythropoietin is about 7–10 hours, and a small but significant fraction, 2–9 percent, is excreted in urine in adult animals over 1–2 days.

Umbilical plasma erythropoietin concentrations were elevated at delivery in 22 of 61 diabetic pregnancies, exceeding the range of 28 controls. Several infants had values three magnitudes above the controls (30,000 versus 30 mU/ml), levels as high as any reported in man. In a subset of subjects, blood elements, plasma glucose, and insulin concentrations were measured in free-flowing umbilical blood. While a significant direct relationship occurred between umbilical plasma insulin and plasma erythropoietin, there was no correlation between umbilical plasma glucose and erythropoietin. No relationships among plasma erythropoietin and red blood cell count, nucleated red blood cells, or reticulocyte counts were found.

In a chronically hyperinsulinemic rhesus fetus model [62], hyperinsulinemia in the absence of hyperglycemia was also associated with significant elevation of plasma erythropoietin levels. In addition, hepatic extramedullary hematopoiesis was affected minimally, but umbilical blood reticulocytes were elevated significantly ($p < 0.007$). This suggested that chronic hyperinsulinemia was associated with fetal hypoxemia.

Using the chronically catheterized fetal sheep, Philipps et al. [63] reported that raised plasma glucose concentrations for 3–11 days were associated with a fall in blood oxygen content and a significant rise in plasma erythropoietin. They concluded that the glucose-induced hypoxemia was responsible for the increase in plasma erythropoietin. The cellular mechanism(s) responsible for the glucose-induced fetal hypoxemia remains to be defined.

In additional human observations, Teramo et al. [64] in Helsinki studied prospectively 25 control and 49 insulin-treated diabetic subjects. There was a direct relationship between amniotic fluid erythropoietin (Ep) and umbilical plasma erythropoietin concentrations, although the erythropoietin concentrations in amniotic fluid were consistently on the average 38 percent lower than those in plasma.

The Ep values in diabetic pregnancies were significantly elevated compared to controls (Fig. 4-3). Because Teramo followed hemoglobin A_{1c} biweekly over the 5-month interval prior to delivery, Widness et al. [65] were able to correlate umbilical plasma and amniotic fluid erythropoietin with maternal Hb A_{1c} determined during the final month of pregnancy ($r = 0.64$, $r = 0.58$, $p < .0001$, respectively). Using forced stepwise multiple regression analysis, additional statistically

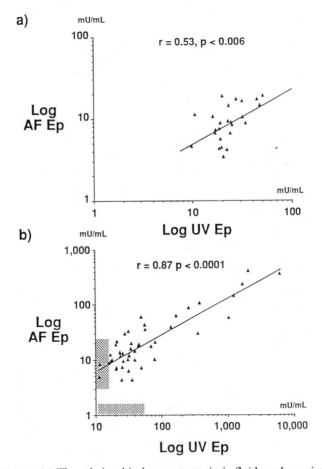

FIGURE 4-3. (a) The relationship between amniotic fluid erythropoietin and umbilical plasma erythropoietin concentrations (log transformed) obtained at elective cesarean section from nondiabetic pregnancies. (b) Similar data obtained from diabetic pregnancies. The shaded areas indicate the normal range for each parameter. Note the scale difference from Figure 4.3a. (Modified from Teramo and Widness. *Obstet Gynecol.* 1987; 69:710, with permission.)

significant contributing factors included umbilical plasma glucose and insulin concentrations but not umbilical plasma C-peptide.

It is clear that hypoxemia may be a significant risk for the fetus of a diabetic pregnancy. Since both fetal hyperglycemia and hyperinsulinemia have been associated with fetal hypoxemia, meticulous metabolic control of the diabetes during pregnancy should reduce the morbidities due to this problem. The hypoxemia appears to be due to increased fetal oxygen consumption in the presence of constant fetal blood flow, which is associated with an increased uptake, primarily of glucose, although amino acids may be involved.

• Polycythemia

Recent studies from Cincinnati [66] indicate a continued significant incidence of polycythemia (hematocrit >65 at 2 hours) in infants of diabetic mothers compared to controls (29.4 versus 5.9 percent). As noted above, the major factor responsible for polycythemia is in utero hypoxemia. Oh [67] has proposed a mechanism for neonatal polycythemia that includes the acute expansion of blood volume due to a placental transfusion occurring either in utero as a result of acute asphyxia or at birth. He has related polycythemia and hyperviscosity to symptoms that include: the central nervous system (jitteriness, irritability), respiratory system (respiratory distress), gastrointestinal system (feeding intolerance), genitourinary system (oliguria), hematologic system (hyperbilirubinemia), and metabolism (hypoglycemia).

Black [68] followed up infants of diabetic mothers at 2 years. She noted less satisfactory motor and neurologic signs than among control children. Importantly, no significant differences were observed between the polycythemic infants and the polycythemic IDMs, although the results showed a consistently greater incidence of problems for the IDMs.

There are inadequate data regarding therapeutic intervention. Thus, no specific recommendation is warranted regarding partial exchange transfusion or partial exchange with fresh frozen plasma. As yet, there is no clear benefit reported from these treatment modalities.

• Bilirubin Metabolism

Hyperbilirubinemia occurs more commonly in infants of diabetic mothers than in controls of comparable weight or gestation [69–71]. Taylor et al. [71] reported that the serum bilirubin values in umbilical cord blood from infants of diabetic mothers were similar to values from controls, but significant differences in bilirubin concentrations between the groups were apparent at 48 hours of age. The 48-hour value for serum bilirubin did not correlate with the value for umbilical cord blood, with the degree of hepatomegaly or splenomegaly, or with the presence of edema. Although the number of nucleated red blood cells was initially high, a sharp drop was found on the second and third day of life. Hematologic studies did not suggest an explanation of the mechanism for this phenomenon. In particular, there was no evidence for increased hemolysis. Olsen et al. [70] drew similar conclusions from 94 surviving infants. Vaginal delivery was associated with a higher incidence of serum bilirubin, above 20 mg/100 ml, than was cesarean section. It was known that complicated vaginal delivery predisposes to hyperbilirubinemia. It is noteworthy that kernicterus apparently is a rare complication of hyperbilirubinemia in these infants even though hypoglycemia, asphyxia, and anoxia are often present and have been considered predisposing factors.

Stevenson et al. [72] have carried out extensive studies of bilirubin metabolism utilizing carbon monoxide excretion (a specific marker for heme catabolism). They reported that bilirubin production is significantly increased in infants of diabetic mothers. They also noted that polycythemic IDMs have a serum bilirubin concentration greater than 10 mg/dl more often than do nonpolycythemic IDMs. Erythropoietin production has been related to macrosomia, polycythemia, and hyperbilirubinemia. While the dynamic set of interacting factors has not yet been established, Stevenson has suggested that ineffective erythropoiesis may be one.

• Renal Vein Thrombosis

Maternal diabetes was first recognized as a predisposing factor to renal vein thrombosis in the infant reported by Avery, Oppenheimer, and Gordon in 1957 [73]. Since then Takeuchi and Benirschke [74] have reported a series of 16 cases, 5 from mothers with diabetes, 7 from prediabetics (presumptive), and 4 from women with unproved diabetic status. The incidence in infants born to diabetic mothers is unknown. However, Francois et al. [75] found 4 of 168 with this complication. The presence of a mass in the flank or abdomen associated with proteinuria and hematuria suggests the diagnosis. Unilateral thrombosis may be treated conservatively or by nephrectomy [76]. The pathogenesis of this complication is speculative at best; polycythemia and local stasis of blood in renal veins, which are possibly secondary to an osmotic diuresis due to hyperglycemia, have been suggested by most authors. This is inadequate to explain the occurrence of thrombosis in infants born to mothers with prediabetes. The mechanism remains obscure. Transient hematuria of unknown origin has also been noted in IDMs and infants of mothers with gestational diabetes (IGDMs) [77].

• Size, Weight, and Water

In addition to their obese, plethoric, and cushingoid appearance, infants from poorly controlled diabetic mothers often have visceromegaly involving the heart, liver, and spleen and hypertrophy of the umbilical cord. Not only are they overweight for gestational age, they have increased length as well. In contrast, the size of the brain and kidneys is unaffected [52]. At 260 days of gestation, the infant of the diabetic mother may be comparable to a normal infant at term with respect to weight and length. Careful obstetric-medical management tends to minimize the excess weight gain. It must be noted, however, that the small-for-gestational age infant is at a greater risk than the larger obese infant.

These infants formerly were thought to be edematous at birth; however, pitting is not noted until after the first day of life. The data indicate that the excessive body weight results from increased body fat, rather than fluid [78–80]. When starved and deprived of water during the initial days after delivery, they lose more weight over a longer period than do normal infants [81]. In the first 48 hours, urine volumes are larger than those from more mature infants of nondiabetic mothers. Renal sodium excretion is also higher when compared with infants of similar weight born to nondiabetic mothers [82]; however, when compared with normal infants of comparable gestation, this difference is insignificant [83]. Early feeding minimizes the weight loss and abolishes the difference when compared with nondiabetic controls [81].

Macrosomia has been one of the hallmarks of the diabetic fetopathy since its recognition over 150 years ago. Although results have been highly variable, macrosomia continues to be a significant problem. Its frequency continues to fluctuate between a minimum of 25 percent [84] to as many as 38 percent [Stys and Tsang, personal communication; 85] of all infants of diabetic mothers.

Evidence has accumulated in the last 50 years to support the original Pedersen hypothesis [28] that many of the pathophysiologic events found in the IDM may be attributed to fetal hyperinsulinemia secondary to inadequate maternal metabolic control. In a recent study in Helsinki [84], a relationship was found between umbilical vein (UV) plasma C-peptide concentration (expressed as log number, LN) and highest maternal hemoglobin A_{1c} (percent) in the third trimester ($r = 0.508$, $p < 0.001$). When body weight in SD units was evaluated relative to LN UV C-peptide for both control infants and IDMs, a positive relationship ($r = 0.547$, $p < 0.0001$) was found (Fig. 4-4). Similar clinical observations have been reported by others [86]. No relationship was found between birth weight and maternal Hb A_{1c}.

C-peptide is the product of posttranslational proteolytic cleavage of dibasic amino acids at position 31,32 and 64,65. It is released into the portal circulation in equimolar quantities with insulin. Since insulin is significantly removed by the liver, C-peptide, which is physiologically inert, has served as an indirect means of assessing insulin secretion. Since insulin assays in umbilical plasma from infants whose mothers have insulin antibodies are difficult to interpret, C-peptide measurements are of value here, as well.

While previous studies have assumed that C-peptide like insulin

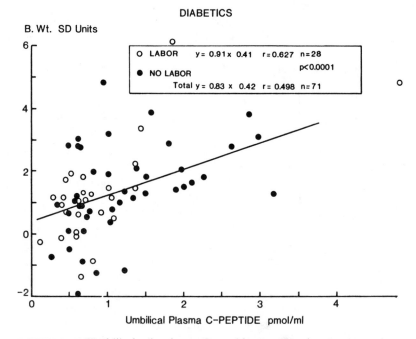

FIGURE 4-4. Umbilical vein plasma C-peptide concentration was natural log transposed because there was not a normal distribution. Birth weight was expressed as standard deviation units compared to a very large contemporary population in Helsinki, Finland. The diabetic and control subjects were studied by Teramo at the Women's Hospital, University of Helsinki. (From Schwartz and Teramo, in Gabbe and Oh (eds.): *Infant of the Diabetic Mother, Report of the 93rd Ross Conference on Pediatric Research.* Columbus, Ohio: Ross Laboratories, 1987, p 40.)

does not cross the placenta, Gruppuso et al. [87] have examined this question by administering ^{125}I-proinsulin or ^{125}I-tyrosylated C-peptide by infusion to normal pregnant rhesus monkeys near term. No transfer of ^{125}I-proinsulin from mother to fetus was found. They concluded that proinsulin, like insulin, does not traverse the placenta. Immunoreactive fragments of C-peptide do cross (Fig. 4-5), because alter-

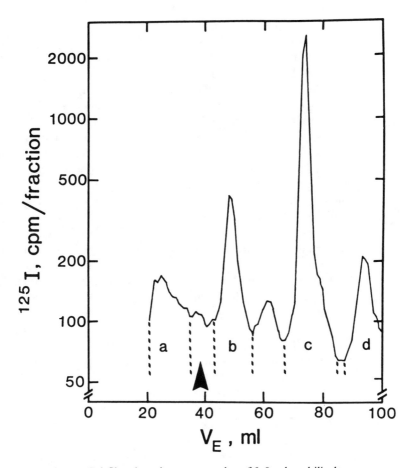

FIGURE 4-5. Gel filtration chromatography of 1.0 ml umbilical venous plasma from a fetal rhesus whose mother received ^{125}I-tyrosylated C-peptide. Immunoprecipitation was carried out on 4 to 6 peak tubes from peaks a–d. The limits used to determine the percentage of total radioactivity per peak are shown by the broken lines. The position at which ^{125}I-tyr-CP elutes is marked by the arrow. (Reproduced from the *Journal of Clinical Investigation.* 1987; 80:1132, by copyright permission of the American Society for Clinical Investigation.)

ations in the metabolism of ^{125}I-tyrosylated C-peptide occur in the placenta.

One may conclude that macrosomia is related in large measure, if not completely, to fetal hyperinsulinism. Fetal hyperglycemia may not be the sole etiologic stimulus for the endogenous fetal hyperinsulinemia. In insulin-treated mothers, maternal antibody may transport insulin to the fetus as well [88]. In a recent study, Menon et al. [89] related macrosomia to maternal antianimal insulin antibodies in cord blood. The mechanism(s) present in human insulin-treated pregnant women was not addressed. Whereas amino acids, especially those that are insulinogenic [90,91], may have a role, this has not been firmly established in the fetus/infant of the diabetic mother.

Insulin is the major anabolic hormone of the fetus, and its role has been evaluated directly over the last 10 years in the normal, third-trimester rhesus monkey [92]. Direct administration of insulin subcutaneously for $2\frac{1}{2}$–3 weeks produced substrate changes including decreased umbilical arterial plasma glucose concentration and plasma total amino acid concentration, but unaltered plasma free fatty acids and 3-hydroxybutyrate. Macrosomia has been a consistent observation at two different insulin doses, providing a physiologic and supraphysiologic level (Fig. 4-6).

A comparison of organ sizes at both insulin doses indicates that macrosomia and cardiomegaly are consistent findings, while enlarged liver, spleen, and placenta only occur at supraphysiologic insulin doses.

Insulinlike growth factor I (IGF-I) (also known as somatomedin-C (SM-C)) and insulinlike growth factor II (IGF-II), because of their structural homology with proinsulin, have received recent attention in the pathogenesis of macrosomia. Inconsistent changes in umbilical plasma IGF-I or -II have been found in IDMs [93]. In the rhesus studies, plasma total somatomedin peptide content was similar in hyperinsulinemic and control fetuses [93].

D'Ercole [94] has recently summarized the data with reference to IGFs and macrosomia in offspring of diabetic mothers. He noted that SM-C/IGF-I concentrations in cord blood from normal infants correlate with birth size. However, SM/IGF concentrations are elevated in some but not all overgrown IDMs. Using a variety of animal models (rabbits, monkeys, pigs, and sheep), the results of IGF measurements have not clearly defined a role in the pathogenesis of macrosomia. The serum SM-C/IGF-I concentrations, however, may not reflect tissue levels, which presumably are the relevant physiologic measure, and the actions of SM-C/IGF-I inhibitors have not been clarified. D'Ercole has concluded that it seems likely that the action of insulin on the synthesis of SM/IGFs is a consequence of the altered metabolic milieu and nutritional status, rather than a direct action. Although

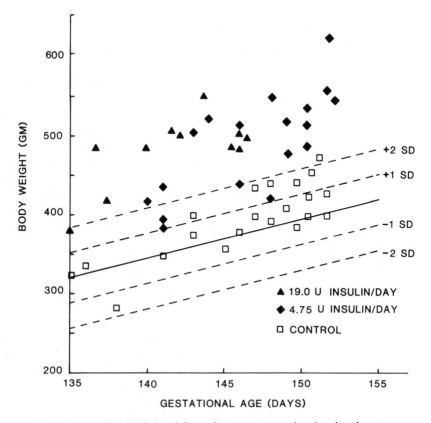

FIGURE 4-6. Body weight at delivery by cesarean section is related to gestational age for rhesus monkeys. The normative data is taken from Cheek and Hill. Controls were implanted with osmotic pumps with vehicle only, while experimentals received sodium insulin in the doses indicated. All animals were delivered by cesarean section. (JB Susa kindly provided these summary data which were previously presented in part in *Diabetes* 1979 28:1058; and the *93rd Ross Conference on Pediatric Research,* 1987 [84].)

speculative, he considers it likely that SM/IGF-I plays some role in the overgrowth of the fetus of the diabetic pregnancy.

Gruppuso et al. [95] also considered the possibility that elevated proinsulin in the fetus of the diabetic mother may act via insulinlike growth factor receptors I and II. The relative activities of IGF-I, insulin, and proinsulin were compared in IGF-I radioreceptor assays using term human placental membranes. Insulin was approximately 0.5 percent as potent as IGF-I, and proinsulin was only 2 percent as potent as insulin or 0.01 percent as potent as IGF-I. They concluded that the binding of proinsulin to IGF-I receptors is not of physiologic significance.

• Respiratory Distress

One of the most serious neonatal complications is respiratory distress. Robert and associates [96] have surveyed 815 diabetic pregnancies from the Joslin Clinic population compared to 10,152 infants of nondiabetic mothers and confirmed the increased risk to these newborns of respiratory distress syndrome (RDS). This study demonstrated an increased risk of RDS in IDMs, irrespective of the gestational age or mode of delivery. Respiratory distress may be due to pulmonary edema, transient tachypnea, or hyaline membrane disease or related to intracranial anomalies or hemorrhage, cardiac failure or aspiration. Pneumothorax or diaphragmatic hernia must also be considered in the differential diagnosis. In addition to a careful physical examination, roentgen and ultrasound studies are necessary to clarify the diagnosis.

Smith et al. [97] have studied lecithin synthesis and cellular growth in monolayer cell cultures from late gestation rabbit fetal lungs. Cortisol enhanced lecithin synthesis and reduced cellular growth. The addition of insulin abolished the stimulatory effect of cortisol on lecithin synthesis but did not affect its growth-inhibiting activity. These observations may provide an important basis for understanding the pathogenesis of the increased frequency of respiratory distress syndrome observed in infants of diabetic mothers.

Chemical analysis of lung fluids has been difficult, because they contain diverse classes of substances consisting of phospholipids and proteins. Both classes are heterogeneous in composition. The biochemistry of the first class, i.e., phospholipids has been defined in detail. The specific enzymes necessary for synthesis and factors that modulate these have been characterized. The effects of corticoids, thyroxine, and catecholamines have been described. As noted below, these events have been critical to understanding the clinical role of phospholipids in surfactant production.

In 1972, King and Clements [98] isolated several fractions, one of which turned out to be a surfactant-associated glycoprotein of molecular weight 30–40,000 daltons which was specific for lung fluid. This apoprotein known as SAP 35 is synthesized from an $M_r = 26,000$ dalton polypeptide precursor which is posttranslationally modified by proteolytic cleavage of a leader sequence and the addition of complex carbohydrate [99]. Smaller molecular weight apoproteins of $M_r = 6,000$, known as SAP 6, have recently been characterized by Whitsett et al. [100]. Both Glasser et al. [101] and Hawgood et al. [102] have identified cDNAs that encode specific apoproteins of lung surfactant. Reconstitution of small molecular weight surfactant proteins with synthetic phospholipids imparts virtually complete surfactantlike properties to the mixture, including rapid surface absorption and surface tension lowering during dynamic compression.

A variety of techniques were found to induce surfactant. The classical studies were made by Liggins [103] in New Zealand. He astutely noted that foetal lambs delivered prematurely after glucocorticoid administration had more mature, partially aerated lungs. Controlled clinical trials by Liggins and Howie [104] then verified that betamethasone administered preterm to the mother could prevent respiratory distress syndrome in premature infants. Notably, infants of diabetic mothers do not respond as well as those of nondiabetic mothers.

A major advance in the diagnosis and management of respiratory distress syndrome was made by Gluck and Kulovich [105] who recognized that lecithin-to-sphingomyelin (L/S) ratios in amniotic fluid were predictive of lung maturation. They noted, however, that diabetics from White's Classes A, B, C (often associated with macrosomia and large placentas) had a significant delay in the appearance of a mature L/S ratio of 2.0 or greater. In contrast, Classes D–F were associated with an accelerated mature ratio. An additional index for predictability of amniotic fluid phospholipids was provided by Hallman et al. [106] who showed that phosphatidylglycerol provided an important indicator of pulmonary maturation. The L/S ratio false mature value in diabetic pregnancies is minimized by analysis of phosphatidylglycerol. Studies in 88 diabetic pregnancies and 65 controls by Hallman and Teramo [107] showed that there were no differences in L/S ratios based on gestational ages. In diabetic pregnancies, phosphatidylglycerol may be absent or low even if the L/S ratio is >2. Respiratory distress syndrome coincided with an L/S ratio of between 2.0 and 3.0 only when phosphatidylglycerol was absent. They concluded that the fetus of the diabetic pregnancy can be safely delivered free of respiratory distress syndrome after phosphatidylglycerol appears, but in its absence RDS may complicate the neonatal course even if the L/S ratio is ≥2. Thus, phosphatidylglycerol may be another important biochemical marker of RDS.

Warburton [108] has studied the effects of chronic hyperglycemia on the flux of surface active material in intratracheal fluid of chronically catheterized fetal lambs at 112–145 days gestation. A mild elevation of serum glucose was associated with an increase in serum insulin and no changes of blood gases or hematocrit. Whereas surface active material began to appear by 123 days' gestation and was present in all controls by 129 days, it did not appear at all in 4 hyperglycemic fetuses at 145 days gestation. In contrast to the controls, there was no rise in tracheal fluid phospholipid content, mixed lecithin content, or disaturated phosphatidyl-choline content. In a later series, cortisol [109] resulted in a 4.8-fold increase in surface active material in tracheal fluid from the controls, but no change in that from glucose-infused animals. These observations have obvious implications regarding management of the diabetic pregnancy and subsequent risk for respiratory distress syndrome.

The above technologies, combined with improved obstetrical and neonatal management, have resulted in an astounding decrease in the incidence of this once-common and overwhelming problem. The occurrence of respiratory distress syndrome in the same institution (Boston Hospital for Women) from 1940 to 1977 decreased dramatically tenfold from 31 to 3 percent.

In the past decade, attention has turned to early treatment of respiratory distress syndrome with surfactantlike materials. Studies in progress include: (1) human surfactant isolated from amniotic fluid, (2) calf lung washing isolates, and (3) synthetic or semisynthetic surfactant. While the lipid components are well characterized, the protein components remain to be finally defined.

From the above, it is evident that no single event has been responsible for the marked improvement in neonatal outcome relative to respiratory distress syndrome. Thus precise quantitative scientific discoveries have been combined with clinical judgment in altering modes of practice to produce the excellent prognosis that exists currently for infants of metabolically well-controlled diabetic mothers.

• Carbohydrate Metabolism

Following delivery, glucose concentrations in offspring of diabetic mothers may decline rapidly to values below those observed in normals. Whereas previously approximately 60 percent of babies from insulin-dependent mothers had glucose concentrations below 30 mg/dl [1.7mM] in the first 6 hours of life [110,111], as compared to a frequency of approximately 15 percent in IGDMs, more recent studies indicate frequencies of less than half of these [112,113]. These differences are mainly attributable to meticulous metabolic control of the mother during pregnancy and delivery. Even so, Landon et al. [114] report an incidence of 19 percent hypoglycemia in infants whose mothers were well controlled.

Observations by McCann et al. [115] and Chen et al. [116] have indicated that infants of diabetic mothers may be subdivided into those from mothers with gestational diabetes and those born of mothers with insulin-dependent diabetes. The infants from mothers with gestational diabetes had, on the average, lower blood sugars and free fatty acids (FFA) at 2 hours of age than did normal infants; however, the values were higher than those found in infants of insulin-dependent mothers. Furthermore, the rate of fall in blood sugar immediately after delivery was slowest in the normal infants, intermediate in the infants of mothers with gestational diabetes, and most rapid in those of insulin-dependent diabetics (Fig. 4-7). Note that these two populations did not receive what would be considered meticulous diabetic management today so that these values represent changes that would occur in the absence of ideal control.

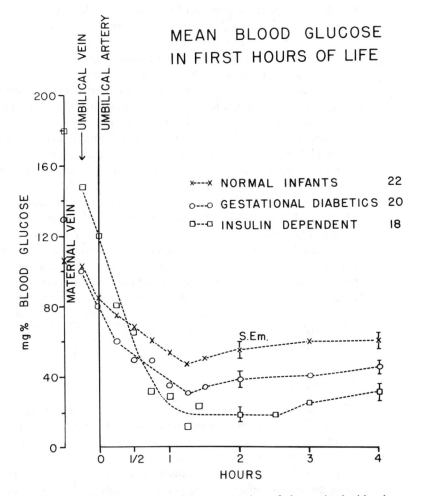

FIGURE 4-7. Serial changes in the concentration of glucose in the blood of infants immediately following delivery. The group from mothers with gestational diabetes had abnormal intravenous glucose tolerance tests during pregnancy but received no insulin therapy. Note initially elevated levels in the mothers. (Adapted from McCann et al., *N Engl J Med.* 1966; 275:1, with permission.)

The initial rate of fall in glucose concentration varied directly with the concentration in maternal blood at the time of delivery, with higher levels resulting in an initial precipitous decline. Light et al. [38] showed in a study of 18 infants of diabetic mothers that the cord blood glucose level was related to the rate of glucose infusion to the mother during delivery, the route of delivery, and the severity of the maternal diabetes. They found that the higher the cord blood glucose level, the more rapid the disappearance of glucose, the lower the level to which the glucose concentration falls, and the greater the prevalence of hypoglycemia during the first hours of life. In many infants, blood sugar rises spontaneously after 4 to 6 hours to values not unlike those found in infants of nondiabetics (see Chapter 2).

The course of changes in the blood sugar level in the hypoglycemic infants usually follows one of three patterns. The majority have a transient, asymptomatic phase soon after birth that lasts between 1 and 4 hours, following which a spontaneous rise occurs. Some have a prolonged initial phase of hypoglycemia (often severe, below 20 mg/dl [1.1 mM]), which may persist for several hours and be associated with symptoms. Others, after an apparently benign initial phase, develop symptomatic hypoglycemia after 12 to 14 hours or as late as 5 days of age [75]. Pennoyer and Hartmann [110] found that only 16 babies had symptoms among 38 with blood sugar values under 30 mg/dl (1.7 mM). Of these, only 5 did not have associated problems that could have contributed to the clinical manifestations. Therefore, clinical manifestations such as apnea, tachypnea, cyanosis, limpness, failure to suck, absent Moro reflex, listlessness, convulsions, and coma, which have been related to hypoglycemia alone, are uncommon in these infants (see Chapter 3). More often, these are secondary to other pathologic conditions associated with low blood glucose levels (see Chapter 3).

Treatment

When clinical manifestations and hypoglycemia coexist at any age, therapy directed at elevating the concentration of glucose in the blood should be initiated. A prompt response to therapy is evidence that hypoglycemia was indeed the cause of the signs and symptoms. However, if the hypoglycemia has been of long duration or if the symptoms are due to other causes, either a partial or delayed response to therapy may occur. During the first hours of life, glucagon in high dosage (300 μg/kg IV or IM to a maximum of 1 mg total dose) can elevate the blood sugar level for 2 to 3 hours in most infants [111] (Fig. 4-8). Wu et al. [117] have minimized the fall in blood glucose in IDMs by the intravenous administration of 300 μg/kg glucagon

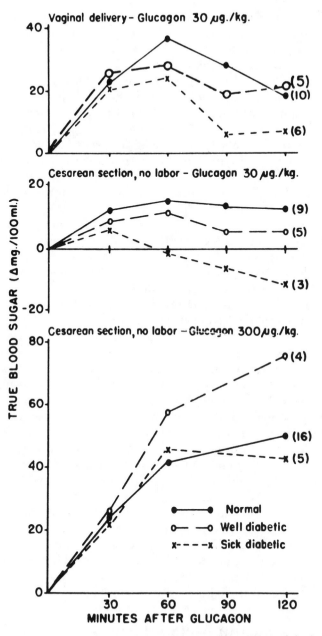

FIGURE 4-8. Relation of labor in the mother and condition of the infant to the concentration of blood sugar following small and large doses of glucagon. All infants were 2 hours of age or younger. Many infants had low blood glucose levels. (From Cornblath et al. Reproduced by permission of *Pediatrics.* 28:592, copyright 1961.)

within 15 minutes after delivery. Glucose administered intravenously is the treatment of choice in the symptomatic infant. Glucagon may be used initially even in the infant who is severely ill until an intravenous line is established.

King et al. [118] have demonstrated that hypoglycemic infants of diabetic mothers respond to low rates of glucose infusion (4–6 mg/kg/min) with a significant rise in plasma glucose concentration. However, symptomatic infants should be treated more vigorously, i.e., given a minibolus (0.25 gm/kg) to avoid insulin stimulation and to promptly raise the blood glucose concentration. This should be followed immediately by a continuous infusion increasing from 6 to 8 to 10 mg/kg/min as indicated. It is important to monitor blood sugar levels at 2–6 hour intervals to be sure that therapy is adequate to maintain blood glucose concentrations in a normal range.

As noted above, meticulous control of maternal glucose during labor and delivery will minimize the frequency of hypoglycemia in the neonate. Various regimens for controlling blood glucose in the infant have been recommended [119] but have not proven to have any advantage over intravenous glucose. Haworth et al. [120] found that a bolus injection of glucose produced marked variation in glucose levels from hyper- to hypoglycemia. Furthermore, epinephrine therapy was of no advantage and even produced serious lactic acidosis. Although two studies [119,121] have demonstrated that intravenous administration of a combination of glucose and fructose, or fructose alone, results in elevation of blood glucose concentration for 2 or more hours, this therapy is not recommended since its advantage over parenteral glucose is, at best, theoretical (less insulin stimulation). Newborns are known to have a transient intolerance to fructose [122] and, rarely, to have undiagnosed hereditary fructose intolerance.

The significance of hypoglycemia without symptoms remains unknown, but to our knowledge there are no convincing data of sequelae, unless the very low blood glucose persists for several days [75]. No specific recommendations for therapy for these asymptomatic infants other than early feeds as tolerated seem justified. However, in those infants with excessively low blood sugar values (under 20 mg/dl [1.1 mM] which persists for an hour or more), conservative management would consist of supporting the blood glucose level.

• Calcium Metabolism

In addition to the electrolyte and acid-base derangement associated with the respiratory distress syndrome, occasional sick infants have other alterations related to calcium metabolism. Hypocalcemia with tetany is now recognized as a significant complication in the infant of the diabetic mother [121, 123–126]. Chvostek's sign, carpopedal spasm, and Trousseau's sign are unreliable indicators of tetany in any newborn infant. Neuromuscular and behavioral alterations have been described, but many of the symptoms and signs are nonspecific and similar to those described for hypoglycemia and hypoxia. Hyperexcitability seems to be a common observation. Gittleman et al. [124] observed that 6 of 22 infants of diabetic mothers had serum calcium levels below 8.0 mg/dl which was considered abnormal on the first day of life. In another group of infants of prediabetic mothers, who had either gestational or noninsulin-dependent diabetes, 7 of 36 infants had similarly low levels. Since most of these infants were delivered preterm, their calcium levels should be compared with those of infants of like gestation and mode of delivery. Previously, Gittleman et al. [127] had shown that many low birth weight infants may have low serum calcium values without symptoms that are related to a variety of factors, e.g., complications of pregnancy, labor, or the immediate postnatal period. In infants delivered by elective cesarean section for cephalopelvic disproportion or for repeat cesarean section, hypocalcemia was noted in 14 percent. A similar incidence, 12 percent, was found for infants delivered by elective cesarean section in well-controlled diabetics. Tsang et al. [125] studied prospectively 28 infants of diabetic mothers with a comparable matched control group. The incidence of hypocalcemia was significantly increased in the infants of diabetic mothers, even when gestational age and perinatal complications were taken into consideration. It is of some interest that the low levels of calcium may persist, as in the two infants of diabetic mothers who were found to have idiopathic hypoparathyroidism [128].

Mimouni et al. [129] prospectively studied 98 infants of diabetic mothers (White's Classes B–RT). Glycemic control of the mothers was aimed at a preprandial blood glucose concentration below 100 mg/dl (5.6 mM) and a 90-minute concentration below 140 mg/dl (7.8 mM). Fifty-one percent (50 infants) had a nadir serum calcium concentration below 8 mg/dl. There was no statistically significant relationship between the lowest serum calcium concentration over the first 72 hours of life and advanced maternal White Class. Weak relationships were present with gestational age ($r = 0.37$, $p < 0.01$) and 1-minute Apgar score ($p = 0.05$). A correlation was found for the lowest serum magnesium concentration and the lowest serum calcium concentration ($r = 0.45$, $p < 0.0002$). There was also a correlation between the lowest serum calcium concentration and the cord calcium concentration ($r = 0.48$, $p < 0.001$). They developed a multiple regression equation which had an $R^2 = 0.37$.

In another study [130], this group evaluated serum magnesium, calcium, parathyroid hormone (PTH), and calcitriol (1,25 dihydroxy vitamin D) in diabetic and nondiabetic pregnant women in three periods from 8 to 38 weeks of gestation. The diabetics had significantly reduced serum magnesium concentrations throughout pregnancy. This was attributed to increased urinary magnesium excretion. Serum calcium and ionized calcium concentrations were not different except in the third trimester when significantly lower levels were found. Furthermore, there was an absence of the normal rise in serum calcitriol with advancing pregnancy. These calcium changes did not elicit a normal maternal parathyroid hormone response. They speculated that maternal hypomagnesemia leads to fetal hypomagnesemia, with subsequent fetal-neonatal impaired PTH secretion and action, resulting in neonatal hypocalcemia. The latter was supported by earlier studies by Tsang et al. [131] in which insignificant increases in serum PTH were found in serum of IDMs who became hypocalcemic postnatally. Amniotic fluid magnesium was significantly lower in the diabetic compared to nondiabetic pregnancy, further adding credence to the hypothesis [132].

One of the consequences of these mineral derangements is a decreased bone mineral content (BMC) in infants of diabetic mothers [133]. Infants of strictly controlled diabetic mothers had BMC similar to controls. The decreased BMC observed in infants of the less well controlled diabetic mothers does not seem to have a significant role in the pathogenesis of neonatal hypocalcemia.

A decrease in serum protein concentrations and calcium binding does not explain the hypocalcemia. Renal studies demonstrated no differences in excretion of calcium, magnesium, and phosphorus in infants of diabetic mothers compared to normal controls [125]. The response of the kidney to exogenous parathormone was normal, as shown by a decrease in calcium and an increase in phosphate excretion.

Although Bergman [121] verified the previously reported incidence of hypocalcemia in infants of diabetic mothers, he noted a significant decrease in ultrafilterable calcium. He also measured plasma parathyroid hormone values in four infants (IDMs); only one had an elevated level, while the others had low values. Calcitonin values in cord blood were in the same range as those of the adult; however, a significant rise occurred by 24 hours after birth in controls as well. In the IDMs, there was a negative correlation between total calcium and calcitonin. Bergman suggested a hypothesis relating hypoglycemia to glucagon secretion, which in turn stimulated calcitonin release. The latter inhibits mobilization of calcium from bone, thereby resulting in hypocalcemia. Unfortunately, this attractive hypothesis is not supported by the studies of Bloom and Johnston [134], who report diminished rather than increased glucagon levels in infants of diabetic mothers.

It has been proposed [135] that hyperinsulinism in IDMs is responsible for the increase in serum 1,25 $(OH)_2D$ observed both at birth and 72 hours postnatally. Thus, two mechanisms, hypomagnesemia and hyperinsulinemia, may be responsible for the complex mineral changes.

The diagnosis of symptomatic hypocalcemia depends upon obtaining a serum calcium and/or ionized calcium determination and must be differentiated from manifestations of central nervous system disease, hypoglycemia, hypoxia, and other metabolic and congenital abnormalities. An electrocardiogram may be helpful in the infant with hypocalcemia since prolongation of the QT interval may be present. Once the diagnosis of hypocalcemic tetany is suspected and blood obtained, intravenous calcium gluconate (5–10 ml as a 10 percent solution) should be given slowly but promptly, with electrocardiogram monitoring to avoid heart block. Thereafter, either calcium lactate, or gluconate in a total dosage of 1 to 2 gm calcium daily, may be given orally. Therapy may be continued by mouth for one week, with repeated determinations of serum calcium concentrations. Therapy should also include feedings of a low-solute milk with added calcium to provide a Ca:P ratio of 2–4:1 (g/g).

• Pathophysiology

The past decade has contributed significant advances in our understanding of the diverse pathophysiologic events occurring in utero and perinatally in the IDM. Recent data have shown interrelationships among hyperinsulinemia, hyperglycemia, hypoxemia, erythropoietin production, surfactant synthesis, and macrosomia, providing a basis for understanding much about the diverse morbidities in these infants. This information elaborates the fundamentally sound concept of the Pedersen hypothesis proposed in 1954 [136].

Previously, attention has been focused primarily on the beta cell hyperplasia and glucose homeostasis. Infants of diabetic mothers often have a rapid fall in the concentration of blood sugar in the period immediately following delivery [110,136,137] which differs from that observed in normal infants (Fig. 4-7) [115].

Hyperinsulinemia utilizing radioimmunoassay techniques has been reported in umbilical cord plasma from infants of mothers with gestational diabetes [138,139]. There is a broad range of values suggesting that this represents a heterogeneous population. In most instances, the elevated insulin level is appropriate for the degree of hyperglucosemia; however, in some cases, there is a dissociation with disproportionately elevated insulin levels [140].

Because of the transfer of maternal antibody to the fetus, radioimmunoassay of plasma from infants of insulin-treated mothers is difficult to interpret and may be unreliable unless maternal antibody is low. Kuhl [141,142] has evaluated this question carefully by analyzing free insulin. His data on nonantibody-bound insulin support the Pedersen hypothesis that hypoglycemia is secondary to fetal/neonatal hyperinsulinemia. Kalhan et al. [143] have shown that human insulin, labelled with iodine-I^{125} administered to either term normal women or diabetic women, does not cross the placenta to the fetus. Bauman and Yalow [88], however, did demonstrate specific transfer of human insulin with human antibody.

An indirect assessment of insulin secretion has been made by Block et al. [144], who observed elevated levels of C-peptide (the connecting segment of the proinsulin molecule) in umbilical plasma from infants of diabetic mothers. Bradley [145] has reported on fetal blood samples by cordocentesis from 20 diabetic pregnancies compared to 56 nondiabetic fetuses. Fetal plasma insulin and C-peptide levels were higher than normal in early pregnancy and rose to even higher levels as pregnancy advanced. Others have noted elevated C-peptide concentrations in amniotic fluid [64,65,86]. Gruppuso et al. have studied radiolabeled human C-peptide transfer from mother to fetus in the normal rhesus near term [87]. Up to 15 percent of C-peptide degradation products were found in fetal plasma due to placental metabolism (Fig. 4-5). These studies make quantitative interpretation of fetal plasma and amniotic fluid C-peptide concentrations difficult.

Elevated proinsulin accounted for a significant cross-reaction in the C-peptide assay in umbilical plasma from infants of diabetic mothers [144]. In a detailed study utilizing sepharose-bound insulin antibodies to remove proinsulin, Heding et al. [146] reported that up to 100 percent of immunoinsulin reactivity in umbilical plasma may be due to proinsulin, mainly bound to anti-insulin antibodies of maternal origin. Differences were also found in infants with high antibody levels. Using gel filtration techniques, Gruppuso et al. (personal communication, 1990) were unable to corroborate these findings. The significance of these observations requires further confirmation and clarification.

Insulin release is usually prompt and increased in infants of gestational diabetic mothers following a variety of stimuli, e.g., oral glucose, IV glucose load, and arginine (Figs. 4-9 and 4-10). This is less apparent with a continuous intravenous glucose infusion [119].

More recently, Kalhan et al. [147] found glucose turnover deter-

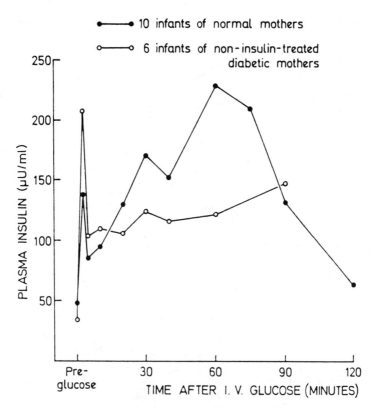

FIGURE 4-9. Mean plasma insulin levels following intravenous glucose (0.5 g/kg body weight). (From Isles, Dickson, Farquhar. *Pediatr Res.* 1968; 2:198, with permission.)

mined with glucose-1-^{13}C to be low in two IDMs (2.8 and 3.2 mg/kg/min) compared to four normals (4.42 ± 0.39, M ± SD) studied at 2 hours of age. They suggest that variable intrauterine hyperglycemia and hyperinsulinemia in the IDM inhibited hepatic glucose production immediately after birth. Cowett et al. [148] made similar observations using ^{13}C-U-glucose, which is a partially recycled tracer. Subsequently, King et al. [149] have evaluated glucose production in infants of diabetic and nondiabetic mothers utilizing 6,6-dideutero glucose which is nonrecycling. Infants of well-controlled mothers were found to have slightly lower plasma glucose levels than normal infants (43.4 ± 3.7 mg/dl versus 65.2 ± 3.6 mg/dl [2.4 ± 0.2 mM versus 3.6 ± 0.2 mM]) at 2–4 hours of age; but glucose production and utilization rates did not differ (3.35 ± 0.26 versus 3.39 ± 0.08 mg/kg/min). As a result, metabolic clearance rates were increased.

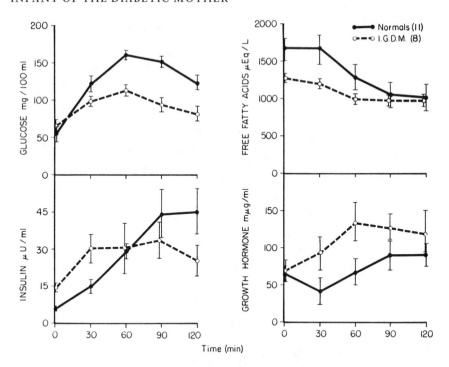

FIGURE 4-10. Blood glucose, plasma insulin, free fatty acids, and growth hormone values (mean ± SE) at fasting and during oral glucose tolerance tests in normal newborns and IGDM. (From Pildes et al. Reproduced by permission of *Pediatrics*. 44:76, copyright 1969.)

Hyperinsulinemia produces a number of metabolic effects on fat and protein metabolism as well. This is manifest by the reduced levels of plasma free fatty acids in the IDM during the first hours after birth [45,150]. The associated elevation in glycerol concentrations [151] has been confirmed but inadequately explained. Plasma ketones (B-OH-B) have also been measured in the first hours of life and do not differ from controls [151].

Plasma amino acids, especially the gluconeogenic amino acids, have been measured to assess the cause and effect of hyperinsulinemia as well as substrate availability. While some umbilical plasma amino acid concentrations correlated positively with maternal levels in IDMs, others did not [152,153]. More importantly, little differences in specific plasma amino acids were found between hypoglycemic IDMs and normoglycemic infants [154,155]. The changes in alanine and glycine were best related to asphyxia rather than hyperinsulinism.

Susa et al. [92] have provided the most direct experimental evidence for the Pedersen hypothesis by producing hyperinsulinemia in normal rhesus monkeys. Utilizing an osmotic pump implanted in a fetal limb in the early third trimester to deliver insulin continuously for 18–24 days, the hyperinsulinemia produced fetal mild hypoglycemia and hypoglucagonemia and increased erythropoietin. There was significant macrosomia and cardiomegaly as well as an increase in adipose tissue grossly. Hepatic concentrations of lipid, protein, DNA, and RNA were not affected, suggesting cellular hyperplasia rather than hypertrophy, whereas activities of hepatic enzymes affecting glucose utilization, glycogen metabolism, and glycolysis did not change. The activity of two gluconeogenic enzymes (PEPCK and glucose-6-phosphatase) were diminished, while those of lipogenic and NADPH-producing enzymes were increased [156]. Thus, the principal effects of in utero hyperinsulinemia were to promote hepatic lipogenesis, while limiting gluconeogenesis.

Freinkel [90] and Milner [91] have expanded the Pedersen hypothesis to include substrates other than glucose, i.e., amino acids and fatty acids. While the evidence for the role of glucose is significant, observations to date of changes in amino acid and fatty acid concentration are limited.

Other hypotheses have been proposed over the years and have not withstood the test of time and experimentation [139,157–161]. These have included a variety of hormones, metabolites, and genetic factors. Recent evidence would support a secondary role for catecholamines [161,162]. Lower plasma glucagon values persist in the first hours of life in IDMs [134]. There is not a normal rise following intravenous glucose [163] or an intravenous bolus of alanine given at one hour of age [164]. These observations raise questions concerning the role of counterregulatory factors in glucose homeostasis in these infants.

The final analysis of this complex problem will require techniques that permit the study of the fetus in utero. While the influence of the maternal environment is evident in overt diabetes, it is less clear in gestational diabetes.

The effects of maternal hyperglycemia or substrate disequilibrium are summarized schematically in Figure 4-11, which represents an expanded pathophysiologic view of the Pedersen hypothesis. This is not all-inclusive, but rather represents those morbidities for which there is reasonable evidence. All evidence strongly supports the effort necessary to achieve the closest approximation of normoglycemia prior to conception and throughout pregnancy in the diabetic mother. The relationship between maternal metabolic control, fetal hyperinsulinemia, and many of the neonatal morbidities are summarized in Figure 4-11.

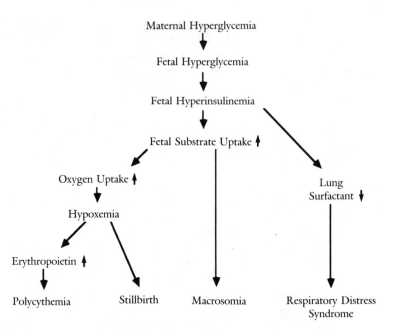

FIGURE 4-11. Flow diagram indicating likely pathogenetic events that result in significant morbidities in the fetus and/or infant of the diabetic mother. (From Schwartz. In: Sutherland, Stowers, Pearson, eds. *Carbohydrate Metabolism in Pregnancy and the Newborn. IV.* London: Springer-Verlag, 1989; 348, with permission.)

• Other Clinical Complications

The sick infant of the diabetic mother may have a variety of other clinical problems, including intracranial, adrenal or renal hemorrhage, or congestive heart failure. One often finds a large heart on roentgen examination in asymptomatic infants (see sections on Congenital Anomalies and Macrosomia); this finding alone is not an indication for digitalization. In the presence of a rapidly enlarging liver, tachypnea, and tachycardia, however, such therapy is suggested. Seratto et al. [165] studied 42 consecutive infants of diabetic mothers, of whom 20 were born to gestational diabetic mothers. Multiple clinical problems were observed, including cardiorespiratory complications. Of 19 patients with tachypnea, 7 had "wet lung" syndrome by x-ray, 7 were in congestive failure, 2 had infiltrates or aspiration pneumonia, and 4 had no abnormal x-ray changes. Abnormal electrocardiograms were observed in 15 patients. Of the 7 infants with congestive heart failure, 1 died and 6 had associated hypoglycemia, while 2 were hypocalcemic.

Neonatal Small Left Colon Syndrome

Davis and Campbell [166] have noted an unusually high incidence of low colonic obstruction and barium enema findings of a uniformly narrowed colon from the splenic flexure to the anus in 8 of 20 symptomatic infants of insulin-dependent mothers. In a prospective analysis, they also observed 6 of 12 asymptomatic IDMs to have similar roentgen findings. The pathogenesis of this lesion is obscure. No surgical intervention is required.

· Long-Term Prognosis

Genetics

With improved survival of insulin-dependent diabetic subjects and especially the improved perinatal mortality and morbidity of offspring of diabetic mothers, significant studies have now been done defining the risk of future diabetes. Warram and associates [7,167] have reported on the extensive series from the Joslin Clinic (1940–1984). In 1,391 offspring of type 1 insulin-dependent mothers who survived the perinatal period, the net cumulative risk of insulin-dependent diabetes mellitus (IDDM) by age 20 years was only 2.1 ± 0.5 percent (SE) which was one-third that reported for the offspring of men with IDDM: 6.1 ± 1.8 percent (Fig. 4-12). While the risk of diabetes in offspring of diabetic mothers was increased significantly in young mothers, it was otherwise independent of risk factors for perinatal mortality. From a careful analysis of early fetal or perinatal loss, no evidence was found for selective loss of diabetes-susceptible fetuses. They speculated that exposure in utero to an affected mother can protect a fetus from developing IDDM later in life. They suggested that induction of immunologic tolerance to the autoantigens of the B cells is a plausible mechanism for this protective effect.

Studies such as those by DiMario et al. [168] of immunologic factors in cord blood should further establish this hypothesis. These investigators have found fully activated T-lymphocytes in cord blood of infants of mothers with IDDM, but not in infants of nondiabetic mothers nor in infants of mothers with non-insulin-dependent diabetes. It should be noted that diabetes in the father has no influence on perinatal outcome although genetic liability is present. Previously, Yssing [169] had observed a 1 percent incidence in 8 of 740 IDMs, representing a 20–30-fold higher incidence than in a comparable Scandinavian population.

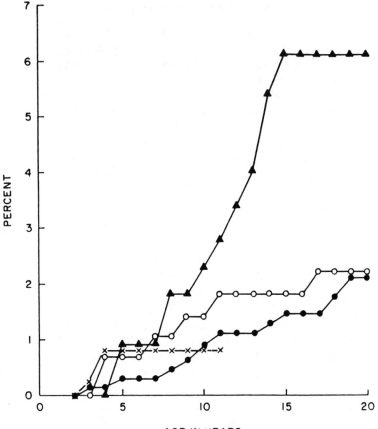

FIGURE 4-12. Cumulative risk of IDDM in offspring of mothers with IDDM, according to year of birth (○, 1940–1960, n = 287; ●, 1961–1974, n = 677; x, 1975–1984, n = 427) contrasted with cumulative risk of IDDM in offspring of fathers with IDDM (▲, n = 244). (From Warram, Krolewski, Kahn. *Diabetes* 1988; 37:1328, with permission.)

Risk for Obesity

Although infants of diabetic mothers may be macrosomic with associated increased adipose tissue, these compositional changes reverse by 4 months of age. Later effects have been inconclusive. In a prospective analysis, Farquhar [170] followed up 329 diabetic pregnancies from 1948–1966 at Edinburgh. In his survivors (251), weights and heights were distributed over a normal range; however, an excess of both boys and girls (9 and 13 percent, respectively) fell below the third percentile for height, while a comparable number fell above the ninety-seventh and below the third percentiles for weight.

Francois et al. [75] evaluated 97 offspring of diabetic mothers between 2 and 16 years of age. Height and weight were normal in all but 8 cases who were above 2 SD in either parameter. In a small series (34 IDMs and IGDMs), Vohr et al. [171] observed a positive relationship between being large for gestational age at birth and having an increased weight-to-height ratio at 7 years for IDMs ($p <$ 0.01). Pettit et al. [172] have reported on the unusual diabetic population of Pima Indians in whom obesity is a major occurrence. Fifty-eight percent of offspring of diabetic mothers were obese by 15 to 19 years of age, with weight equal or greater than 140 percent of ideal body weight. This adolescent obesity was directly related to maternal diabetes but not to maternal obesity. Whether these implications of an intrauterine influence in this unique population can be extrapolated to a more general population remains to be clarified.

Neurodevelopmental Outcome

The interpretation of behavior assessment is confounded in part by the improvements that have occurred in the past two decades in perinatal care. Originally, Yssing advantageously utilized the unique pregnant diabetic population that had been carefully studied by Pedersen and his associates over two decades [3]. For example, she evaluated outcome relative to maternal estriol excretion in 154 pregnancies that resulted in 158 surviving children [173]. At follow-up between 1 year, 8 months and 10 years, 1 month, major congenital abnormalities and cerebral damage were significantly more frequent in infants from mothers with subnormal estriol excretion. Several studies reported in the past 20 years are summarized by Vohr [174] in Table 4-3. The largest series from Copenhagen concern the extensive population (749 children ages 1½ to 26 years at follow-up) of the late Jørgen Pedersen. Yssing [169] reported a 36 percent frequency of cerebral dysfunction or related conditions. Among 12 problems, behavior disturbances, reading difficulties and squint accounted for 10 percent each, while enuresis was present in 9 percent, as were speech disturbances. Mental retardation was found in 5 percent. The latter did not differ from the incidence in the normal population. She analyzed for associated events and noted that a high incidence of major cerebral dysfunction was related to genetic factors, high or low maternal age in pregnancy, maternal White Class D and F, low gestational age, and low birth weight.

As noted above, Persson and Gentz [85] reported an absence of any major neurologic abnormality or developmental delay. The series

TABLE 4-3. Neurologic and developmental sequelae of infants of diabetic mothers

STUDY	N	YEARS OF FOLLOW-UP	MAJOR NEUROLOGIC ABNORMALITY* (%)	DEVELOPMENTAL DELAY (IQ ≤ 84) (%)
Yssing, 1975	740	1.5–26	11	7
Stehbens et al., 1977	50	5	6	13
Haworth et al., 1976	37	4.5	8	8
Cummins and Norrish, 1980	51	4–13	3.9	13.7
Persson and Gentz, 1984	73	5	0	0

(From Vohr, in Gabbe and Oh (eds.): *Infant of the Diabetic Mother, Report of the 93rd Ross Conference on Pediatric Research*. Columbus, Ohio: Ross Laboratories, 1987 [174].)
*Cerebral palsy, blindness, deafness, seizures.

is sufficiently small (94 infants) as to make small differences from the control population difficult to ascertain. The combined series presented above indicate a variable, but likely low frequency. Petersen [175] has carefully evaluated the status of 90 children of insulin-dependent diabetic mothers born between October 1980 and January 1983 in Copenhagen. After 4–5 years, poor performance in three noncognitive fields suggested a neurological immaturity or sequelae to some adverse influence on the development of the fetal brain. These infants/children should be considered at risk for psychomotor developmental problems even in the presence of optimal obstetrical management.

Hypoglycemia has not been directly implicated in the neurodevelopmental outcome of these infants.

• Summary

Diabetes during pregnancy not only affects maternal metabolism but also has diverse effects on the fetus and newborn. Congenital anomalies of the fetus are more common. Anatomic alterations may include increased body fat with selective organomegaly and macrosomia. Increased islet cells with beta cell hyperplasia are associated with hyperinsulinemia which produces hypoxemia, hypererythropoietinemia, increased hematopoiesis, and polycythemia. Other effects of hyperinsulinemia include hypoglycemia and diminished surfactant production with subsequent respiratory distress syndrome.

Current management includes prepregnancy counseling and rigid normalization of maternal metabolic control throughout pregnancy. Optimal control has produced major improvement in fetal and neonatal mortality and morbidity. The delivery is individualized according to lung maturation. Ideally, delivery should occur in a tertiary center where an intensive care team is available to manage untoward events. Prognosis has improved remarkably in the past two decades.

REFERENCES

1. FARQUHAR JW. The child of the diabetic woman. *Arch Dis Child.* 1959;34:76.
2. MILLS JL, SIMPSON JL, DRISCOLL SG, et al. National Institute of Child Health and Human Development—Diabetes in Early Pregnancy Study. *N Engl J Med.* 1988;319:1617.
3. PEDERSEN J, MØLSTED-PEDERSEN L, ANDERSEN B. Perinatal foetal mortality in 1245 diabetic pregnancies. *Acta Chir Scand Suppl.* 1973;433:191.
4. O'SULLIVAN JB, CHARLES D, MAHAN CM, DANDROW RV. Gestational diabetes and perinatal mortality rate. *Am J Obstet Gynecol.* 1973; 116:901.
5. WHITE P. Diabetes mellitus in pregnancy. *Clin Perinatol.* 1974;1:331.
6. KYLE GC. Diabetes and pregnancy. *Ann Inter Med.* 1963;59:No. 1, pt. 2 (Suppl. 3).
7. WARRAM JH, KROLEWSKI AS, KAHN CR. Determinants of IDDM and perinatal mortality in children of diabetic mothers. *Diabetes.* 1988; 37:1328.
8. PERSSON B, STANGENBERG M, HANSSON V, NORDLANDER E. Gestational diabetes mellitus (GDM). Comparative evaluation of two treatment regimens, diet versus insulin and diet. *Diabetes.* 1985;34(2):101.
9. HANSON V, PERSSON B, STANGENBERG M. Factors influencing neonatal morbidity in diabetic pregnancy. *Diabetes Res* 1986;3:71.
10. REECE EA, COUSTAN DR, eds. *Diabetes Mellitus in Pregnancy.* New York: Churchill Livingstone, 1988.
11. SUTHERLAND HW, STOWERS JM, PEARSON DWM, eds. *Carbohydrate Metabolism in Pregnancy and the Newborn. IV.* London: Springer-Verlag, 1989.
12. BRUDENELL M, DODDERIDGE MC, eds. *Diabetic Pregnancy.* Edinburgh: Churchill Livingstone, 1989.
13. HARE JW, WHITE P. Gestational diabetes and the White classification. *Diabetes Care.* 1980;3:394.
14. MILLER HC. Offspring of diabetic and prediabetic mothers. *Adv Pediatr.* 1956;8:137.
15. CARRINGTON ER. Diabetes in pregnancy. *Clin Obstet Gynecol.* 1973; 16:28.
16. O'SULLIVAN JB. Gestational diabetes. Unsuspected, asymptomatic diabetes in pregnancy. *N Engl J Med.* 1961;264:1032.
17. CARPENTER MW. Testing for gestational diabetes. In: Reece EA, Coustan DT, eds. *Diabetes Mellitus in Pregnancy.* New York: Churchill Livingstone, 1988;423.
18. O'SULLIVAN JB. Natural history of diabetes. *Adv Metab Disord.* 1970; (Suppl.) 1:385.
19. FREINKEL N, METZGER BE. Gestational diabetes: problems in classification and implications for long-range prognosis. *Adv Exp Med Biol.* 1985;189:47.

20. TYSON JE, FELIG P. Medical aspects of diabetes in pregnancy. *Med Clin North Am.* 1971;55:947.

21. SURMACZYNSKA BZ, NITZAN M, METZGER BE, FREINKEL N. XII. The effect of oral glucose on plasma concentrations of human placental lactogen and chorionic gonadotropin during late pregnancy in normal subjects and gestational diabetics. *Isr J Med Sci.* 1974;10:1481.

22. PEDERSEN J, MØLSTED-PEDERSEN L, ANDERSEN B. Assessors of fetal perinatal mortality in diabetic pregnancy. *Diabetes.* 1974;23:302.

23. WIDNESS JA, COWETT RM, COUSTAN DR, CARPENTER MW, OH W. Neonatal morbidities in infants of mothers with glucose intolerance in pregnancy. *Diabetes.* 1985;34(2):61.

24. JOVANOVIC L, DRUZIN M, PETERSON CM. Effect of euglycemia on the outcome of pregnancy in insulin-dependent diabetic women as compared with normal subjects. *Am J Med.* 1981;71:921.

25. COUSINS L. Obstetric complications. In: Reece EA, Coustan DR, eds. *Diabetes Mellitus in Pregnancy. Principles and practice.* New York: Churchill Livingstone, 1988;455.

26. ROSZKOWSKI I, JANCZEWSKA E. The daily glycemia profile in pregnancy. *Am J Obstet Gynecol.* 1964;88:204.

27. BODDY K, DAWES GS. Fetal breathing. *Br Med Bull.* 1975;31:3.

28. PEDERSEN J. *The Pregnant Diabetic and Her Newborn. Problems and Management.* Copenhagen, Munksgaard, 1967.

29. PERSSON B, LUNNELL NO, CARLSTROM K, FURUHJELM M. Urinary estriol excretion in strictly controlled diabetic pregnancies. *Acta Obstet Gynecol Scand.* 1970;49:379.

30. OAKLEY W. The Treatment of Pregnancy in Diabetes Mellitus. In: Leibel BS, Wrenshall GA, eds. *On the Nature and Treatment of Diabetes.* Amsterdam: Excerpta Medica Foundation, 1965;673.

31. PHILIPSON EH, KALHAN SC, EDELBERG SC, WILLIAMS TG. Maternal obesity as a risk factor in gestational diabetes. *Am J Perinat.* 1985;2:268.

32. SUTHERLAND HW, BREWSHER PD, CORMACK JD, HUGHES CRT, REID A, RUSSELL G, STOWERS JM. Effect of moderate dosage of chlorpropamide in pregnancy on fetal outcome. *Arch Dis Child.* 1974;49:283.

33. STOWERS JM, SUTHERLAND HW. Use of sulphonylureas, biguanides, and insulin in pregnancy. In: Sutherland HW, Stowers JM, eds. *Carbohydrate Metabolism in Pregnancy and the Newborn.* New York: Churchill Livingstone, 1975;205.

34. KEMBALL ML, MCIVER C, MILNER RDG, NOURSE CH, SCHIFF D, TIERNAN JR. Neonatal hypoglycaemia in infants of diabetic mothers given sulphonylurea drugs in pregnancy. *Arch Dis Child.* 1970;45:696.

35. SELTZER HS. Drug-induced hypoglycemia. A review based on 473 cases. *Diabetes.* 1972;21:955.

36. NITOWSKY HM, MATZ L, BERZOFSKY JA. Studies on oxidative drug metabolism in the full-term newborn infant. *J Pediatr.* 1966;69:1139.

37. GLUCK L, KULOVICH MV. Lecithin/sphingomyelin ratios in amniotic fluid in normal and abnormal pregnancy. *Am J Obstet Gynecol.* 1973; 115:539.

38. LIGHT IJ, KEENAN WJ, SUTHERLAND JM. Maternal intravenous glucose administration as a cause of hypoglycemia in the infant of the diabetic mother. *Am J Obst Gynecol.* 1972;113:345.

39. SCHWARTZ HC, KING KC, SCHWARTZ AL, EDMUNDS D, SCHWARTZ R. Effects of pregnancy on hemoglobin A_{1c} in normal, gestational diabetic and diabetic women. *Diabetes.* 1976;25:1118.

40. LESLIE RDG, PYKE DA, JOHN PN, WHITE JM. Hemoglobin A₁ in diabetic pregnancy. *Lancet.* 1979;ii:958.

41. MILLER E, HARE JW, CLOHERTY JP, et al. Elevated maternal hemoglobin A$_{1c}$ in early pregnancy and major congenital anomalies in infants of diabetic mothers. *N Engl J Med.* 1981;304:1331.

42. YLINEN K, AULA P, STENMAN U-H, KESANIEMI-KUDKKANEN T, TERAMO K. Risk of minor and major fetal malformations in diabetics with high haemoglobin A$_{1c}$ values in early pregnancy. *Br Med J.* 1984;289:345.

43. FUHRMANN K, REIHER H, SEMMLER K, FISCHER F, FISCHER M, GLOCKNER E. Presention of congenital malformations in infants of insulin-dependent diabetic mothers. *Diabetes Care.* 1983;6:219.

44. FUHRMANN K, REIHER H, SEMMLER K, GLOCKNER E. The effect of intensified conventional insulin therapy before and during pregnancy on the malformation rate in offspring of diabetic mothers. *Exp Clin Endocrinol.* 1984;83:173.

45. MILLS JL, KNOPP RH, SIMPSON JL, et al. Lack of relation of increased malformation rates in infants of diabetic mothers to glycemic control during organogenesis. *N Engl J Med.* 1988;318:671.

46. MILLS JL, BAKER L, GOLDMAN AS. Malformations in infants of diabetic mothers occur before the seventh gestational week. *Diabetes.* 1979; 28:292.

47. PINTER E, REECE EA. Diabetes-associated congenital malformations: epidemiology, pathogenesis, and experimental methods of induction and prevention. In: Reece EA, Coustan DR, eds. *Diabetes Mellitus in Pregnancy.* New York: Churchill-Livingstone, 1988;205.

48. ERIKSSON UJ, KARLSSON MG, STYRUD J. Mechanisms of congenital malformations in diabetic pregnancy. *Biol Neonate.* 1987;51:113.

49. FREINKEL N. Diabetic embryopathy and fuel-mediated organ teratogenesis: lessons from animal models. *Horm Metabol Res.* 1988;20:463.

50. GELLIS SS, HSIA DYY. The infant of the diabetic mother. *Am J Dis Child.* 1959;97:1.

51. MILLER HC. The effect of diabetic and prediabetic pregnancies on the fetus and newborn infant. *J Pediatr.* 1946;29:455.

52. NAEYE RL. Infants of diabetic mothers: a quantitative morphologic study. *Pediatrics.* 1965;35:980.

53. SINGER DB. Hepatic erythropoiesis in infants of diabetic mothers. *Pediatr Pathol.* 1986;5:471.

54. MIMOUNI F, MIODOVIK M, SIDDIQI TA, et al. Neonatal polycythemia in infants of insulin-dependent diabetic mothers. *Obstet Gynecol.* 1986;68:370.

55. CARSON BS, PHILLIPS AF, SIMMONS MA, BATTAGLIA FC, MESCHIA G. Effects of a sustained insulin infusion upon glucose uptake and oxygenation of the ovine fetus. *Pediatr Res.* 1980;14:147.

56. MILLEY JR, ROSENBERG AA, PHILLIPS AF, MORTENI RA, JONES MD JR, SIMMONS MA. The effect of insulin on ovine fetal oxygen extraction. *Am J Obstet Gynecol.* 1984;149:673.

57. MILLEY JR, PAPACOSTAS JS, TABATA BK. Effect of insulin on uptake of metabolic substrates by the sheep fetus. *Am J Physiol.* 1986; 251:E349.

58. PHILIPPS AF, DUBIN JW, MATTY PJ, RAYE JR. Arterial hypoxemia and hyperinsulinemia in the chronically hyperglycemic fetal lamb. *Pediatr Res.* 1982;16:653.

59. PHILIPPS AF, PORTE PJ, STABINSKY S, ROSENKRANTZ TS, RAYE JR. Effects

of chronic fetal hyperglycemia upon oxygen consumption in the ovine uterus and conceptus. *J Clin Invest.* 1984;74:279.

60. PHILIPPS AF, ROSENKRANTZ TS, RAYE JR. Consequences of perturbations of fetal fuels in ovine pregnancy. *Diabetes.* 1985;34:32.

61. PHILIPPS AF, ROSENKRANTZ TS, PORTE PJ, RAYE JR. The effects of chronic fetal hyperglycemia on substrate uptake by the ovine fetus and conceptus. *Pediatr Res.* 1985;19:659.

62. WIDNESS JA, SUSA JB, GARCIA JF, et al. Increased erythropoiesis and elevated erythropoietin in infants born to diabetic mothers and in hyperinsulinemic rhesus fetuses. *J Clin Invest.* 1981;67:639.

63. PHILIPPS AF, WIDNESS JA, GARCIA JF, RAYE JR, SCHWARTZ R. Erythropoietin elevation in the chronically hyperglycemic fetal lamb. *Proc Soc Exp Biol Med.* 1982;170:42.

64. TERAMO KA, WIDNESS JA, CLEMONS GK, VOUTILAINEN P, MCKINLAY S, SCHWARTZ R. Amniotic fluid erythropoietin correlates with umbilical plasma erythropoietin in normal and abnormal pregnancy. *Obstet Gynecol.* 1987;69:710.

65. WIDNESS JA, TERAMO KA, CLEMONS GK, et al. Direct relationship of antepartum glucose control and fetal erythropoietin in human type 1 (insulin-dependent) diabetic pregnancy. Diabetologia. 1990;33:378.

66. MIMOUNI F, MIODOVIK M, SIDDIQI TA, BUTLER JB, HOLROYDE J, TSANG RC. Neonatal polycythemia in infants of insulin dependent diabetic mothers. *Obstet Gynecol.* 1986;68:370.

67. OH W. Pathophysiology of polycythemia in infants of diabetic mothers. In: Gabbe SG, Oh W, eds. *Infant of the Diabetic Mother. Report of the 93rd Ross Conference on Pediatric Research.* Columbus, Ohio: 1987;133.

68. BLACK VD. Polycythemia and the infant of the diabetic mother. In: Gabbe SG, Oh W, eds. *Infant of the Diabetic Mother. Report of the 93rd Ross Conference on Pediatric Research.* Columbus, Ohio: 1987;142.

69. ZETTERSTRÖM R, STRINDBERG B, ARNHOLD RG. Hyperbilirubinemia and ABO hemolytic disease in newborn infants of diabetic mothers. *Acta Paediat.* 1958;47:238.

70. OLSEN BR, OSLER M, PEDERSEN J. Neonatal jaundice in infants born to diabetic mothers. *Dan Med Bull.* 1963;10:1.

71. TAYLOR PM, WOLFSON JH, BRIGHT NH, BIRCHARD EL, DERINOZ MN, WATSON DW. Hyperbilirubinemia in infants of diabetic mothers. *Biol Neonate.* 1963;5:289.

72. STEVENSON DK. Bilirubin metabolism in the infant of the diabetic mother: an overview. In: Gabbe SG, Oh W, eds. *Infants of the Diabetic Mother. Report of the 93rd Ross Conference on Pediatric Research.* Columbus, Ohio: 1987;109.

73. AVERY ME, OPPENHEIMER EH, GORDON HH. Renal-vein thrombosis in newborn infants of diabetic mothers. *N Engl J Med.* 1957;265:1134.

74. TAKEUCHI A, BENIRSCHKE K. Renal venous thrombosis of the newborn and its relation to maternal diabetes. *Biol Neonate.* 1961;3:237.

75. FRANCOIS R, PICAUD JJ, RUITTON-UGLIENGO A, DAVID L, CARTAL MY, BAUER D. The newborn of diabetic mothers. *Biol Neonate.* 1974;24:1, and International Congress of Pediatrics, Buenos Aires, Argentina, Oct. 1974.

76. TVETERÅS E, RUDSTROM P. Renal thrombosis of the newborn; Report of a primary case successfully treated by surgery. *Acta Paediatr.* 1956;45:545.

77. WARRNER RA, CORNBLATH M. Infants of gestational diabetic mothers. *Am J Dis Child.* 1969;117:678.

78. GARN SM. Fat, body size and growth in the newborn. *Hum Biol.* 1958;30:265.

79. OSLER M, PEDERSEN J. The body composition of newborn infants of diabetic mothers. *Pediatrics.* 1960;26:985.

80. FEE BA, WEIL WB JR. Body composition of infants of diabetic mothers by direct analysis. *Ann NY Acad Sci.* 1963;110:869.

81. FARQUHAR JW, SKLAROFF SA. The post-natal weight loss of babies born to diabetic and non-diabetic women. *Arch Dis Child.* 1958;33:323.

82. COOK CD, O'BRIEN D, HANSEN JDL, BEEM M, SMITH CA. Water and electrolyte economy in newborn infants of diabetic mothers. *Acta Paediatr.* 1960;49:121.

83. OSLER M. Renal function in newborn infants of diabetic mothers. *Acta Endocrinol.* 1960;34:287.

84. SCHWARTZ R, TERAMO KA. Primary hyperinsulinemia and macrosomia in infants of diabetic mothers. In: Gabbe SG, Oh W, eds. *Infant of the Diabetic Mother. Report of the 93rd Ross Conference on Pediatric Research.* Columbus, Ohio: 1987;40.

85. PERSSON B, GENTZ J. Follow-up of children of insulin-dependent and gestational diabetic mothers. Neuropsychological outcome. *Acta Paediatr Scand.* 1984;73:349.

86. TSCHOBROUTSKY G, HEARD I, TSCHOBROUTSKY C, ESCHWEGE E. Amniotic fluid c-peptide in normal and insulin-dependent diabetic pregnancies. *Diabetologia.* 1980;18:289.

87. GRUPPUSO PA, SUSA JB, SEHGAL P, FRANK BN, SCHWARTZ R. Metabolism and placental transfer of ^{125}I-proinsulin and ^{125}I-tyrosylated c-peptide in the pregnant rhesus monkey. *J Clin Invest.* 1987;80:1132.

88. BAUMAN WA, YALOW RS. Transplacental passage of insulin complexed to antibody. *Proc Natl Acad Sci USA.* 1981;78:4588.

89. MENON RK, COHEN RM, SPERLING MA, CUTFIELD WS, MIMOUNI F, KHOURY JC. Transplacental passage of insulin in pregnant women with insulin-dependent diabetes mellitus. Its role in fetal macrosomia. *N Engl J Med.* 1990;323:309.

90. FREINKEL N, METZGER BE. Pregnancy as a tissue culture experience: the critical implications of maternal metabolism for fetal development. *Ciba Foundation Symposium.* 1979;63:3.

91. MILNER RDG. Amino acids and beta cell growth in structure and function. In: Merkatz IR, Adam PAJ, eds. *The Diabetic Pregnancy: A Perinatal Perspective.* New York: Grune and Stratton, 1979;145.

92. SUSA JB, MCCORMICK KL, WIDNESS JA, et al. Chronic hyperinsulinemia in the fetal rhesus monkey. Effects on fetal growth and composition. *Diabetes.* 1979;28:1058.

93. SUSA JB, WIDNESS JA, HINTZ R, LIU R, SEHGAL P, SCHWARTZ R. Somatomedins and insulin in diabetic pregnancies: effects on fetal macrosomia in the human and rhesus monkey. *J Clin Endocrinol Metab.* 1984;58:1099.

94. D'ERCOLE AJ. Somatomedins/insulin-like growth factors: relationship to insulin and diabetes. In: Gabbe SG, Oh W, eds. *Infant of the*

Diabetic Mother. Report of the 93rd Ross Conference on Pediatric Research. Columbus, Ohio: 1987;50.

95. GRUPPUSO PA, FRANK BH, SCHWARTZ R. Binding of proinsulin and proinsulin conversion intermediates to human placental IGF-1 receptors. *J Clin Endocrinol Metab.* 1988;67:194.

96. ROBERT MF, NEFF RK, HUBBELL JP, TAEUSCH HW, AVERY ME. Association between maternal diabetes and the respiratory distress syndrome in the newborn. *N Engl J Med.* 1976;294:357.

97. SMITH BT, GIROUD CJP, ROBERT M, AVERY ME. Insulin antagonism of cortisol action on lecithin synthesis by cultured fetal lung cells. *J Pediatr.* 1975;85:953.

98. KING RJ, CLEMENTS JA. Surface active materials from dog lung. II. Composition and physiological correlations. *Am J Physiol.* 1972;223:715.

99. WEAVER TE, ROSS G, DAUGHERTY C, WHITSETT JA. Synthesis of surfactant-associated protein, 3500 daltons in fetal lung. *J Appl Physiol.* 1986;61:694.

100. WHITSETT JA, HULL WM, OHNING B, ROSS G, WEAVER JE. Immunological identification of a pulmonary surfactant associated protein of molecular weight = 6000 daltons. *Pediatr Res.* 1986;20:744.

101. GLASSER SW, KORFHAGEN TR, WEAVER TE, et al. cDNA, deduced polypeptide structure and chromosomal assignment of human pulmonary surfactant proteolipid, SPL (pVal). *J Biol Chem.* 1988;263:9.

102. HAWGOOD S, BENSON BJ, SCHILLING J, DAMM D, CLEMENTS JA, WHITE RT. Nucleotide and amino acid sequences of pulmonary surfactant protein SP18 and evidence for cooperation between SP18 and SP28-36 in surfactant lipid adsorption. *Proc Natl Acad Sci USA.* 1987;84:86.

103. LIGGINS GC. Premature delivery of foetal lambs infused with glucocorticoids. *J Endocrinol.* 1969;45:515.

104. LIGGINS GC, HOWIE RN. A controlled trial of antepartum glucocorticoid treatment for prevention of the respiratory distress syndrome in premature infants. *Pediatrics.* 1972;50:515.

105. GLUCK L, KULOVICH MW. Lecithin/sphingomyelin ratios in amniotic fluid in normal and abnormal pregnancy. *Am J Obstet Gynecol.* 1973;115:539.

106. HALLMAN M, FELDMAN BH, KIRKPATRICK E, GLUCK L. Absence of phosphatidyl glycerol (PG) in respiratory distress syndrome in the newborn. *Pediatr Res.* 1977;11:714.

107. HALLMAN M, TERAMO K. Amniotic fluid phospholipid profile as a predictor of fetal maturity in diabetic pregnancies. *Obstet Gynecol.* 1979;54:703.

108. WARBURTON D. Chronic hyperglycemia reduces surface active material flux in tracheal fluid of fetal lambs. *J Clin Invest.* 1982;71:550.

109. WARBURTON D. Chronic hyperglycemia with secondary hyperinsulinemia inhibits the maturational response of fetal lamb lungs to cortisol. *J Clin Invest.* 1983;72:433.

110. PENNOYER MM, HARTMANN AF SR. Management of infants born of diabetic mothers. *Postgrad Med.* 1955;18:199.

111. CORNBLATH M, NICOLOPOULOS D, GANZON AF, LEVIN EY, GORDON MH, GORDON HH. Studies of carbohydrate metabolism in the newborn infant. IV. The effect of glucagon on the capillary blood sugar in infants of diabetic mothers. *Pediatrics.* 1961;28:592.

112. DUFFTY P, LLOYD DJ. The infant of the diabetic mother: recent experience. In: Sutherland JW, Stowers JM, Pearson DWM, eds. *Carbohydrate Metabolism in Pregnancy and the Newborn. IV.* London: Springer-Verlag, 1989;329.

113. PERSSON B, HANSON U. Impact of maternal blood glucose control on neonatal morbidity in diabetic pregnancies. In: Lindblad BS, ed. *Perinatal Nutrition.* New York: Academic Press, Inc., 1988;291.

114. LANDON MB, GABBE SG, PIANA R, MENNUTI MT, MAIN EK. Neonatal morbidity in pregnancy complicated by diabetes mellitus: predictive value of maternal glycemic profiles. *Am J Obstet Gynecol.* 1987;156:1089.

115. MCCANN ML, CHEN CH, KATIGBAK EB, KOTCHEN J, LIKLY BF, SCHWARTZ R. The effects of fructose on hypoglucosemia in infants of diabetic mothers. *N Engl J Med.* 1966;275:1.

116. CHEN CH, ADAM PAJ, LASKOWSKI DE, MCCANN ML, SCHWARTZ R. The plasma free fatty acid composition and blood glucose of normal and diabetic pregnant women and of their newborns. *Pediatrics.* 1965; 36:843.

117. WU PYK, MODANLOV H, KARELITZ M. Effect of glucagon on blood glucose homeostasis in infants of diabetic mothers. *Acta Paediatr Scand.* 1975;64:441.

118. KING KC, TSERNG K-Y, KALHAN SC. Regulation of glucose production in newborn infants of diabetic mothers. *Pediatr Res.* 1982;16:608.

119. MCCANN ML, ADAM PAJ, LIKLY BF, SCHWARTZ R. The prevention of hypoglucosemia by fructose in infants of diabetic mothers. *N Engl J Med.* 1966;275:8.

120. HAWORTH JC, DILLING LA, VIDYASAGAR D. Hypoglycemia in infants of diabetic mothers. Effect of epinephrine therapy. *J Pediatr* 1973;82:94.

121. BERGMAN L. Studies on early neonatal hypocalcemia. *Acta Paediatr Scand.* (Suppl.) 1974;248:5.

122. SCHWARTZ R, GAMSU H, MULLIGAN PB, REISNER SH, WYBREGT SH, CORNBLATH M. Transient intolerance to exogenous fructose in the newborn. *J Clin Invest.* 1964;43:333.

123. CRAIG WS. Clinical signs of neonatal tetany: With especial reference to their occurrence in newborn babies of diabetic mothers. *Pediatrics.* 1958;22:297.

124. GITTLEMAN IF, PINCUS JB, SCHMERZLER E, ANNECCHIARICO F. Diabetes mellitus or the prediabetic state in the mother and the neonate. *Am J Dis Child.* 1959;98:342.

125. TSANG RC, KLEINMAN LI, SUTHERLAND JM, LIGHT IJ. Hypocalcemia in infants of diabetic mothers. *J Pediatr.* 1972;80:384.

126. TSANG RC, CHEN IW, FRIEDMAN MA, GIGGER M, STEICHEN J, KOFFLER H. FENTON L, BROWN D, PRAMANIK A, KEENAN W, STRUB R, JOYCE T. Parathyroid function in infants of diabetic mothers. *J Pediatr.* 1975;86:399.

127. GITTLEMAN IF, PINCUS JB, SCHMERZLER E, SAITO M. Hypocalcemia occurring on the first day of life in mature and premature infants. *Pediatrics.* 1956;18:721.

128. KUNSTADTER RH, OH W, TANMAN F, CORNBLATH M. Idiopathic hypoparathyroidism in the newborn. *Am J Dis Child.* 1963;105:499.

129. MIMOUNI F, LOUGHEAD J, MIODOVNIK M, KHOURY J, TSANG RC. Early neonatal predictors of neonatal hypocalcemia in infants of diabetic mothers: an epidemiologic study. *Am J Perinatol.* 1990;7:203.

130. MIMOUNI F, TSANG RC, HERTZBERG VS, NEUMANN V, ELLIS K. Parathyroid hormone and calcitriol changes in normal and insulin-dependent diabetic pregnancies. *Obstet Gynecol.* 1989;74:49.

131. TSANG RC, CHEN IW, FREIDMAN MA, et al. Parathyroid function in infants of diabetic mothers. *J Pediatr.* 1975;86:399.

132. MIMOUNI F, MIODOVNIK M, TSANG RC, CALLAHAN J, SHAUL P. Decreased amniotic fluid magnesium concentration in diabetic pregnancy. *Obstet Gynecol.* 1987;69:12.

133. MIMOUNI F, STEICHEN JJ, TSANG RC, HERTZBERG V, MIODOVNIK M. Decreased bone mineral content in infants of diabetic mothers: improvement by strict management of diabetes during pregnancy in a randomized, prospective trial. *Am J Perinatol.* 1988;5:339.

134. BLOOM SI, JOHNSTON DI. Failure of glucagon release in infants of gestational diabetic mothers. *Br Med J.* 1972;4:453.

135. MIMOUNI F, TSANG RC. Diabetes in pregnancy: perinatal magnesium metabolism. In: Gabbe SG, Oh W, eds. *Infant of the Diabetic Mother. Report of the 93rd Ross Conference on Pediatric Research.* Columbus, Ohio; 1987;124.

136. PEDERSEN J, BOJSEN-MØLLER B, POULSEN H. Blood sugar in newborn infants of diabetic mothers. *Acta Endocrinol.* 1954;15:33.

137. FARQUHAR JW. Hypoglycaemia in newborn infants of normal and diabetic mothers. *S Afr Med J.* 1968;42:237.

138. JORGENSEN KR, DECKERT T, MØLSTED-PEDERSEN L, PEDERSEN J. Insulin, insulin antibody and glucose in plasma of newborn infants of diabetic women. *Acta Endocrinol.* 1966;52:154.

139. JOASSIN G, PARKER ML, PILDES RS, CORNBLATH M. Infants of diabetic mothers. *Diabetes.* 1967;16:306.

140. SCHWARTZ R. Islet responsiveness of the human fetus *in utero.* In: Camerini-Davalos RS, Cole HS, eds. *Early Diabetes in Early Life.* New York: Academic Press, Inc., 1975;231.

141. KUHL C, WINKEL S, SKOVBY S, MOLSTED-PEDERSEN L, PEDERSEN J. Plasma glucose, insulin, and glucagon concentrations over the first 12 hours in infants of diabetic mothers (1977). Cited in Pedersen J, ed. *The Pregnant Diabetic and Her Newborn.* Baltimore: Williams & Wilkins, 1977;150.

142. KUHL C, ANDERSEN GE, HERTEL J, MØLSTED-PEDERSEN L. Metabolic events in infants of diabetic mothers during the first 24 hours after birth. I. Changes in plasma glucose, insulin and glucagon. *Acta Paediatr Scand.* 1982;71:19.

143. KALHAN SC, SCHWARTZ R, ADAM PAJ. Placental barrier to human insulin-I[125] in insulin dependent diabetic mothers. *J Clin Endocrinol Metab.* 1975;40:139.

144. BLOCK MB, PILDES RS, MOSSABHOY NA, STEINER DF, RUBENSTEIN AH. C-peptide immunoreactivity (CPR): A new method for studying infants of insulin-treated diabetic mothers. *Pediatrics.* 1974;53:923.

145. BRADLEY RJ. Cited in: Brudenell M, Doddridge MC, eds. *Diabetic pregnancy,* pg. 142; in series by Lind T, ed. *Current Reviews in Obstetrics and Gynaecology,* Edinburgh: Churchill Livingstone, 1989.

146. HEDING LG, PERSSON B, STANGENBERG M. Beta cell function in newborn infants of diabetic mothers. *Diabetologia.* 1980;19:427.

147. KALHAN SC, SAVIN SM, ADAM PAJ. Attenuated glucose production rate in newborn infants of insulin-dependent diabetic mothers. *N Engl J Med.* 1977;296:375.

148. COWETT RM, SUSA JB, GILETTI B, et al. Glucose kinetics in infants of diabetic mothers. *Am J Obstet Gynecol.* 1983;146:781.

149. KING KC, TSERNG K-Y, KALHAN SC. Regulation of glucose production in newborn infants of diabetic mothers. *Pediatr Res.* 1982;16:608.

150. MELICHAR V, NOVAK M, HAHN P, KOLDOVSKÝ O. Free fatty acids and glucose in the blood of various groups of newborns. Preliminary report. *Acta Paediatr.* 1964;53:343.

151. PERSSON B, GENTZ J, KELLUM M. Metabolic observations in infants of strictly controlled diabetic mothers. *Acta Paediatr Scand.* 1973; 62:465.

152. COCKBURN F, BLAGDEN A, MICHIE EA, FORFAR JO. The influence of pre-eclampsia and diabetes mellitus on plasma free amino acids in maternal, umbilical vein and infant blood. *J Obstet Gynecol Br Comm.* 1971;78:215.

153. PERSSON B, PSCHERA H, LUNELL N-O, BARLEY J, GUMAA KA. Amino acid concentrations in maternal plasma and amniotic fluid in relation to fetal insulin secretion during the last trimester of pregnancy in gestational and type I diabetic women and women with small-for-gestational-age infants. *Am J Perinatol.* 1986;3:98.

154. SOLTESZ G, SCHULTZ K, MESTYAN J, HORVATH I. Blood glucose and plasma amino acid concentrations in infants of diabetic mothers. *Pediatrics.* 1978;61:77.

155. HERTEL J, ANDERSEN GE, BRANDT NJ, CHRISTENSEN E, KUHL C, MOLSTED-PEDERSEN L. Metabolic events in infants of diabetic mothers during the first 24 hours after birth. *Acta Paediatr Scand.* 1982;71:33.

156. MCCORMICK KL, SUSA JB, WIDNESS JA, SINGER DB, ADAMSONS K, SCHWARTZ R. Chronic hyperinsulinemia in the fetal rhesus monkey. Effects on hepatic enzymes active in lipogenesis and carbohydrate metabolism. *Diabetes.* 1979;28:1064.

157. FARQUHAR JW. The possible influence of hyperadrenocorticism on the foetus of the diabetic woman. *Arch Dis Child.* 1956;31:483.

158. MIGEON CJ, NICOLOPOULOS D, CORNBLATH M. Concentrations of 17-hydroxycorticosteroids in the blood of diabetic mothers and in blood from umbilical cords of their offspring at the time of delivery. *Pediatrics.* 1960;25:605.

159. SMITH EK, REARDON HS, FIELD SH. Urinary constituents of infants of diabetic and non-diabetic mothers. I. 17-hydroxycorticosteroid excretion in premature infants. *J Pediatr.* 1964;64:652.

160. KALKHOFF R, SCHALCH DS, WALKER JL, BECK P, KIPNIS DM, DAUGHADAY WH. Diabetogenic factors associated with pregnancy. *Tr A Am Physicians.* 1964;77:270.

161. STERN L, RAMOS A, LEDUC J. Urinary catecholamine excretion in infants of diabetic mothers. *Pediatrics.* 1968;42:598.

162. YOUNG JB, COHEN WR, RAPPAPORT EB, LANDSBERG L. High plasma norepinephrine concentrations at birth in infants of diabetic mothers. *Diabetes.* 1979;28:697.

163. LUYCKX AS, MASSI-BENEDETTI F, FALORNI A, LEFEBVRE PJ. Presence of pancreatic glucagon in the portal plasma of human neonates. Differences in the insulin and glucagon responses to glucose between normal infants and infants from diabetic mothers. *Diabetologica.* 1972;8:296.

164. WILLIAMS PR, SPERLING MA, RACASA Z. Blunting of spontaneous and

alanine-stimulated glucagon secretion in newborn infants of diabetic mothers. *Am J Obstet Gynecol.* 1979;133:51.

165. SERRATTO M, CANTEZ T, HARRIS V, YEH T, PILDES R. Cardiac pulmonary and metabolic findings in infants of diabetic mothers. Presented to International Pediatric Conference, Buenos Aires, Argentina, 1974.

166. DAVIS WS, CAMPBELL JB. Neonatal small left colon syndrome. *Am J Dis Child.* 1975;129:1024.

167. WARRAM JH, KROLEWSKI AS, GOTTLIEB MS, KAHN CR. Differences in risk of insulin-dependent diabetes in offspring of diabetic mothers and diabetic fathers. *N Engl J Med.* 1984;311:149.

168. DiMARIO U, DOTTA F, GARGIULO P, et al. Immunology in diabetic pregnancy: activated T cells in diabetic mothers and neonates. *Diabetologia.* 1987;30:66.

169. YSSING M. Long-term prognosis of children born to mothers diabetic when pregnant. In: Camerini-Davalos RA, Cole HS, eds. *Early Diabetes in Early Life.* New York: Academic Press, Inc., 1975;575.

170. FARQUHAR JW. Prognosis for babies born to diabetic mothers in Edinburgh. *Arch Dis Child.* 1969;44:36.

171. VOHR B, LIPSITT LP, OH W. Somatic growth of children of diabetic mothers with reference to birth size. *J Pediatr.* 1980;97:196.

172. PETTIT DJ, BAIRD HR, ALECK KA, et al. Excessive obesity in offspring of Pima Indian women with diabetes during pregnancy. *N Engl J Med.* 1983;308:242.

173. YSSING M. Oestriol excretion in pregnant diabetics related to long-term prognosis of surviving children. *Acta Endocrinol.* 1974;(Suppl. 185) 75:95.

174. VOHR BR. Long-term follow-up of the infant of the diabetic mother. In: Gabbe S, Oh W, eds. *Report of the 93rd Ross Conference on Pediatric Research.* Columbus, Ohio: Ross Laboratories, 1987;159.

175. PETERSEN MB. Status at 4–5 years in 90 children of insulin-dependent diabetic mothers. In: Sutherland JW, Stowers JM, Pearson DWM, eds. *Carbohydrate Metabolism in Pregnancy and the Newborn. IV.* London: Springer-Verlag, 1989;353.

C H A P T E R 5

RECURRENT OR PERSISTENT NEONATAL HYPOGLYCEMIA

Although the least common of all types of hypoglycemia, the recurrent or persistent (>7 days) types of neonatal hypoglycemia are associated with the highest mortality and morbidity (Table 5-1). A precise pathophysiologic classification can usually be defined even though specific molecular defects are not yet known for each type. Those syndromes associated with hypoglycemia resulting either from hormone deficiencies or hormone excess, such as hyperinsulinemia, are presented here. For the hereditary defects in carbohydrate metabolism, see Chapters 7–9, and for those in amino acid or fatty acid metabolism, see Chapter 10. This classification provides one approach for diagnosis and therapy. Those manifestations unique to the newborn or neonate will be emphasized.

This category of neonatal hypoglycemia is defined as that which requires either infusions of large amounts of glucose (>12 mg/kg/min) at any time after birth to establish normoglycemia or which persists or recurs frequently beyond the first 7 to 14 days of life. These infants require specific diagnostic determinations, as well as a rapid trial of therapeutic-diagnostic agents to determine specific etiology and therapy [1,2].

Although the diagnosis of hypoglycemia mandates prompt restoration of normoglycemia, a diagnostic blood sample should be taken for the determination of plasma glucose, insulin, and beta-hydroxybutyrate concentrations (Table 5-2). This plasma sample should also be analyzed for growth hormone, ACTH, cortisol, T4, glucagon,

---

TABLE 5-1. Recurrent or persistent hypoglycemia

HORMONE DEFICIENCIES

Multiple Endocrine Deficiencies or Congenital Hypopituitarism, p. 180

"Aplasia" anterior pituitary	Hypothalamic hormone deficiencies
Hypoplastic pituitary	Midline CNS malformations
Congenital optic nerve hypoplasia	

Primary Endocrine Deficiency, p. 191

Growth hormone: isolated	Thyroid
ACTH: ACTH unresponsiveness	Epinephrine
Cortisol: (a) hemorrhage, (b) adrenogenital syndrome	Glucagon

---

HORMONE EXCESS HYPERINSULINISM

EMG syndrome of Beckwith-Wiedemann, p. 206
Islet cell adenoma, p. 193
Beta cell hyperplasia or dysplasia, p. 193
Adenomatosis, p. 193

HEREDITARY DEFECTS IN CARBOHYDRATE METABOLISM

Glycogen storage disease, type I, p. 251
Fructose intolerance, p. 327
Galactosemia, p. 299
Glycogen synthase deficiency, p. 282
Fructose, 1-6 diphosphatase deficiency, p. 357

HEREDITARY DEFECTS IN AMINO ACID METABOLISM

Maple syrup urine disease, p. 378
Propionic acidemia, p. 379
Methylmalonic acidemia, p. 379
Tyrosinosis, p. 381
3-hydroxy, 3-methyl glutaryl CoA lyase deficiency, p. 370

HEREDITARY DEFECTS IN FATTY ACID METABOLISM

Dehydrogenase—medium and long chain deficiency, p. 365

---

somatomedins (IGF-I and II), and other substrates such as lactate, pyruvate, uric acid, quantitative amino acids, especially glutamine and alanine. Blood samples obtained both before and after glucagon administration at the time when the patient is hypoglycemic can be diagnostic [2]. Urine collections for the determination of catecholamines, amino acids, organic acids, and specific reducing sugars should

TABLE 5-2.   The critical blood sample in hypoglycemia

SUBSTRATES	HORMONES
Glucose	Insulin
Beta-hydroxybutyrate	hGH
FFA	Cortisol
Lactate	Glucagon
Amino acids	TSH, T4, T3
alanine, glutamine	
Uric acid	

be done promptly. Specific intolerances to galactose (Chapter 8), fructose (Chapter 9), or leucine (Chapter 10) can be documented by eliminating these substances from the diet for 2 or 3 days [3] while definitive diagnostic tests are done. Glycogen storage disease, Type I (p. 251), and the exomphalos-macroglossia-gigantism syndrome of Beckwith-Wiedemann (p. 206) and leprechaunism (p. 208) usually have diagnostic physical stigmata, as do many neonates with congenital hypopituitarism (p. 187).

Along with infusions of glucose, the diagnostic-therapeutic trial should be initiated, as indicated in Table 5-3. As additional therapeutic courses are added, it is not necessary to discontinue the previous unsuccessful agent; e.g., the patient with hyperinsulinemic hypoglycemia may be given hydrocortisone, growth hormone, and diazoxide concurrently. During therapeutic trials, all blood samples collected to monitor glucose should also be assayed for insulin. With this approach, infants with serious resistant and intractable hypoglycemia due to hyperinsulinemia can benefit from definitive surgery as soon

TABLE 5-3.   Therapeutic-diagnostic trial for recurrent or persistent neonatal hypoglycemia

IN ADDITION TO IV GLUCOSE AT 12–14 MG/KG/MIN AND, IN SEQUENCE:

Trial	Agent	Dosage	Duration
1	Hydrocortisone (or)	15 mg/kg/day PO or IV	24 hours
	Prednisone	2 mg/kg/day PO	
2	Human growth hormone	1 U/day IM	2–3 days
3	Diazoxide	10–25 mg/kg/day PO TID	3–5 days
4	Somatostatin	8 μg/kg/hr IV	1–7 days
5	Glucagon	100 μg/kg IV or IM	2–3 hours
6	Susphrine	0.01 ml/kg/6 hours IM	12–24 hours
7	Surgery	For proven hyperinsulinism	

as medical failure is evident or as early as 2 to 3 weeks after birth. As soon as an endocrine deficiency or metabolic error is identified, specific therapy can be initiated promptly.

• Hormone Deficiencies

Multiple Hormone Deficiencies or Congenital Hypopituitarism Syndromes

Multiple hormone deficiencies have been associated with severe, even fatal, hypoglycemia during the first days of life, and the concepts of their origin and pathogenesis have expanded significantly within this past decade. Previously, the congenital hypopituitarism was attributed to either hypothalamic hormone deficiencies [4,5] or "aplasia" [6], or hypoplasia [7–10] of the anterior pituitary gland. It is now well established from a number of case reports [11–15] and series [16–22] that a similar clinical picture can be associated with congenital optic nerve hypoplasia (CONH), both unilateral and bilateral, with or without agenesis of the septum pellucidum or other structural abnormalities of the brain (compare Tables 5-4 and 5-5). Currently, advanced imaging techniques of the CNS, pituitary, and optic nerves, as well as the specificity and ready availability of sensitive endocrine hormone assays have resulted in the recognition of a number of syndrome complexes associated with a variety of pituitary malfunctions.

A source of case finding is the universal newborn screening currently used to detect phenylketonuria (PKU), hypothyroidism, galactosemia, and maple syrup urine disease (MSUD) [43]. Over a 10-year period, the Northwest Regional Screening Program (NRSP) screened 850,431 infants for hypothyroidism [43]. They detected 192 infants with primary hypothyroidism (1:4,500) and 8 with hypopituitary hypothyroidism (1:100,000). In addition, 11 other infants were recognized clinically and diagnosed as congenital hypopituitarism. Of this total of 19, there were 12 females and 7 males, and 16 had multiple pituitary hormone deficiencies. Of note, all who were tested were found to be hGH deficient. Fourteen (~75 percent) had hypoglycemia, and 7 (~40 percent) had persistent jaundice. Of the 7 males, 5 (~70 percent) had microgenitalia. Seven infants (~35 percent) had CONH, of whom 6 fit into the syndrome of septo-optic dysplasia. Cleft lip or cleft palate was present in 5 patients (~25 percent), 4 of whom also had midface hypoplasia. Thus, congenital hypopituitarism detected by screening for hypothyroidism represents a complex problem.

In this study population, then, the frequency of congenital hy-

TABLE 5-4. Congenital optic nerve hypoplasia (CONH)
(septo-optic dysplasia [23,24], septo-optic-pituitary dysplasia [20])

YEAR	AUTHOR, SUMMARY
1864–1970	
1864 [25]	Newman, absent optic discs
1941 [23]	Reeves, septo-optic dysplasia
1956 [24]	De Morsier, septo-optic dysplasia plus agenesis septum pellucidum
1970–1980	
1970 [11]	Kaplan, Grumbach, Hoyt, *growth failure*
1975 [13]	Patel et al., clinical constellations: neonatal apnea, *hypoglycemia,* jaundice, seizures, hypotonia
1979 [14,15]	Friesen, Holmgaard; Gendrel, Chaussin, Job, variations in visual acuity, asymmetric nerve atrophy, multiple associated CNS and/or neuro-endocrine abnormalities: hypoglycemia, jaundice, midline abnormalities
1980–present	
1984 [16]	Skarf, Hoyt, CONH 41-bilateral blind-78% nonocular developmental involvement: *neonatal hypoglycemia* (6%), 11-unilateral and 41-bilateral segmental—good vision—21% nonocular; abnormal development (25%)
1984 [17]	Margalith et al., "young mothers," toxemia, *40 = AGA, 4 = SGA, 7 = LGA, 6 = hypoglycemia, 10 = jaundice, 9 = seizures;* 19 = no problems; cerebral palsy (29), mental retardation [(36) 15 = severe and profound], neuroradiological findings; 35 of 38 abnormal
1985 [18]	Margalith et al., hypothalamic—pituitary, abnormalities in 16 of CONH group [17]; hypoglycemia in 80%; GH deficient 75%
1986 [20]	Morishima, Aranoff, 4 cases diverse presentation, 2 of 4 neonatal hypoglycemia; reviewed 191 bilateral septo-optic-pituitary case reports: 60% CT abnormalities; 62% hypopituitarism; 30% both abnormal CT and hypopituitarism

popituitarism was 1:45,000. However, in Oregon, Hanna et al. [43] estimated a frequency of 1:29,000, based on 5 infants detected by the NRSP and 10 by clinical presentation of a total of 430,000 screened. This represents almost a fourfold increase over the frequency of 1:100,000 estimated at the Second International Conference on Neonatal Screening [48].

The clinical presentation of this variety of syndromes clearly indicates the need for an endocrine-metabolic workup in every neonate, infant, and child with optic nerve hypoplasia or a congenital abnormality detected by a computed tomography (CT) scan, MRI, or ultrasound of the brain. A CT scan and a careful retinal examination should be performed in anyone diagnosed with hypopituitarism as a

TABLE 5-5. Hypopituitarism (aplasia, hypoplasia, familial, congenital, perinatal)

YEAR	AUTHOR, SUMMARY
Before 1960	
1953	Steiner [26], rare dwarfism, chronic *hypoglycemia* (1965 [27] autopsy age 17 years) aplasia
1956	Mosier [10], twin girl, hypoplasia
	Blizzard, Alberts [28], aplasia, microphallus
1957	Brewer [29], aplasia
	Erhlich [9], ectopic pituitary
1960–1975	
1960	Reid [30], congenital absence
1964	Cornblath [7], male, *hypoglycemia*, jaundice, exchange hypoplasia pituitary, adrenal, testes, died 17 months of endocardial fibroelastosis
1966	Dunn [31], aplasia of pituitary and adrenal
1972	Moncrieff et al. [32], aplasia, micropenis as marker
	Willard et al. [33,34], 2 brothers, aplasia—familial
1973	Johnson et al. [8], 3 patients, jaundice, exchange, blind (1)
1974	Sadeghi-Nejad, Senior [6], familial, estriol for prenatal diagnosis, *prior neonatal death*, suggest congenital hypopituitarism, CONH, septo-optic-dysplasia, multiple CNS abnormalities, anencephaly, a continuum
1975	Lovinger, Kaplan, Grumbach [4], showed hypothalamic hormone deficiency
1975	Herman et al. [35], emphasized conjugated *hyperbilirubinemia*

neonate or infant. The association of elevated bilirubin values and particularly conjugated bilirubin with intractable or recurrent hypoglycemia [13] and hypopituitarism or septo-optic-pituitary dysplasia should alert physicians and prevent delays in diagnosis [42] and specific therapy, and even deaths [39].

Central nervous system, midline (medial cleft palate syndrome [15]), genital (microphallus in the male), optic, and growth abnormalities usually do not require immediate attention. Nevertheless, the severe recurrent hypoglycemia, often unresponsive to intravenous glucose alone, the persistent jaundice primarily due to conjugated bilirubin, and the frequently associated hypothyroidism [43] emphasize the importance of early recognition and therapy.

Congenital Optic Nerve Hypoplasia (CONH)

CONH/septo-optic-pituitary dysplasia appear to reflect a large number of syndromes of varying severity including DeMorsier syndrome, septo-optic pituitary dysplasia, and absent septum pellucidum syn-

TABLE 5-5. Continued

YEAR	AUTHOR, SUMMARY
After 1975	
1978	Lanes et al. [36], with conjugated hyperbilirubinemia, giant cell transformation liver biopsy (1)
	Hall [37], hypoplasia in Russell-Silver syndrome
1979	Drop et al. [38], liver functions abnormal for 5–8 months, *hypoglycemia for months*
	Kauschansky et al. [39], female association with hypoglycemia and hypothyroidism
1980	von Petrykowski et al. [40], septo-optic with hypopituitarism
1981	Copeland et al. [41], emphasis on hyperbilirubin
	Gendrel et al. [15], 14 patients includes optic atrophy (7), hypoglycemia (8), micropenis (5 of 10)
1984	Salisbury, Leonard [42], "lesson of week" in *BMJ:* 2 males with micropenis, *recurrent hypoglycemia* diagnosed 4 months (1), hypoglycemia worse with thyroid RX—finally HGH
1986	Hanna et al. [43], utilizing Northwest Regional Screening Program; data on hypopituitary hypothyroidism: 8 infants (1:100,000) 1975–1985; 11 others recognized; both resulted in 1:29,000 frequency; 7 males, 12 females; 7 CONH or septo-optic dysplasia
1988	Costello, Gluckman [22], increasing numbers, 50% CONH; craniofacial and neurological features, especially seizures; hyperbilirubinemia, hypoglycemia, microphallus
	Ruvalcaba [44], with CHARGE association
	Kristjansson et al. [45], with Johanson-Blizzard syndrome
1989	McQueen, Copeland [46], free water intolerance and lack of thymic involution
	Lischka, Herkner, Pollak [47], hypoglycemia, micropenis, GH deficiency and peripheral androgen insensitivity

dromes. It is beyond the scope of this book to include all of these associations [see 16,17,20,21 for recent reviews].

A number of hypotheses have been proposed as to the etiology and pathogenesis of the CONH [13,16,17,21]. Most appear to be idiopathic in origin. Correlations to varying degrees, however slight, have been found with young mothers, firstborn infants, in utero cytomegalic infections, genetic factors, congenital cysts or tumors of the anterior visual pathways, and porencephalic cysts. Maternal use of quinine, LSD, anticonvulsants (mainly phenytoin), or alcohol and other illicit drugs has also been implicated, along with maternal diabetes mellitus, toxemia, polyhydramnios, anaphylactoid shock [17], and blunt trauma [17], as causative factors in optic nerve hypoplasia. The high frequency (33 percent) of perinatal asphyxia in these infants suggests that some cases may be secondary to untoward perinatal events.

Originally, the insult was presumed to occur at about 4 to 6 weeks gestation (13–15 mm stage of embryogenesis) with failure of the differentiation of retinal ganglion cells, along with the development of the septum pellucidum and pituitary gland. However, autopsy material and extensive neuroradiological studies indicate that many other areas of the brain, in addition to the midline structures, may be involved as well. In contrast, many now support Friesen and Holmegaard's [14] hypothesis proposed in 1978 that CONH should be considered a secondary atrophic process of optic nerve fibers occurring any time before full development of the visual pathways and the eye. This theory suggests that embryogenesis of the retina proceeds normally, and at a later stage, either coincident with or after the normal phase of ganglion cell death, a far greater number than normal degenerate as a result of a nonspecific insult or insults to the brain. This presumably prevents the ganglion cells from forming or maintaining appropriate connections at their target sites and can be manifest as optic nerve hypoplasia.

Anomalies, other than those of the CNS, have also been reported in these syndromes, adding to the complexity of understanding causation. Unilateral CONH or segmented bilateral atrophy with good vision and either no other CNS anomalies or those attributed to perinatal asphyxia support the possibility that perinatal degeneration of optic-nerve axons and the ganglion cells in the retina does occur [16,17,20,21]. Margalith et al. [17] concluded: "Obviously, the degree of CONH and the associated CNS and/or other malformations would be determined by the time during embryogenesis when the insult occurs and by the aetiological factors producing the insult."

The clinical presentation of CONH depends on the severity of the loss of vision, the associated anomalies in the CNS and elsewhere, the presence of hypopituitarism, with either isolated or multiple deficiencies, and the age of the patient.

In 1975, in one of the first reports emphasizing the association among CONH, hypopituitarism, hypoglycemia, and hyperbilirubinemia, Patel et al. [13] provided a useful guide to the clinical picture at different ages.

> In the newborn period there may be apnea, hypotonia, hypoglycemia, with or without seizures, and hyperbilirubinemia. . . .
>
> At the age of 3 months, patients have hypotonia, psychomotor retardation, defective visual fixation, and seizures. A firm, nontender liver may be palpable, and, in one case, there was mild jaundice. A receding lower jaw, and occasionally, a high-arched palate may be present. The general appearance is otherwise nor-

mal. The fasting blood glucose level may be mildly depressed, and results of the liver function tests may be abnormal.

The older child in this series had psychomotor retardation, growth failure, defective vision, and seizures.

Margalith et al. [17], in 1984, analyzed the prenatal course, labor and delivery, neonatal course, and outcome of 51 children with CONH, of whom 48 had bilateral hypoplasia. Presenting symptoms included impaired vision (60 percent), searching eye movements (29 percent), and strabismus (8 percent), often in combination. In contrast, 29 percent presented with nonocular symptoms, including a stormy neonatal course and neurological or endocrine problems. Thirty-seven (72 percent) were diagnosed during the first year of life, but only four, during the neonatal period, indicated the need for a higher index of suspicion for this entity in neonates with unusual problems (see Case Report 5-1, p. 192).

Maternal age was known in only 33 patients and parity in 46. Of these, half were less than 20 years of age and half were primipara. Abnormalities of gestation in 48 included toxemia, bleeding, drug and alcohol abuse, premature (<37 wks) and postmature (>42 wks) delivery. Only 13 of 48 had an uneventful pregnancy.

None of the abnormalities of labor and delivery in 48 pregnancies occurred in a greater frequency than that of all deliveries in British Columbia in 1980.

More than half of a total of 44 had neonatal problems including resuscitation, apneic and cyanotic spells, respiratory difficulties, and electrolyte disturbances. Six (14 percent) had hypoglycemia diagnosed at a mean age of 16 hours (range 8–36 hours) *with blood glucose concentrations of 9 to 27 mg/dl (0.5 to 1.5 mM)*. Hypoglycemia was associated with seizures in four patients and with maternal diabetes in one. Seizures unrelated to hypoglycemia occurred in five additional neonates. Jaundice was noted in ten infants and was treated by phototherapy in four infants and by exchange transfusions in one. No apparent cause for the jaundice could be found.

Systemic congenital anomalies such as dysmorphic features were common, occurring in a third of the children. Major malformations were seen in only two cases, one with arthrogryposis multiplex congenita and one with neurofibromatosis. While only six infants had neonatal hypoglycemia (supra vide), 75 percent of the entire group had neuropsychiatric and developmental handicaps. Of the 51 children, 29 had cerebral palsy of every type, 36 were mentally retarded (15 profoundly and 8 moderately), and 19 had epilepsy. This is not surprising in view of the large number of abnormal neuroradiological findings in this group as well as those reported in the literature (see recent summary [21] and review [20]). Of 38 patients studied, 90 percent had abnormalities, including the expected anterior midline developmental defects, in addition to encephaloclastic lesions of the developing brain. The latter included hydranencephaly, porencephaly, cerebral and cerebellar atrophy. Other abnormalities included gross brain malformations, cerebral infarcts, and congenital communicating hydrocephalus.

Of 51 children, 31 had growth retardation and one, precocious puberty. Twenty-one had an endocrine workup, and 19 were found to be abnormal. Three (one with IDDM and two with acquired hypothyroidism) may have been unrelated to CONH. The other 16 [18] included a wide variety of abnormalities, more from deficiencies than from hypersecretion of trophic hormones. Three children had single and six had multiple trophic hormone deficiencies. Eleven were growth hormone deficient, two had central diabetes insipidus, and six had panhypopituitarism.

Additional studies in considering a differential diagnosis included: normal karyotypes in 13 chromosomal studies; no abnormalities in the concentrations of plasma amino acids or urine amino acids, sugars, ketoacids, and mucopolysaccharides in 22; torch titers were positive in 1 and STS in none of 14 children investigated. One had a significantly high titer for cytomegalovirus (CMV) and a high value for specific IgM.

In another study, 93 children referred to a Children's Eye Clinic between July 1977 and May 1982 were diagnosed with optic nerve hypoplasia and became participants in a prospective study utilizing CT scans and neurologic and endocrine evaluations, with a complete laboratory investigation of endocrine function after the first birthday. This report is from the Department of Ophthalmology only [16]. The patients were divided into 3 groups: 41 in Group 1 had bilateral CONH, poor vision, and nystagmus; 11 in Group 2 had unilateral CONH; and 41 in Group 3 had bilateral segmental CONH and/or good vision. The pertinent findings in this study are summarized in Table 5-4 and Figure 5-1. The endocrine, neurological, and other nonocular CNS abnormalities were associated with the more severe involvement in Group 1, as reported by others. The 46 percent frequency of developmental delay, 41 percent of endocrine abnormalities, and 10 percent of neonatal hypoglycemia do not differ significantly from those reported from Vancouver [17,18]. These complications occurred less frequently in Groups 2 and 3.

Recognizing the importance of bilateral CONH, Morishima and Aranoff summarized the frequency of associated CNS abnormalities and hypopituitarism in 195 such patients reported since 1980, including 4 of their own [20]. Sixty percent had CT abnormalities, 62

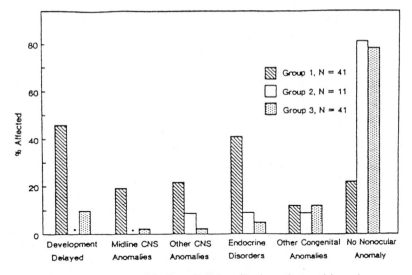

FIGURE 5-1. Summary of findings in 93 pediatric patients with optic nerve hypoplasia. Group 1 included patients with bilateral optic nerve hypoplasia, nystagmus, and poor vision; group 2, unilateral hypoplasia; and group 3, segmental hypoplasia and/or good visual acuity without nystagmus. Percentage of patients in each group with specific developmental disorders is indicated by height of bars. Asterisk indicates that no patients in that column were affected. (From Skarf and Hoyt. *Arch Ophthalmol* 1984; 102:65. Copyright 1984, American Medical Association.)

percent had hypopituitarism, and approximately 30 percent had a combination of both CT abnormalities and hypopituitarism.

With CONH, the frequency of hypoglycemia appears to be associated with the severity of the hormone deficiencies, usually derived from hypothalamic pituitary insufficiency. The high incidence of neurologic and developmental disabilities is related to the underlying cerebral developmental anomalies. The contribution of hypoglycemia to outcome appears to be minimal.

Congenital Hypopituitarism Syndromes

Congenital hypopituitarism syndromes now should include the caveat "without optic nerve hypoplasia" to distinguish these patients from the groups discussed above (Table 5-4). Beginning with less specific presenting symptoms than blindness and nystagmus, these infants and children appear to be fewer in number than those with the CONH complex. However, to further complicate matters, congenital hypopituitarism has been reported in association with a number of other syndromes, e.g., Russell-Silver [37,49], midline craniofacial defect with

CHARGE association [44], peripheral androgen insensitivity [47], and Johanson-Blizzard syndrome of aplasia of the alae nasi, deafness, dwarfism, and hypothyroidism (see [45] for review) (Table 5-5). Discussion of these entities are beyond the scope of this book. It should be emphasized that recurrent hypoglycemia, which is difficult to control, deserves an endocrine workup measuring growth hormone, cortisol, thyroid and insulin hormones during the episode of low blood glucose concentration. A detailed CT scan or MRI of the CNS to detect congenital anomalies is also indicated.

Congenital hypopituitarism alone or in combination with other anomalies has been more readily recognized during this past decade. Yet its etiology and pathogenesis still remain unclear. While aplasia of the gland may be a continuation of the process implicated in CONH (supra vide), the causes of hypoplasia or isolated hormone deficiency or the hypothalamic defects are essentially unknown. The recent statistical implication of untoward perinatal events such as breech births, forceps deliveries, abnormal birth weights and male gender as etiological factors in children with symptomatic growth hormone deficiency in England, Wales [50], and the Netherlands [51] does not appear relevant in this group of neonates. The presence of the microphallus, for example, in some 65 percent of the males would imply intrauterine problems dating to the second trimester. The high frequency of hyperbilirubinemia, often with an elevated conjugated component, implicates both hGH and thyroid deficiencies of some duration prior to birth [52]. These deficiencies together can explain both the hyperbilirubinemia and the giant cell transformation of the liver noted at biopsy [36].

In contrast, a number of additional problems have been identified with reasonable frequency in these babies to alert the physician to the possibility of hypopituitarism (Fig. 5-2). Infants with symptomatic hypoglycemia, hyperbilirubinemia (often conjugated [53]), microphallus in males [54], and midline defects especially in girls [15] have often been LGA (25 percent > 95th percentile) [55,56]. They also have thrombocytopenia alone or associated with other hematologic abnormalities, and tested abnormal on the neonatal screen for T4 [43,55,56]. Recently, free water intolerance and a lack of thymic involution was noted as well [46]. A critical blood sample (Table 5-2) during a hypoglycemic episode, followed by a prompt response to the Diagnostic-Therapeutic Trial (Table 5-3) after the addition of cortisol and biosynthetic hGH, should establish the diagnosis.

Therapy consists of adequate amounts of parenteral glucose (10–12 mg/kg/min), to which is added cortisol when the glucose values cannot be maintained over 50 mg/dl (2.8 mM) with glucose alone. If

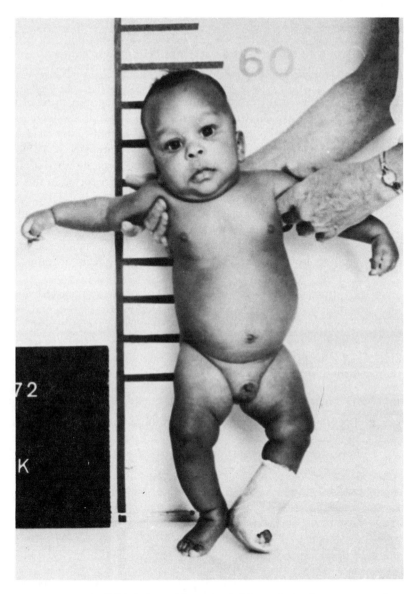

FIGURE 5-2. An LGA infant with congenital hypopituitarism at one week of age. Note the microphallus and club foot.

hypoglycemia still recurs, biosynthetic GH is added to the regimen. It is noteworthy that recurrent hypoglycemia has been reported even after cortisol was added to the therapy, and normoglycemia was restored only after the addition of GH.

Prognosis

As noted previously, whether considering these entities separately or as a continuum, the prognosis is guarded at best [22,55]. In the CONH septo-optic dysplasia series, systemic congenital anomalies such as dysmorphic features were common, occurring in a third of the children. Neuropsychiatric and developmental handicaps were present in approximately 75 percent of patients. Cerebral palsy of every type, mental retardation, and epilepsy were common (see p. 185).

This is not surprising in view of the large number of abnormal neuroradiological findings in this group and reported in the literature (see recent summary and review by Morishima and Aranoff [20]). These include anterior midline developmental defects, encephaloclastic lesions of the developing brain (hydranencephaly, porencephaly, cerebral and cerebellar atrophy), and other abnormalities such as gross brain malformations, cerebral infarcts, and congenital communicating hydrocephalus.

In the 17 cases of congenital hypopituitarism reviewed since 1975, 3 patients died (18 percent). Several show developmental and intellectual problems at various ages after diagnosis, in addition to their multiple endocrine deficiencies.

The poor prognosis reported is not unexpected as these syndromes become more carefully defined through the use of CT scans, MRI, and PET scanning. The numerous congenital malformations of the brain, macro- and microscopic, being recognized by the neuroradiologist and the pathologist are impressive. The recurrent symptomatic hypoglycemia, inadequately treated without GH therapy, also may affect the outcome.

Future Studies

Early recognition, close coupling with the hypothyroid screening programs, rapid diagnosis, and adequate therapy should improve the outcome for these patients.

Studies to better understand the etiology and pathogenesis of the multitude of these syndromes is clearly needed. Certainly, every neonate, infant, or child considered to have congenital hypopituitarism must have a thorough ophthalmologic, neurologic, and neuroradiologic examination to rule out CONH or septo-optic dysplasia. Similarly, all infants diagnosed as having CONH or any midline abnormality must have a thorough evaluation of their pituitary function and glucose homeostasis.

Primary Endocrine Deficiency

An isolated deficiency of almost every endocrine secretion directly involved in carbohydrate homeostasis or energy metabolism has been associated with or implicated in neonatal hypoglycemia. However, in the majority of infants, the hypoglycemia was often mild and transient and provided a clue suggesting the need for an endocrinologic investigation. This form of hypoglycemia has been reported in patients with isolated growth hormone deficiency [56,57] or hypothyroidism or with adrenal medullary or cortical insufficiency [58–61]. In contrast, patients with congenital glucagon deficiency have recurrent or persistent neonatal hypoglycemia [62,63]. Children with isolated growth hormone deficiency [57,64–66] have an increased frequency of hypoglycemia later in infancy, as do those with congenital ACTH unresponsiveness [67,68], but rarely in the neonatal period.

On the other hand, adrenal insufficiency regardless of etiology [58–60,68,69,70] has been associated with neonatal hypoglycemia. This is especially true in those neonates with adrenal hemorrhage or born to mothers on high-dose corticosteroid treatment during pregnancy. Defective catecholamine responses to hypoglycemia have also been observed in both the neonate [71] and throughout infancy [65,66,70].

Recent reviews [72] and reports [73] have elucidated the specific areas on the chromosomes involved in the genetic transmission, as well as the basic gene defects in a variety of adrenogenital syndromes [72] and in familial forms of isolated growth hormone deficiency [73].

Glucagon Deficiency

Although previous reports [74,75] had postulated glucagon deficiency as a cause of hypoglycemia, Vidnes and Oyasaeter [62] established the fact that glucagon deficiency does occur and was responsible for recurrent neonatal hypoglycemia in a boy born to closely related Pakistani parents. While the neonatal hypoglycemia was easily managed with parenteral glucose, severe hypoglycemia recurred at 3 months of age and required parenteral glucagon to control. Glucagon (0.1 mg zinc protamine glucagon per kg body weight) increased the rate of gluconeogenesis and lipolysis, while the concentrations of alanine in plasma decreased. Another male infant, also born in 1975, was subsequently reported from Amsterdam [63] with a similar course and response to zinc-protamine-glucagon. Glucagon levels were significantly low on several occasions. The response to glucagon was dramatic, and a relapse occurred when glucagon was discontinued by the parents. At age 16 months, motor development was that of an 11-month-old. Both reports establish glucagon deficiency as an entity that must be considered in the differential diagnosis of persistent or recurrent hypoglycemia in the neonate.

Case Report (Patient 5-1): CONH with Hypopituitarism Complicated by Severe Respiratory Distress

B.J. was a full-term female infant born to a 25-year-old white primipara. Pregnancy was complicated by intrauterine growth retardation. Labor and delivery were uneventful. After a spontaneous vaginal delivery, she had Apgar scores of 5 and 8 at 1 and 5 minutes. There was meconium staining. While the weight (2,550 gm) and length (45 cm) were less than the tenth percentile, head circumference (35.8 cm) was at the ninetieth percentile. Mild hydro-cephalus was noted. Her father had a congenital arrested hydrocephalus.

At one hour after birth, a Dextrostix (read by reflectance meter) was 16 mg/dl (0.9 mM) with a laboratory serum glucose of 26 mg/dl (1.4 mM). Parenteral glucose was given at 8 mg/kg/min shortly after birth. She devel-oped respiratory distress that became rapidly and progressively more severe. A trial of surfactant was ineffective. At 12 hours of age, she was transferred from the local hospital to a level 3 NICU for further evaluation and care.

On admission, physical examination revealed bilateral colobomata, low-set ears, an anteriorly displaced anus and hepatosplenomegaly. An ultrasound of the head indicated absence of the corpus callosum with moderately en-larged ventricles. Repeated glucose screening values were below 30–45 mg/dl (1.7–2.5 mM), finally requiring 18 mg/kg/min of glucose to avoid hypo-glycemia. Values of serum glucose below 25 mg/dl (1.4 mM) were not unu-sual at lower rates of glucose infusion. Jaundice was noted, with a maximum serum total bilirubin of 13.8 mg/dl at 5 days of age.

The respiratory distress and pulmonary failure continued to progress relentlessly even with ventilator support, the use of pressor agents, and vol-ume expanders over the next few days. Arterial blood gases continued to deteriorate and, in spite of high PIP, oxygenation could not be sustained. She required ECMO support for a period of 5 days, but remained ventilator dependent for 50 days and then was gradually weaned to room air.

Cardiovascular instability persisted as well. She was treated for poor perfusion with pressor agents and volume expanders on several occasions. She had a patent ductus arteriosus ligation at 17 days of age.

In view of the serious respiratory and cardiac problems, further investi-gation of the etiology of the recurrent hypoglycemia was delayed.

Routine neonatal metabolic screening was abnormal for T4 (< 2 mcg/dl [normal > 6.5]) and TSH (< 2.1 μU/ml). This prompted an extensive endocrine investigation, which revealed the following results: serum glucose 23 mg/dl (1.3 mM), serum Na 145 mEq/L, cortisol 3 mcg/dl (normal > 15 with low glucose level), growth hormone 0.15 ng/ml, cholesterol 172 mg/dl (normal 0–132), triglycerides 207 mg/dl and concentrations of plasma amino acids were normal. Urine amino acids and organic acids were not abnormal. Urine specific gravity varied between 1.002 and 1.006. Chromosome studies were normal. A CT scan of the head showed the absence of the corpus cal-losum and moderate diffuse cerebral atrophy.

Her clinical course, in addition to her cardiopulmonary problems, was complicated by feeding intolerance, requiring total parenteral nutrition (TPN) for some 6 weeks, as well as the high infusion rate of glucose (18 mg/kg/min). She also had seizures, both with and without hypoglycemia, temperature instability, and two suspected episodes of sepsis that were treated with antibiotics. The lumbar punctures provided clear cerebrospinal fluid with only an elevated protein content. All cultures were negative.

The diagnosis of panhypopituitarism was based on low TSH, cortisol, and growth hormone values and clinical evidence of persistent, recurring hypoglycemia and hypothyroidism. She was treated with both thyroid and steroid replacement but was not treated with growth hormone.

She responded promptly and within days tolerated oral feedings of Pregestimil and was weaned off her intravenous glucose infusion. An ophthalmologic examination confirmed bilateral colobomata with extensive involvement of the choroid, retina, and optic nerve. A repeat EEG was normal and showed no seizure activity. Still hospitalized at 57 days of age, she continued to improve slowly.

Comment

This infant illustrates the complex problems that the newborn with congenital optic nerve hypoplasia, absent corpus callosum, and panhypopituitarism may present in the hours and days after birth. The recurrent and resistant hypoglycemia in the presence of optic anomalies, hepatomegaly, and hyperbilirubinemia should have prompted obtaining the critical blood sample before and after glucagon (see p. 178) at one of the times when the infant was hypoglycemic. Analysis of the concentrations of hormones in that sample could have established the diagnosis. However, the life-threatening cardiopulmonary problems that required constant surveillance and finally ECMO support clearly assumed priority over any other considerations.

This patient represents the fourth seen in consultation in the past 3 years whose diagnosis of congenital hypopituitarism was first suspected when the routine newborn screening test for thyroid function was abnormal.

• Hyperinsulinemic (Organic) Hypoglycemia

For over 50 years, infants with recurrent or intractable hypoglycemia have presented as difficult diagnostic and therapeutic problems. While advances in diagnosis and aggressive therapy have occurred during the past two decades, challenges still remain in understanding the pathogenesis, in identifying the disorder and in developing pharmacologic agents or better surgical techniques to minimize ongoing problems. While survival has improved dramatically, definitive studies of prognosis remain to be done.

Table 5-6 identifies major events in the history of this complex neonatal problem. Subtotal pancreatectomy was introduced by Graham and Hartmann [76] but was reserved for infants who could not be managed by the medical techniques of the time. Hyperinsulinism was inferred from histological studies and physiologic parameters such as excessive glucose requirements to prevent seizures. On this basis, Talbot and associates [77] administered alloxan, a beta-cytotropic agent, but side effects were sufficiently marked to discourage further use. Later, a similar agent, streptozotocin, was used in adult pancreatic islet carcinoma [78], but not in infants and children.

The major advance in diagnosis occurred in 1960 when Yalow and Berson [79] described the radioimmunoassay of insulin, thus setting the stage for micro (50 µl) and subsequently rapid analysis of plasma insulin concentration in infants. The simultaneous analysis of plasma glucose and insulin has permitted rapid diagnosis (within 1–2 days) and thus early use of definitive therapy.

Medical therapy initially depended upon agents such as epinephrine, susphrine, and ephedrine to suppress insulin secretion. Subsequently, the most effective has been diazoxide, the insulin-inhibiting effect of which was recognized by Wolff and Parmeley in 1963 [80]. Pharmacologic agents such as somatostatin and/or glucagon have permitted preoperative stabilization but have not provided long-term effective therapy.

As surgical outcome improved, due in large measure to pediatric anesthesia and supportive perioperative care, major infections long after the surgery were recognized as a problem in splenectomized patients. In 1966, Ellis and Smith [81] described the role of the spleen in immunity and as protection against the risk of sepsis. Thereafter, preservation of the spleen became an important additional goal of surgery. Because subtotal pancreatectomy was not consistently successful, Harken et al. [82] in 1971 strongly recommended near-total

---

TABLE 5-6. Time line for hyperinsulinemic hypoglycemia

1934	Subtotal pancreatectomy recommended by Graham and Hartmann
1948	Chemical ablation of the beta cells by alloxan by Talbot et al.
1960	Radioimmunoassay for insulin developed by Yalow and Berson
1963	Diazoxide discovered as inhibitor of insulin secretion by Wolff and Parmeley
1966	Recognition of the role of the spleen in immunity by Ellis and Smith
1971	Near-total pancreatectomy emphasized by Harken et al.
1980 +	Newer pharmacologic agents (somatostatin, glucagon) as adjunctive therapy

(95–99 percent) or total pancreatectomy. In the subsequent 15 years, this form of aggressive therapy has become accepted at early stages (weeks) after diagnosis and failed medical therapy.

During the past decade, the use of immunohistochemistry and electron microscopy has required a revision in the interpretation of the pathologic diagnosis. In contrast, the advances in diagnostic radiologic techniques have been disappointing.

The frequency of hyperinsulinemic hypoglycemia is unknown. While a number of medically managed patients treated with diazoxide exist unreported, the numbers are probably significantly less than those treated surgically. Thomas [83] thoroughly analyzed the reported surgical experiences from 1934–1977 and from 1977–1987. His populations included infants with an onset from birth to one year. Prior to 1965, neonates were not included in the surgical experience, whereas in the past decade they have predominated. Birth weights have been normal or increased. Both sexes are affected, and familial occurrence has been reported. These characteristics occur independently of the pathological diagnosis. Thus, the summary of Rich et al. [84] of distinct islet-cell adenoma (31 cases) is similar to those with "nesidioblastosis"[1] or islet cell adenomatosis [83].

Aggressive, early surgical intervention is no assurance of a successful outcome. In the past decade, of 12 infants who have been operated on as early as 5–18 days after birth, 10 were reported with normal mental status. However, 5 had seizures, 1 was retarded, and another died [83]. This limited outcome may relate to the severity and duration of the hypoglycemia or to other congenital factors. There are inadequate data to quantify these relationships.

There has been an evolution of interpretation of the microscopic findings associated with hyperinsulinemic hypoglycemia. Following the description by Laidlaw in 1938 [85] of "nesidioblastosis" and by Yakovac et al. in 1971 [86] of "beta cell nesidioblastosis," the predominate diagnosis for these problems has become "nesidioblastosis." This pathologic term has also been used indiscriminately for the clinical entity. In recent years, pediatric pathologists utilizing immunohistochemistry, quantitative histochemistry, and electron microscopy have reassessed this problem with appropriate age-matched controls [87]. The predominant opinion currently is that "nesidioblastosis" is a normal developmental stage in the maturation of the pancreas. (See below for details of pathology.)

---

[1]In view of the controversy concerning the significance of nesidioblastosis, this term will be given in quotation marks throughout this text.

Diagnostic Studies

Diagnostic studies must document the hypoglycemia and the hyper-insulinemia. This is best achieved by analyzing simultaneously obtained plasma samples for insulin and glucose concentrations at the time of clinical manifestations as well as pre- and postfeeding on multiple occasions. Hypoglycemia rarely poses problems in interpretation. In those reported, the blood glucose levels were less than 35 mg/dl (1.9 mM) and frequently were 20 mg/dl (1.1 mM) or less. In contrast, hyperinsulinemia may be relative rather than absolute. Thus, a slight elevation of fasting plasma insulin concentration with a markedly reduced plasma glucose concentration may be diagnostic. This relationship has been quantified by the insulin (μU/ml) to glucose (mg/dl) ratio which does not exceed 0.30 in the normal infant, child, or adult under basal conditions [88]. For example, a plasma glucose of 10 mg/dl (0.56 mM) associated with a plasma insulin of 6 μU/ml (36 pM, a level considered normal) results in a ratio of 0.60 which is clearly abnormal. The Minnesota group [84] has suggested that modifying the ratio has improved its discrimination: corrected insulin/ glucose ratio: $\dfrac{\text{insulin } \mu\text{U/ml} \times 100}{\text{glucose mg/dl} - 20}$. The normal ratio does not exceed 100. This assumes that insulin secretion in infants normally ceases below a blood glucose concentration of 20 mg/dl (1.1 mM). This ratio is difficult to interpret in the affected neonate whose blood glucose concentration is often below 20 mg/dl (1.1 mM). Recently, two reports [89,90] have suggested I/G ratios of >0.38–0.40 on repeated samples for the diagnosis of hyperinsulinemic hypoglycemia. There are inadequate data to interpret any of these ratios definitively in the neonate. However, the simple ratio has repeatedly been reported to be useful in the past 10 years.

The analysis of immunoreactive insulin in plasma includes free insulin as well as proinsulinlike components (PLC) which cross-react with the insulin antibodies. Using gel filtration techniques, islet cell tumors in adults have been associated with significant elevations of PLC (normally less than 25 percent of total immunoreactivity) [91]. There are few data in infants with hyperinsulinemic hypoglycemia. Aynsley-Green et al. [92] evaluated three such neonates and found a two- to threefold increase in plasma proinsulin in one.

If the plasma insulin levels are elevated absolutely (>200 μU/ml [>1200 pM]), it is critical to obtain a C-peptide level to establish its endogenous origin as well as to rule out the administration of exogenous insulin [93]. Recently, we have been consulted on four infants with "abnormal" hyperinsulinemia. Three were very low birth weight (VLBW) infants being given total parenteral nutrition (TPN) in the

NICU and one, a 6-month-old with a recent onset of profound hypoglycemia (plasma glucose concentrations between 10 and 20 mg/dl (0.56 and 1.1 mM) at the time of symptoms). The VLBW infants, two of whom were being given small quantities of insulin for symptomatic hyperglycemia (see p. 000) and one of whom was on TPN without insulin, had apparently been given excessive quantities of insulin in their TPN feeds by error. The 6-month-old infant had extremely high plasma insulin concentrations (>400–500 μU/ml [2400–3000 pM]) both before and after a 95 percent pancreatectomy. An exogenous source of the insulin was subsequently detected. Insulin was apparently being injected into the central venous line. C-peptide determinations would have established the exogenous source of the insulin in all four instances. In three, analyses of the parenteral fluid established the source of the insulin.

Hyperinsulinemia is associated with suppression of both lipolysis and ketone formation. Thus, plasma beta hydroxybutyrate concentrations are very low or unmeasurable [94]. While hypoketonemic hypoglycemia is consistent with hyperinsulinemia, it also occurs with defects in fatty acid or ketone body metabolism, as in 3-hydroxy, 3-methyl glutaryl Co A lyase deficiency (see Chapter 10).

Hypoglycemia associated with absolute or relative elevation of plasma insulin, together with low concentrations of plasma ketones (beta-hydroxybutyrate and/or acetoacetate), are diagnostic of hyperinsulinemic hypoglycemia. If, in addition, there is a requirement for high rates of parenteral dextrose (>12 mg/kg/min) to achieve normoglycemia and a failure to maintain normoglycemia with diazoxide, surgical intervention is indicated.

Diagnostic Localization

In adults, islet cell tumors have been localized by ultrasound, pre- and intraoperatively, scintiscan or celiac axis arteriography. Kirkland et al. [95] in 1978 reported a hypoglycemic infant whose islet cell tumor was diagnosed at 45 days of age by selective angiography. However, the risks and rate of success of this procedure have not been well defined as yet. In 1978, Ingemansson et al. [96] introduced percutaneous transhepatic portal vein catheterization and transfemoral portal and caval catheterization under local anesthesia and blood sampling for insulin assay as a diagnostic and localization procedure in two adult patients with insulinoma and two with islet cell hyperplasia. Intraoperative biochemical localization by insulin assay requires a long intraoperative wait for assay results. The insulin assays have been modified for rapid turnaround time. Teichmann et al. [97] reported an assay time of 30 minutes with successful localization in six adults:

five with pancreatic adenoma and one with carcinoma. To date, there has been little or no experience or success with this approach in the neonate. In adults, angiography is more diagnostic than either CT or ultrasonography [98].

While these techniques are not currently recommended for infants, they may be feasible in older children and adolescents.

An informal query of pediatric radiologists confirmed that the new imaging modalities have not been diagnostic in searching for small pancreatic tumors in infants. The current recommendation is to use ultrasonography, enhanced CT, and MRI sequentially. These are not likely to reveal a lesion.

Medical Therapy

The primary objective of treatment is to stabilize the blood glucose concentration to the normal range (>45 mg/dl [2.5 mM] plasma). A symptomatic infant should receive an immediate bolus of 0.25–0.5 gm/kg as a concentrated dextrose[2] solution (10–25 percent). In order to avoid rebound hypoglycemia, which may occur within 30 minutes, a continuous dextrose infusion at 8–10 mg/kg/min must be given immediately following the bolus. This rate may be insufficient to maintain a normal blood glucose concentration, as evident in low blood glucose determinations made initially at hourly intervals. If hypoglycemia persists, the infusion rate should be increased by 2 mg/kg/min increments until normoglycemia is achieved. High volume rates carry the risk of fluid overload manifest in pulmonary edema and/or heart failure. This can be minimized by the use of a central venous catheter and concentrated solutions (25 percent dextrose). After the initial 24 hours, maintenance electrolytes should be added: Na^+ at 2–3 mEq/kg/day; K^+ at 1–2 mEq/kg/day; Cl^- at 3–4 mEq/kg/day.

In the event that very high dextrose infusion rates are required (16–24 mg/kg/min), a course of intravenous synthetic cyclic somatostatin may be effective in suppressing insulin secretion and sustaining normoglycemia [99]. In addition to hyperinsulinemia, Bloomgarden et al. [100] also observed diminished plasma glucagon levels and a failure to correct the hypoglycemia with somatostatin alone. They supplemented the somatostatin infusion with glucagon and noted a rise in plasma glucose levels to normal. This therapy permitted a reduction in glucose concentration in the parenteral fluids. Both the patient of Hirsch [99] and that of Bloomgarden [100] required pancreatectomy as definitive treatment. Pollak et al. [101] have developed

---

[2]Dextrose, the pharmaceutical form of glucose, is the monohydrate and has a molecular weight of 198 compared to glucose at 180.

a somatostatin sensitivity test (SST) for diagnosis and preoperative management. It is apparent that somatostatin and/or glucagon should be considered as adjuncts in therapy. Glucagon alone may exacerbate the hyperinsulinemia, since glucagon is an insulin secretagogue. Neither glucagon nor somatostatin alone is recommended in the ongoing medical management of hyperinsulinemic hypoglycemia, but may be useful diagnostically and for short-term therapy.

If hyperinsulinemia has been documented, then pharmacologic agents that suppress insulin secretion should be used. These include diazoxide, epinephrine, susphrine, or ephredrine. Diazoxide [80,102] is preferred and may be given orally at 5–30 mg/kg/day in three divided doses. The other agents tend to have too transient an effect to be useful. Side effects occur with all these agents and must be monitored carefully. Patients who respond to Diazoxide should be monitored at home with prefeed capillary blood glucose determinations, as well as home glucose monitoring screens. Raw cornstarch has proven to be a useful adjunctive therapy in some patients [103].

When medical therapy is not effective, i.e., hypoglycemia persists intermittently and high infusion rates (>12 mg/kg/min) are required, pancreatectomy must be considered. In the past, surgery has been reserved for late in the course of management. However, the previously noted significant risk of complications and ultimate mental retardation has advanced surgery to an earlier position in the course of therapy. If there is no significant progress within 2 weeks, then surgery becomes an important consideration.

Surgical Therapy

Pancreatectomy should be performed by a skilled, experienced pediatric surgeon in a tertiary care center. Historically, the operation tended to be two-thirds or subtotal pancreatectomy (often >80 percent) and included splenectomy, with the later complication of sepsis. In addition, perioperative morbidity and mortality were significant. The high failure rate of a standard two-thirds pancreatectomy and the advances in pediatric anesthesia and surgery have allowed a more extensive pancreatic resection of 80–90 percent as the safe initial surgical approach.

In 1971, Harken et al. [82] first reported using "total" pancreatectomy for the surgical failure to control the recurrent severe hypoglycemia of 10 infants with a subtotal pancreatectomy in the previous 15 years; in 5, initial surgery failed to control hypoglycemia which recurred in 1 day to 2 weeks. When reinstated medical therapy was inadequate, total pancreatectomy was performed by excision of the residual pancreatic tissue. There were no postoperative surgical complications, and hypoglycemia was eliminated in all. "Total" pancreatectomy was well tolerated by these growing infants. Insulin was necessary in three children, and four required oral pancreatic enzymes for adequate intestinal absorption.

Reviewing all reports of surgical treatment for persistent hypoglycemia between 1934 and 1976, Thomas and associates [104] summarized 87 cases, including 6 of their own. Onset of symptoms varied from day 1 to 6 months of age; surgery was performed as early as 19 days and as late as 72 months of age following failure of medical therapy. Twelve patients had near-total pancreatectomy. Of the 87 subjects, the pancreas was normal in 26, adenoma was present in 14, hyperplasia in 29, "nesidioblastosis" in 15, and unknown in 3. Outcome in 72 neonates undergoing subtotal pancreatectomy is summarized in Table 5-7. Sepsis was the major cause of death in 5 of 7 patients.

During this era, less than half of the surviving infants were mentally normal. Hypoglycemic relapses also occurred in some 40 percent of infants following surgery.

In a follow-up study during this past decade (1977–1987), Thomas et al. [83] summarized 165 patients, including 6 of their own. The increased frequency reflects early recognition and ready availability of glucose and insulin measurements in many centers. They reviewed initial evaluation and surgical management for intractable hypoglycemia, pathophysiology, and clinical findings. The results of pancreatectomy for intractable hypoglycemia in 165 neonates and infants have been summarized in Figure 5-3. Compared to previous results (Table 5-7), many more survivors were normal mentally in all three groups (80 percent versus 46 percent). While mortality remained unchanged with more extensive surgery during this past decade, both seizures and the need for subsequent insulin therapy have been significantly reduced by near-total pancreatectomy (95 to 98 percent).

The optimal time for surgical intervention has not been defined [105–108]. Medical therapy must be reviewed continuously, and obvious failure is an indication for surgery. The treatment of choice currently is near-total pancreatectomy, retaining the spleen and duodenum. This is a safe procedure, well-tolerated by infants and children, and should be considered early for the correction of hypoglycemia of infancy. This procedure is unique because (1) the common bile duct is preserved, (2) the duodenal arterial supply is preserved, and (3) remnants of the pancreas are left around the duodenal vessels (Fig. 5-4).

Immediately postoperatively, glucose control commonly becomes erratic because of secondary diabetes. The principles used in managing new type I diabetes mellitus apply here [109,110]. However, because the source of glucagon has also been removed, there may be

TABLE 5-7. Outcome of 72 neonates and infants undergoing subtotal pancreatectomy for intractable hypoglycemia, 1934–1976

PATHOLOGIC DIAGNOSIS	MENTALLY NORMAL	MENTALLY RETARDED	REQUIRED POSTOPERATIVE MEDICAL THERAPY	TOTAL DEATHS	LOST TO FOLLOW-UP
Normal pancreas	9	9	7	2(2)*	2
Hyperplasia	6	11	7	3(2)	1
"Nesidioblastosis"	5	4	4	...	1
Adenoma	5	4	1	1	1
Unknown	...	1	1	1(1)	...
Total	25	29	20†	7(5)	5‡

(From Thomas et al. *Ann Surg.* 1977; 185:505, with permission.)
*Number in parentheses indicates number of patients who died of sepsis.
†Mental status of six not reported.
‡No results given for these patients.

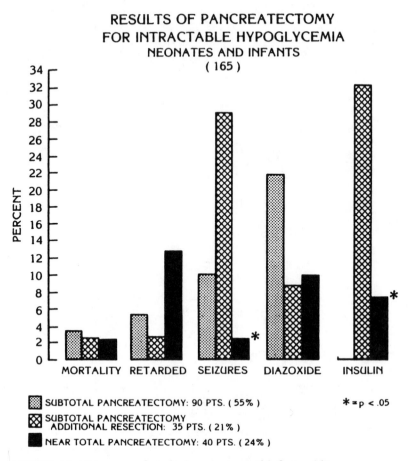

**RESULTS OF PANCREATECTOMY
FOR INTRACTABLE HYPOGLYCEMIA**
NEONATES AND INFANTS
(165)

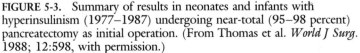

FIGURE 5-3. Summary of results in neonates and infants with
hyperinsulinism (1977–1987) undergoing near-total (95–98 percent)
pancreatectomy as initial operation. (From Thomas et al. *World J Surg.*
1988; 12:598, with permission.)

insulin sensitivity. It is unusual to see ketoacidosis in this situation.
The degree and persistence of the hyperglycemia is highly variable
and usually transient.

In some patients, the secondary diabetes may persist or recur
subsequently, especially with "total" pancreatectomy or reoperation
following subtotal pancreatectomy. The use of near-total pancreatectomy (95 percent or more) has been associated with less-than-
expected secondary diabetes mellitus, perhaps related to (1) amount
of residual pancreatic tissue and (2) regeneration of the pancreas.
Careful control depends upon frequent home blood glucose monitoring in order to avoid induced symptomatic hypoglycemia. Ketonuria
rarely occurs, even with infections.

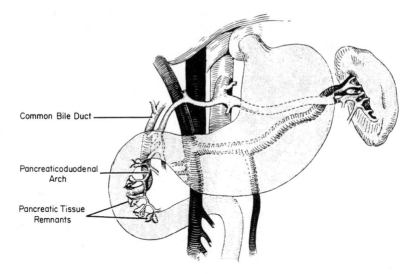

Common Bile Duct

Pancreaticoduodenal
Arch

Pancreatic Tissue
Remnants

FIGURE 5-4. Anatomy after near-total pancreatectomy. (From Moazam et al. *Arch Surg.* 1982; 117:1151. Copyright 1982, American Medical Association.)

Another postoperative complication may be malabsorption due to a deficiency of pancreatic enzymes. Absorption problems, particularly fat, have been described. Thus pancreatic enzymes have been recommended. However, there have been patients both with normal stools and normal growth and development who have not required enzyme therapy. This must be assessed individually.

Morphological Findings

Recent studies emphasize the difficulty in establishing a morphologic basis for hyperinsulinemic hypoglycemia. The extensive control material containing "nesidioblastosis" makes this a questionable diagnosis in these cases. The macroscopic aspect of the pancreas is unremarkable in most cases of hyperinsulinemic hypoglycemia. The pathologic diagnosis relies entirely on precise histologic and immunohistologic assessment of the specimen.

In 1980, Jaffe summarized the pathologic findings in hyperinsulinemic hypoglycemia (Table 5-8) and concluded as follows: "Persistent hyperinsulinemic hypoglycemia appears to be a syndrome with varying causes and a correspondingly wide range of pathological findings in the pancreas" [111, 112].[3]

---

[3]Reference numbers from the original text have been adjusted to fit this text.

TABLE 5-8. Pancreatic findings in infants with hyperinsulinemic hypoglycemia

FINDING	ASSOCIATION	INCIDENCE* (%)
No pathologic change		10
Endocrine cell dysplasia		70
Adenomatosis		20
Focal		
Multifocal	MEA	
Diffuse	Beckwith-Wiedemann	
Adenoma		rare

(From Jaffe. In: Wigglesworth and Singer, eds. *Textbook of Fetal and Perinatal Pathology.* Boston: Blackwell Scientific Publications, 1991, p. 1043, with permission.)
*Compiled from reinterpretation of previous cases.

It is clear that intimate knowledge of normal development of the pancreas in the human fetus, neonate, and infant is necessary to interpret any abnormal pathology. In fact, some infants show no pathologic findings. For a detailed discussion, see Jaffe in Singer and Wigglesworth [112]. The following extract has been reproduced from this book.

> "Nesidioblastosis" was the term used by Laidlaw for the islet cell tumor of the pancreas, the nesidioblast being the duct-derived cell giving rise to islets [85]. Previously, B-cell hyperplasia, "nesidioblastosis," a diffuse or disseminated neoproliferation of islets from ducts, and "beta cell nesidioblastosis," single cells and small packets of 2–6 beta cells around small ducts or in glandular acini, were used to describe the pancreas surgically removed from hypoglycemic infants. More recently, "nesidioblastosis" and "beta cell nesidioblastosis" have been found to be normal situations in the newborn, and inappropriate terms to describe the pathologic features seen in most hyperinsulinemic infants [113,114].
>
> Currently, endocrine cell dysplasia [111], nesidiodysplasia [113], and islet cell dysmaturation syndrome [112] are the terms used to describe the panoply of pathologic features noted in the pancreas of infants with hyperinsulinism and hypoglycemia. These findings are seen only on immunostained sections of pancreas and include a loss of the normal centrilobular congregation of large islets, and an increased number of small islet cell clusters arranged haphazardly in the lobule instead of in the usual peripheral distribution. There appears to be wide case to case variation in the extent of the endocrine proliferation in endocrine cell dysplasia. An overall excess of endocrine tissue may occur, but is not re-

quired for the diagnosis. The qualitative change in endocrine distribution is more constant.

Adenomas are extraordinarily rare in infants. Adenomas are well demarcated and differ from adenomatosis in being devoid of admixed acinar tissue. The adenoma may contain more than one cell type, but the islet-like arrangement is not seen. Most previous descriptions of adenomas in infants appear to be instances of adenomatosis when the illustrations are reviewed.

Adenomatosis is an excessive proliferation of islet cells (usually more than 40% of all cells in a given area) pushing the exocrine elements aside or haphazardly incorporating them. Focal adenomatosis is restricted to one or more discrete areas, but not generalized throughout the pancreas.

Multifocal adenomatosis occurs in multiple discrete sites throughout the pancreas. Diffuse adenomatosis is the occurrence of adenomatosis not in discrete sites but throughout the pancreas. This is characteristic of the Beckwith-Wiedemann syndrome, though not specific.

Summary

Severe and persistent hypoglycemia in the neonate is associated with high risk for both short- and long-term morbidity and mortality. Diagnostic studies at onset for hormones and substrates may provide the basis for the etiology. For example, low values for GH and cortisol associated with prolonged jaundice, midline defects, micropenis, and recurrent hypoglycemia indicate congenital hypopituitarism. In contrast, high plasma insulin and C-peptide concentrations, macrosomia, and inability to maintain normoglycemia with high rates of parenteral dextrose administration support the diagnosis of organic hyperinsulinemic hypoglycemia. Aggressive medical therapy is indicated with parenteral dextrose, hormones, and pharmacologic agents. In organic hyperinsulinemic hypoglycemia, the failure of medical therapy mandates prompt surgical intervention, usually with near-total pancreatectomy.

Outcome for survival has improved significantly. However, while prognosis for neurologic and mental outcome has improved, a significant risk still remains.

Beckwith-Wiedemann (BWS) or Exomphalos-Macroglossia-Gigantism (EMG) Syndrome

In 1963–1964, Beckwith and his colleagues [115,116] and Wiedemann [117] described a syndrome characterized by omphalocele, muscular macroglossia, gigantism, visceromegaly, hypoglycemia, mild microcephaly, as well as diffuse cytomegaly of the adrenal fetal cortex, and hyperplasia of the kidneys, pancreas, and gonadal interstitial cells. Additional major findings included postnatal gigantism with increased bone age, abnormal insertion of the diaphragm, flame nevus of the face, earlobe anomalies [118], hepatomegaly, genitourinary anomalies, nephromegaly, seizures and apnea, and hemihypertrophy. Over 500 patients have been reported and extensive reviews of the syndrome published [118–120]. A variety of minor clinical findings (<20 percent frequency) include cardiac anomalies, microcephaly, splenomegaly, skeletal and gastrointestinal anomalies, somatic asymmetry, and mental retardation. Laboratory findings may include hypoglycemia and polycythemia, with hypocalcemia and hypercholesterolemia occurring less frequently. The syndrome has been diagnosed prenatally by ultrasound. More recent reports have emphasized the endocrine and metabolic problems in these neonates [121–124], which are summarized here.

Hypoglycemia

Hypoglycemia is not a constant finding and varies in severity and duration. The frequency has been 30–63 percent in two recent large series; yet the consequences are such that blood glucose concentrations should be monitored from birth in any infant suspected of having the EMG syndrome. It is particularly important to measure plasma glucose and serum insulin values during the first 24 hours of life and for the first 3 days. The importance of early recognition and continuous therapy of the hypoglycemia in the EMG syndrome has been repeatedly reemphasized [120,123,124]. Much of the neonatal mortality and subsequent morbidity, which consist of microcephaly and mental retardation, have been attributed to untreated hypoglycemia, although the evidence is far from conclusive.

Course

Schiff et al. [123] performed longitudinal studies on an infant with Beckwith-Wiedemann syndrome during the first 2 years of life. From age 47 hours to 25 months, eight glucose tolerance tests showed fasting plasma glucose levels varying from 14–80 mg/dl (0.8–4.4 mM), while plasma insulin concentrations were 0–28 μU/ml (0–168 pM). Calculated I/G varied from 0.53 initially to 0 after the first year of life. Peak insulin was greater than 400 μU/ml (2400 pM). Hyperresponsiveness was also noted to glucagon and tolbutamide but not to arginine or leucine. This child failed to respond to diazoxide therapy alone but was controlled by a combination of diazoxide and susphrine (long-acting epinephrine). These observations support the recommendation that such patients be studied frequently with plasma glucose and insulin measurements until a stable metabolic state is established.

The carbohydrate tolerance tests, serum insulin values, and pancreatic hyperplasia all support the concept that hyperinsulinemia is probably responsible for the low blood glucose concentrations. The features of the pancreas are those of diffuse adenomatosis, some nodules of which may form large or even palpable masses. Besides the proliferation of pancreatic endocrine cells maintaining a normal topographical distribution of β versus non-β cells, the pancreas of patients with the Beckwith-Wiedemann syndrome may have undergone abnormal development, with a consequent lack of segregation of glucagon and pancreatic polypeptide cells to different parts of the gland. The unusual appearance and size of the Beckwith-Wiedemann pancreas should not be confused with the pancreatoblastoma [125], an embryoma that may arise in association with the syndrome. Even though hypoglycemia is transient, Sotelo-Avila and Singer [126] found islet cell hyperplasia at autopsy in seven children with the Beckwith-Wiedemann syndrome who died later in life with neoplasms.

Pathogenesis

Speculation concerning the pathogenesis has extended to include the insulinlike growth factors (IGF-I and -II). Since duplications of the short arm of chromosome 11 have been found in a high proportion of subjects [127], the location of the IGF-II gene to this region has made IGF-II a major factor. The IGFs are important growth factors during the first trimester and may primarily act locally. Perinatal measurements of plasma IGFs have yielded conflicting data [128–130]. There is inadequate information to implicate growth factors other than insulin. There have now been many reports of the Beckwith-Wiedemann syndrome association with duplication of chromosomal region 11p15 noted above. Dosage analyses have been performed for insulin and IGF-II genes which also map to 11p15 in somatic DNAs. In each of seven patients studied by Spritz et al. [131], they observed apparent diploid representation of these genes. They suggested that BWS was not frequently associated with small duplications of 11p15 material that embed the insulin and IGF-II genes.

Therapy

Therapy has varied with the degree of the hypoglycemia and response of the patient. Originally, zinc glucagon, diazoxide, and cortisol [121] were found to be effective. Subsequently, depending upon the severity of the hypoglycemia, diazoxide alone [132] or with susphrine [123] or pancreatectomy as early as 24 days of life [133] has been required to maintain a normal blood sugar level in affected children.

Prognosis

Prognosis is guarded since the multiple anomalies can result in an increased mortality [126] and morbidity [133]. Failure to recognize and treat the hypoglycemia may contribute to mental retardation. Survival with normal mentality and physical growth and development has occurred [126,134].

Leprechaunism Syndrome

In 1948, Donohue first described an infant (age 27 days) with unusual features and multiple endocrine dysfunction, which he termed dysendocrinism [135]. Shortly thereafter, he reported two sisters born to a consanguineous marriage. These infants had very low birth weight and growth retardation at seven months in utero. Because of an elf-inlike facies, the name "leprechaunism" was applied.

Subsequently, further cases [136,137] were described, and the following features of leprechaunism were compiled:

1. Prenatal growth retardation, lack of adipose tissue, and low birthweight.
2. Abnormal facies with "elfin" appearance (prominent eyes, wide nostrils, thick lips, and large ears).
3. Breast hyperplasia.
4. Large phallus.
5. Leydig cell hyperplasia in the male, cystic ovaries, and hyperplasia of the islets of Langerhans.
6. Hirsutism (body and facial).
7. Mental retardation.
8. Severe failure to thrive and death in infancy.

Striking cutaneous abnormalities have been described, including hypertrichosis, pachyderma, acanthosis nigricans, and prominent rugal skin around the body orifices. Additionally, dysplastic nails have also been reported.

Metabolic dysfunction is manifest primarily in disordered carbohydrate metabolism expressed as postprandial hyperglycemia, fasting hypoglycemia, insulin resistance, and notable hyperinsulinemia. Other endocrinopathies reported include congenital lipodystrophy, Cushing's syndrome, and acromegaly. In many patients reported, the serum concentrations of thyroid hormones, estrogens, androgens, glucocorticoids, and growth hormones have been normal.

Over 40 infants have been reported [138]. The data are consistent with an autosomal recessive inheritance. No specific pancreatic histology other than islet hyperplasia has been described.

A Canadian Indian male infant with typical features had hyperinsulinemia (660–2,480 µU/ml [4,000–15,000 pM]) and variable blood glucose concentrations (13–219 mg/dl [0.7–12.2 mM]) without symptomatic hypoglycemia [137]. Gel filtration of serum showed 13 percent proinsulinlike material and 87 percent insulin. No anti-insulin antibodies were found. The insulin peak was lyophilized, reconstituted, and assayed in the glucose oxidation bioassay in isolated rat adipocytes. The biological activity (relative to porcine insulin standard) was 70 percent of the immunoreactivity. Studies of cultured fibroblasts indicated a profound and selective deficiency of insulin binding, indicating a primary defect of insulin receptors.

In another infant, cultured fibroblasts were studied for a variety of metabolic events [139]. Doubling time was prolonged (90 versus 29 hours) and morphology was abnormal. ^{3}H-Glucose uptake was minimal compared to controls at low insulin levels but comparable at high concentrations. Stimulation of ^{3}H-aminoisobutyric acid uptake by insulin, epidermal growth factor (EGF), multiplication-stimulating activity, and somatomedin-C (SMC) in leprechaun cells was diminished relative to controls at all concentrations studied. Stimulation of ^{3}H-thymidine incorporation by EGF, SMC, and fibroblast growth factor was also subnormal. Normal binding to ^{125}I-insulin and ^{125}I-somatomedin C had been demonstrated previously for this patient. They concluded that it is likely that the defect in these cells is at the postreceptor level, perhaps involving a metabolic pathway common to the action of multiple growth factors since receptors for three of the peptides were apparently normal.

With recent advances in technology that permit characterization of the insulin receptor, clarification of a variety of insulin resistant states has been possible. Elsas et al. [140] studied an affected female and both parents. In vivo responses to a standard oral glucose tolerance test showed marked hyperinsulinemia (plasma insulin concentration = 4,210 µU/ml [25,000 pM]); the father had mild hyperinsulinemia (240 µU/ml [1,440 pM]); while the mother was normal. They also studied monolayers of intact fibroblasts and found complex kinetics with ^{125}I-insulin binding which were interpreted with a two-receptor model. The proband had no high-affinity binding but normal low-affinity binding. Uptake of 2-methylamino-isobutyric acid was normal, but 2-deoxyglucose uptake was increased only when insulin was increased 100-fold over control observations. Affinity cross-linking studies were also carried out. They concluded that, in this family, two different recessive mutations impair high-affinity, insulin-receptor binding and that the proband with leprechaunism is a compound heterozygote for these mutations. The two mutations produced structural changes in the receptor that altered subunit interactions and caused loss of high-affinity binding and cellular responsivity.

Studies are currently directed to molecular genetics of the insulin receptor in a variety of insulin-resistant states, including non-insulin-dependent diabetes mellitus and ranging to those with severe insulin resistance such as type A syndrome, the Rabson-Mendenhall syndrome, lipoatrophic diabetes, and leprechaunism. Kadowaki et al. [141] cloned insulin-receptor-complementary DNA from the patient noted above (leprechaun/Ark-1). They concluded that the patient is a compound heterozygote, having inherited two different mutant alleles of the insulin receptor gene. One allele contains a missense mutation encoding the substitution of glutamic acid for lysine at position 460 in the A subunit of the receptor. The second allele has a nonsense mutation causing premature chain termination after amino acid 671 in the A subunit, thereby deleting both the transmembrane and tyrosine kinase domains of the receptor. Interestingly, the father is heterozygous for this nonsense mutation and exhibits a moderate degree of insulin resistance. This raises the possibility that mutations in the insulin receptor gene may account for the insulin resistance in some patients with non-insulin-dependent diabetes mellitus.

Shortly thereafter, Moller and Flier [142] improved on techniques involved in screening of genomic and cDNA libraries by the use of the polymerase chain reaction (PCR) which permits rapid amplifications of specific genetic sequences without the need for library construction, cloning, or screening. They prepared RNA from a patient with type A insulin resistance from cultured fibroblasts and lymphocyte cell lines transformed by Epstein-Barr virus. A small amount of the patient's cellular RNA served as the initial template for the PCR to amplify and sequence a 1,268 subunit base pair (bp) region that encodes for the intracellular B subunit of the insulin receptor. Two single base changes in the insulin receptor gene of this patient were detected, one which encoded a substitution of serine for tryptophan at a site within the tyrosine kinase domain of the receptor, resulting in defective receptor autophosphorylation (Fig. 5-5).

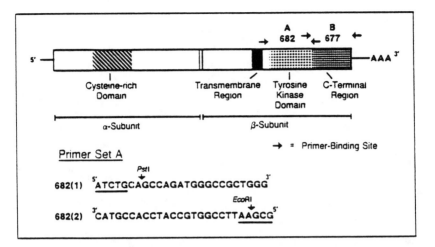

FIGURE 5-5. Schematic representation of the human insulin-receptor cDNA sequence, which encodes a single α- and β-subunit precursor protein (top panel). Several important domains are noted by the variously shaded areas. Two regions (A and B) chosen for PCR amplification are indicated by arrows showing the binding sites for primer pairs. The direction of the arrows indicates the 5' to 3' orientation of the primers. The length (in base pairs) of each region chosen for amplification is noted above its respective location. The bottom panel shows the DNA sequence of PCR oligonucleotide primer set A. Additional nonhomologous bases (which are underlined) that were added to the 5' end of each primer to create recognition sites for restriction enzymes (arrows) are indicated. (From Moller and Flier. Reprinted by permission of the *New England Journal of Medicine,* 319:1526, 1988.)

The differences in the molecular genetics observed to date in these two patients (one with leprechaunism, the other with type A syndrome) indicate that further studies will be necessary to determine the specific molecular abnormalities in insulin receptor defects.

Case Report (Patient 5-2): Focal Adenomatosis, Failure of Drug Therapy, and a Two-Stage Pancreatectomy Resulting in Transient Diabetes Mellitus [110]

J.T., a 4.88-kg, 55.5-cm female, was born after a 43-week gestation. The mother was gravid II and not a gestational diabetic. The firstborn was normal. The infant was macrosomic and plethoric at birth and tachypneic and jittery by 45 minutes of age. Serum glucose level was 20 mg/dl (1.1 mM). Dextrose infusions at rates up to 16 mg/kg/min were inadequate to maintain the plasma glucose concentration above 36 mg/dl (2.0 mM). On the third day of life, the first immunoreactive insulin (IRI) determinations revealed marked hyperinsulinemia. Over the first week of life (Fig. 5-6), diazoxide in doses up to 25 mg/kg/day PO and subcutaneous susphrine were inadequate to allow a decrease in the rate of dextrose administration.

RECURRENT OR PERSISTENT NEONATAL HYPOGLYCEMIA

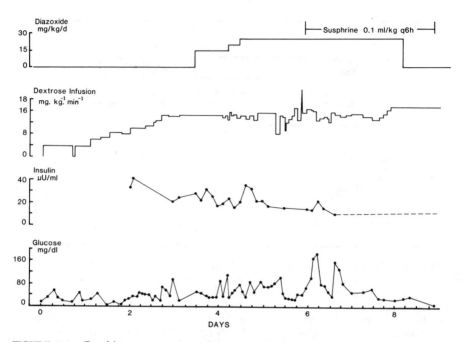

FIGURE 5-6. Graphic representation of the patient's course from birth to 8 days of age. Shown are medical therapy, rate of dextrose administration, and plasma insulin and glucose concentrations. Note the failure of medical therapy, including high glucose infusion rates. (From Gruppuso et al. *Acta Paediatr Scand.* 1985; 74:311, with permission.)

At 9 days of age, angiography of the pancreas was normal. The following day, the patient had a subtotal (90 percent) pancreatectomy. At surgery, the pancreas appeared normal in size and consistency, and on pathologic examination, including immunostaining, the specimen was indistinguishable from normal.

Plasma glucose concentration rose to 149 mg/dl (8.3 mM) during the procedure. After 10 hours, however, dextrose at rates above 14 mg/kg/min were again required. Over the next 6 days, plasma glucose concentration ranged between 40 mg/dl (2.2 mM) and 79 mg/dl (4.4 mM) with dextrose infusions via a central venous catheter at 25 mg/kg/min. Diazoxide again proved ineffective. Plasma insulin concentrations were variable just before the near-total pancreatectomy. Twelve paired plasma glucose and insulin measurements had an average insulin-to-glucose ratio of 0.35 (SD 0.21), with a range from 0.07–0.66. Normal infants have an I/G of <0.30 (mean ratio = 0.11; SD ± 0.09; and a range = 0.03–0.28). At 16 days of age, the patient had a near-total pancreatectomy. The second surgical specimen consisted of normal pancreatic tissue and a nonencapsulated firm mass 0.5 cm in diameter. Microscopic examination of immunostained sections of the nodule revealed large, polyhedral islet cells. Immunostaining demonstrated that, as in normal islets, glucagon and somatostatin positive cells were at the periphery. "Nesidioblastosis" was quite prominent. This was considered to represent a focal adenomatosis of the pancreas.

The second postoperative period (Fig. 5-7) was characterized by wide fluctuations in the plasma glucose concentration between 20 mg/dl (1.1 mM) and 504 mg/dl (28 mM). Initial intravenous insulin therapy with 0.05 to 0.1 U/kg/h resulted in hypoglycemia. Stable glucose concentrations were achieved by 48 hours postoperatively with intravenous insulin, 0.01 U/kg/h, and dextrose, 13 mg/kg/min. This extreme insulin sensitivity waned over the ensuing 10 days, after which time therapy was begun with subcutaneous regular insulin, 0.2 to 0.3 U per dose q 6 h. Once stable on NPH insulin, 0.8 U, q 12 h, the patient was discharged at 5 weeks of age. Blood glucose levels (Chemstrip bG, Bio-Dynamics, Inc.) ranged from 79–239 mg/dl (4.4–13.3 mM) over the first postoperative month. Glycemic control further improved over

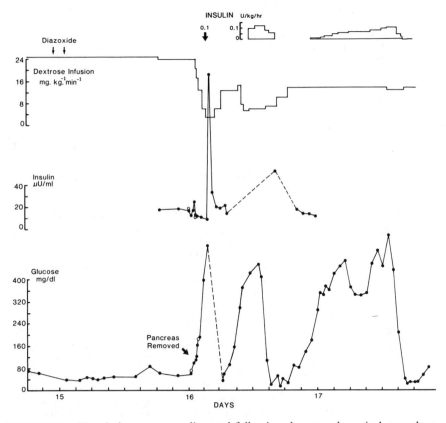

FIGURE 5-7. Hospital course preceding and following the second surgical procedure, near-total pancreatectomy. Shown are insulin dose, dextrose infusion rate, and plasma insulin and glucose concentrations. Open circles represent portal vein samples obtained at the start and end of pancreatectomy (second operation). The erratic blood glucose control postoperatively stabilized after the third day. (From Gruppuso et al. *Acta Paediatr Scand.* 1985; 74:311, with permission.)

the next 4 months, and insulin was gradually decreased and discontinued 5 months after the near-total pancreatectomy. Prior to the second operation, plasma C-peptide concentration averaged 0.542 ± 0.166 pmol/ml, $n = 12$. On days 17 and 18 (1–2 days post-near-total pancreatectomy), C-peptide was not detectable in plasma. However, at 3.5 months of age, plasma C-peptide concentration was 0.55 pmol/ml and remained detectable thereafter, reaching a peak or normal value of 0.93 pmol/ml at 15 months. Thereafter, random blood sugar concentrations by Chemstrip bG all ranged from 80–160 mg/dl (4.4–8.8 mM), while length and weight continued along the fiftieth to seventy-fifth percentile. At 15 months of age, psychological testing revealed skills commensurate with chronological age. Intake of an elemental formula and the addition of cereals, vegetables, and meats have been tolerated well and not associated with malabsorption. A Hb A_{1c} determination at 9 months of age was normal at 6.2 percent.

At age 5 years, she continued to develop normally, with weight above the fiftieth percentile and height at the twenty-fifth percentile. Except for a diet limited in fats, her nutrition is normal. She attends school and is psychosocially normal as well. Currently, there is no evidence of carbohydrate or glucose intolerance.

Comment

This infant presented immediately after birth and was diagnosed promptly. She did not respond to medical therapy but finally responded to a two-stage pancreatectomy. Her diabetes was easily managed and was transient. Her subsequent course was benign.

Case Report (Patient 5-3): Familial "Nesidioblastosis," Recurrent Hypoglycemia Requiring Multiple Therapies [143]

This 7-year-old white girl was the 4,564-gm product of a full-term pregnancy in a 26-year-old woman (gravida VIII, para II, abortus VI). On day 1 of life, she was noted to have a plasma glucose concentration of 18 mg/dl (1.0 mM) and plasma insulin of 25 μU/ml (150 pM); T4 was 9.4 ng/dl, growth hormone 19 ng/ml, and cortisol 14 ng/dl. I/G ratio was 1.4. Initial therapy included intravenously administered dextrose, diazoxide, and glucocorticoid drugs. At 23 days of age, a 95 percent pancreatectomy was performed. Histopathology indicated findings consistent with "nesidioblastosis." Postoperative plasma insulin values were 17–37 μU/ml (102–222 pM). Hypoglycemia recurred, and the patient required hourly nasogastric feedings until the age of 6 months, and then a regimen of feedings every 3 hours, supplemented with dextrose orally when hypoglycemia was apparent. Developmental milestones occurred early. The family performed blood glucose monitoring and learned to give glucose intravenously when needed.

At 20 months of age, early-morning hypoglycemia was documented in the hospital. An oral glucose tolerance test (1.7 gm/kg) revealed a peak glucose concentration of 205 mg/dl (11.4 mM) and insulin of <10 μU/ml (<60 pM) at 120 minutes. An oral leucine tolerance test (150 mg/kg) demonstrated a glucose concentration of 33 mg/dl (1.8 mM) and insulin of 8.2 μU/ml (49 pM) at 60 minutes. These results suggested inappropriate insulin release. Glucagon secretion was also inappropriate, with no response during spontaneous hypoglycemia (basal concentration 220 pg/ml, hypoglycemia 220 pg/ml). Leucine restriction and diazoxide therapy orally (10 to 12 mg/kg/day) were begun with moderate improvement, but the patient continued to have occasional seizures with documented hypoglycemia. Although these hypoglycemic episodes were associated with electroencephalographic changes, this patient had a normal EEG in the euglycemic state and normal neurologic and physical development.

Family History. A prior male sibling, born at term and weighing 5,115 gm, evidenced poor feeding and seizures, and died at 4 days of age; no autopsy was performed. A female sibling born after the patient, at term and weighing 5,400 gm, had hypoglycemia (17 mg/dl [0.9 mM]) and elevated insulin levels (75 μU/ml [450 pM]) in cord blood (growth hormone 22.5 ng/ml). Management was identical to that in her sibling, including 95 percent pancreatectomy at 23 days. The diagnosis based on histopathologic findings was also reported to be consistent with "nesidioblastosis." Subsequently, she remained hypoglycemic and required nasogastric feedings, dextrose orally, and diazoxide. However, she appeared neurologically damaged from birth, continued to do poorly, and died at age 5 months.

Both the mother and father described episodes consistent with hypoglycemia occurring after fasting longer than 6–8 hours. Evaluation of the mother during her eighth pregnancy revealed preprandial plasma glucose values between 40 and 50 mg/dl (2.2 and 2.8 mM). An oral glucose tolerance test (100 gm) was interpreted as showing mild carbohydrate intolerance (glucose 189 mg/dl [10.5 mM], insulin 137 μU/ml [822 pM] at 60 minutes) and symptomatic hypoglycemia (glucose 37 mg/dl [2.1 mM], insulin 6 μU/ml [36 pM] at 240 minutes). The father has had episodes of syncope associated with documented hypoglycemia, usually occurring in the morning before food intake.

Zinc Protamine Glucagon (ZPG) Therapy. At 2¼ years of age, diazoxide therapy was discontinued because of marked hirsutism and continuing episodes of hypoglycemia. Intramuscular injections of zinc protamine glucagon (kindly provided by Novo Industries, Copenhagen) were begun. Assay by Novo of this preparation revealed 80–125 percent of the stated glucagon potency, with minimal levels of related peptides. It was stored in lyophilized form in vials containing 10 mg zinc glucagon, and was reconstituted with 5 ml vehicle (containing protamine sulfate, zinc chloride, sodium acetate, glycerin, and methylparaben) before administration. Initial doses were 0.8 mg twice per day. Subsequently, doses ranged between 1.2 and 1.6 mg/day, divided into two doses. During therapy, the patient continued a low leucine diet and dextrose supplements between meals and at bedtime. With this regimen, there were continued but considerably less frequent episodes of severe hypoglycemia.

At 6½ years of age, plasma glucose and insulin levels were monitored while the patient continued the basic regimen. Glucose peaks of 175 mg/dl (9.7 mM) after dextrose supplements and troughs to 28 mg/dl (1.6 mM) in the early morning were found (Fig. 5-8a). Variation in glucose concentrations was great (48-hour coefficent of variation 56.8 percent). Insulin levels as measured by a double antibody radioimmunoassay were found to be spuriously elevated because insulin antibodies, which were present in high titer, interfered with the assay. Assay of the ZPG preparation showed significant insulin immunoreactivity (79.8 μU/ml [479 pM]).

Starch Therapy. At age 6½ years, starch therapy was begun in an effort to decrease the wide variability in glucose levels and to avoid nighttime hypoglycemia. Tapioca starch (chosen because tapioca has a low leucine content) was given orally every 8 hours (each dose as follows: 1.5 gm raw starch per kilogram body weight, prepared as a suspension in tap water at room temperature, weight/volume ratio 1:2). Dextrose supplements were discontinued. During the first 24 hours, this regimen immediately improved the stability of nighttime plasma glucose values, all of which were >60 mg/dl (3.3 mM). The intramuscular dose of ZPG was tapered over the subsequent 4 months, then discontinued. After this, the insulin antibody titer gradually decreased.

Three months after complete discontinuation of ZPG and 7 months after starting starch therapy, hourly plasma glucose levels were monitored for 48 hours. At this time, glucose values were consistently between 60 and 120 mg/dl (3.3 and 6.7 mM) (Fig. 5-8b). Glucose concentrations at night (in the absence of food or leucine intake) were higher than during the day. The variation in glucose levels was much less (half) than that during the prior study (48-hour coefficient of variation 23.6 percent).

Maintenance therapy has included a low leucine diet and oral starch (regimen described above), with no additional medications for a total of 18 months. The mother states that additional leucine intake has been tolerated since starch therapy. When a viral illness interfering with oral intake of starch has occurred, intravenous glucose has still been required. However, the oral regimen has been well tolerated and has generally been successful in preventing hypoglycemic episodes. The family's sleep patterns have improved, and anxiety about possible hypoglycemia has diminished.

The child has progressed well, both neurologically and developmentally, even though she experienced multiple episodes of hypoglycemia in early infancy. She was selected for a summer program for exceptionally bright children at Johns Hopkins University at age 7 years.

Comment

Recurrent, persistent hyperinsulinemic hypoglycemia is not always a well-defined definitive diagnosis either pathophysiologically or by pathologic examination of the resected pancreas ("nesidioblastosis"). This case reports the multiplicity of therapeutic modalities that may be required to prevent hypoglycemia. The introduction of raw, uncooked tapioca starch provided a stable plasma glucose concentration with discontinuation of other forms of treatment.

Her neurologic, psychologic, and intellectual development have been advanced throughout. This is noteworthy in view of her severe and recurrent episodes of symptomatic hypoglycemia since birth.

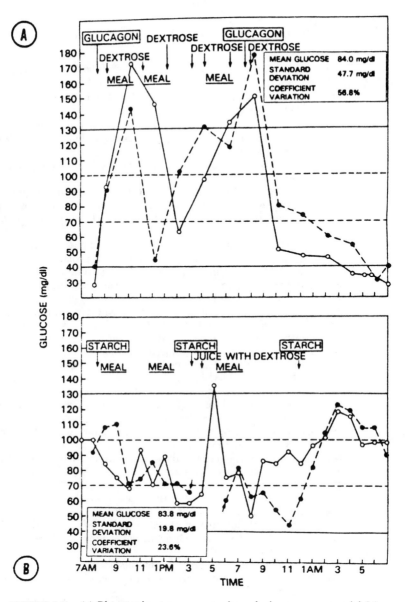

FIGURE 5-8. (a) Plasma glucose concentrations during two sequential 24-hour periods at age 6½ years while patient was receiving long-acting zinc protamine glucagon intramuscularly (0.6 mg two times per day), with three meals per day and seven supplements of orally administered dextrose solution at times indicated. (b) Plasma glucose concentrations during two sequential 24-hour periods at age 7 years while patient was receiving uncooked tapioca starch (6 tablespoons three times a day). Dextrose was given orally in the afternoon on one day at time indicated. Dashed lines represent normal range; solid lines, "safe" range. (From Rose et al. *J Pediatr.* 1986; 108:97, with permission.)

REFERENCES

1. CORNBLATH M. Hypoglycemia in infancy and childhood. *Pediatr Ann.* 1981;10:356.

2. CORNBLATH M, POTH M. Hypoglycemia. In: Kaplan SA, ed. *Clinical Pediatric and Adolescent Endocrinology.* Philadelphia: WB Saunders, 1983;157.

3. MILNER RDG. Neonatal hypoglycaemia: A critical reappraisal. *Arch Dis Child.* 1972;47:679.

4. LOVINGER RD, KAPLAN SL, GRUMBACH MM. Congenital hypopituitarism associated with neonatal hypoglycemia and microphallus: Four cases secondary to hypothalamic hormone deficiencies *J Pediatr.* 1975; 87:1171.

5. KAPLAN SL, GRUMBACH MM, FRIESEN HG, COSTOM BH. Thyrotropin releasing factor (TRF) effect on secretion of prolactin and thyrotropin in children and in idiopathic hypopituitary dwarfism: Further evidence for hypophysiotropic hormone deficiencies. *J Clin Endocrinol Metab.* 1972;35:825.

6. SADEGHI-NEJAD A, SENIOR B. A familial syndrome of isolated "aplasia" of the anterior pituitary. *J Pediatr.* 1974;84:79.

7. CORNBLATH M. Neonatal hypoglycemia and growth hormone deficiency with or without other endocrine abnormalities. Advances in Human Growth Hormone Research DHEW Publication No. (NIH) 74-612; 809, Oct. 1973.

8. JOHNSON JD, HANSEN RC, ALBRITTON WL, WERTHEMANN U, CHRISTIANSEN RO. Hypoplasia of the anterior pituitary and neonatal hypoglycemia. *J Pediatr.* 1973;82:634.

9. EHRLICH RM. Ectopic and hypoplastic pituitary with adrenal hypoplasia. *J Pediatr.* 1957;51:377.

10. MOSIER HD. Hypoplasia of the pituitary and adrenal cortex: Report on occurrence in twin siblings and autopsy findings. *J Pediatr.* 1956; 48:633.

11. KAPLAN SL, GRUMBACH MM, HOYT WF. A syndrome of hypopituitary dwarfism, hypoplasia of the optic nerves and malformation of the prosencephalon: report of six patients. *Pediatr Res.* 1970;4:480.

12. WALTON DS, ROBB RM. Optic nerve hypoplasia. *Arch Ophthalmol.* 1970;84:572.

13. PATEL H, TZE WJ, CRICHTON JU, McCORMICK AQ, ROBINSON GC, DOLMAN CL. Optic nerve hypoplasia with hypopituitarism. *Am J Dis Child.* 1975;129:175.

14. FRIESEN L, HOLMEGAARD L. Spectrum of optic nerve hypoplasia. *Br J Ophthalmol.* 1978;62:7.

15. GENDREL D, CHAUSSAIN JL, JOB JC. Les hypopituitarismes congénitaux par anomalie de la lignè médiane. *Arch Fr Pediatr.* 1981;38:227.

16. SKARF B, HOYT CS. Optic nerve hypoplasia in children. Association with anomalies of the endocrine and CNS. *Arch Ophthalmol.* 1984; 102:62.

17. MARGALITH D, JAN JE, McCORMICK AQ, TZE WJ, LAPOINTE J. Clinical spectrum of congenital optic nerve hypoplasia: review of 51 patients. *Dev Med Child Neurol.* 1984;26:311.

18. MARGALITH D, TZE WJ, JAN JE. Congenital optic nerve hypoplasia with hypothalamic-pituitary dysplasia. *Am J Dis Child.* 1985;139:361.

19. LACEY DJ. Agenesis of the corpus callosum. *Am J Dis Child.* 1985; 139:953.

20. MORISHIMA A, ARANOFF GS. Syndrome of septo-optic-pituitary dysplasia: the clinical spectrum. *Brain & Development.* 1986;8:233.

21. NELSON M, LESSELL S, SADUN AA. Optic nerve hypoplasia and maternal diabetes mellitus. *Arch Neurol.* 1986;43:20.

22. COSTELLO JM, GLUCKMAN PD. Neonatal hypopituitarism: A neurological perspective. *Develop Med Child Neurol.* 1988;30:190.

23. REEVES DL. Congenital absence of the septum pellucidum. *Bull Johns Hopkins Hosp.* 1941;69:61.

24. DEMORSIER G. Etudes sur les dystrophies cranioencephaliques. III. Agenesie due septum lucidum avec malformation du tractus optique: la dysplasie septo-optique. *Schweiz Arch Neurol Neurochir Psychiatr.* 1956;77:267.

25. NEWMAN W. Absence of optic disc and retinal vessels: congenital blindness in two sisters. *Ophthal Hosp Rep.* 1864;4:202.

26. STEINER MM. Rare dwarfism with chronic hypoglycemia and convulsions: Observations with (1) ACTH and cortisone, (2) ACTH and thyroid. *J Clin Endocrinol Metab.* 1953;13:283.

27. STEINER MM, BOGGS JD. Absence of pituitary gland, hypothyroidism, hypoadrenalism and hypogonadism in a 17 year old dwarf. *J Clin Endocrinol Metab.* 1965;25:1591.

28. BLIZZARD RM, ALBERTS M. Hypopituitarism, hypoadrenalism and hypogonadism in the newborn infant. *J Pediatr.* 1956;48:782.

29. BREWER DB. Congenital absence of the pituitary gland and its consequences. *J Pathol Bacteriol.* 1957;73:59.

30. REID JD. Congenital absence of the pituitary gland. *J Pediatr.* 1960; 56:658.

31. DUNN JM. Anterior pituitary and adrenal absence in a live-born normocephalic infant. *Am J Obstet Gynecol.* 1966;96:893.

32. MONCRIEFF MW, HILL DS, ARTHUR LJH. Congenital absence of pituitary gland and adrenal hypoplasia. *Arch Dis Child.* 1972;47:251.

33. WILLARD D, SACREZ R, MESSER J, KORN R, KRUG JP, VORS J. La dysgénesie antéhypophysaire primitive. *Nouv Presse Med.* 1972;1:2237.

34. WILLARD D. Primary pituitary dysgenesis. *Pediatrics.* 1973;73:586.

35. HERMAN SP, BAGGENSTOSS AH, CLOUTIER MD. Liver dysfunction and histologic abnormalities in neonatal hypopituitarism. *J Pediatr.* 1975;87:892.

36. LANES R, BLANCHETTE V, CHANDRA E, et al. Congenital hypopituitarism and conjugated hyperbilirubinemia in two infants. *Am J Dis Child.* 1978;132:926.

37. HALL JG. Microphallus, growth hormone deficiency and hypoglycemia in Russell-Silver syndrome. *Am J Dis Child.* 1978;132:1149. (Letter to the Editor.)

38. DROP SLS, COLLE E, GUYDA HJ. Hyperbilirubinemia and idiopathic hypopituitarism in the newborn period. *Acta Paediatr Scand.* 1979; 68:277.

39. KAUSCHANSKY A, GENEL M, SMITH GJW. Congenital hypopituitarism in female infants: Its association with hypoglycemia and hypothyroidism. *Am J Dis Child.* 1979;133:165.

40. VON PETRYKOWSKI W, SAUER M, OTTO M, OLIVER D. Septo-optic dysplasia with congenital hypopituitarism. *Klin Paediatr.* 1980;192:336.

41. COPELAND KC, FRANKS RC, RAMAMURTHY R. Neonatal hyperbilirubinemia and hypoglycemia in congenital hypopituitarism. *Clin Pediatr.* 1981;20:523.

42. SALISBURY DM, LEONARD JV, DEZATEUX CA, SAVAGE MO. Micropenis: an important early sign of congenital hypopituitarism. *Br Med J.* 1984; 288:621.

43. HANNA CE, KRAINZ PL, SKEELS MR, MIYAHIRA RS, SESSER DE, LAFRANCHI SH. Detection of congenital hypopituitary hypothyroidism: Ten-year experience in the Northwest Regional Screening Program. *J Pediatr.* 1986;109:959.

44. RUVALCABA RHA. Pituitary deficiency in midline craniofacial defect (CHARGE association). *J Pediatr Endocrinol.* 1988;3:63.

45. KRISTJANSSON K, HOFFMAN WH, FLANNERY DB, COHEN MJ. Johanson-Blizzard syndrome and hypopituitarism. *J Pediatr.* 1988;113:851.

46. MCQUEEN MC, COPELAND KC. Congenital hypopituitarism with free water intolerance and lack of thymic involution. *Clin Pediatr.* 1989;28:579.

47. LISCHKA A, HERKNER K, POLLAK A. Diagnosis of peripheral androgen insensitivity in a male infant. Excretion analysis. *Arch Androl.* 1989; 22:49.

48. FISHER DA. Second international conference on neonatal screening: progress report. *J Pediatr.* 1983;102:653.

49. CASSIDY SB, BLONDER O, COURTNEY VW, RATZAN SK, CAREY DE. Russell-Silver syndrome and hypopituitarism: patient report and literature review. *Am J Dis Child.* 1986;140:155.

50. RONA RJ, TANNER JM. Aetiology of idiopathic growth hormone deficiency in England and Wales. *Arch Dis Child.* 1977;52:197.

51. STEENDIJK R. Diagnostic and aetiologic features of idiopathic and symptomatic growth hormone deficiency in the Netherlands. A survey of 176 children. *Helv Paediat Acta.* 1980;35:129.

52. GARTNER LM, ARIAS IM. Hormonal control of hepatic bilirubin transport and conjugation. *Am J Physiol.* 1972;222:1091.

53. HAAGEN M, AKKURT I, BLUNCK W. Hypoglykamie und cholestatischer ikterus bei konnatalem panhypopituitarismus. *Monatsschr Kinderheilkd.* 1989;137:678.

54. GOUMY P, DALENS B, MALPUECH G. Association d'une dysraphie de la ligne mediane et d'une insuffisance antehypophysaire congenitale avec micropenis et hypoglycemie neonatale. *Pediatrie.* 1978;33:551.

55. CORNBLATH M, SCHWARTZ R. *Disorders of Carbohydrate Metabolism in Infancy, 2nd ed.* Philadelphia: W.B. Saunders, 1976;177.

56. Patient summaries provided by DRS. L BAKER, Philadelphia; LP PLOTNIK, Baltimore; AL DRASH, Pittsburgh; and NRM BUIST, Portland, Oregon. 1966–1989.

57. GOODMAN HC, GRUMBACH MM, KAPLAN SL. Growth and growth hormone. II. A comparison of isolated growth-hormone deficiency and multiple pituitary hormone deficiencies in thirty-five patients with idiopathic hypopituitary dwarfism. *N Engl J Med.* 1968;278:57.

58. ROCHICCIOLO P, RIBOT C, DUTAU G, DALOUS A. Hypoglycemie par deficit cortico et/ou medullo-surrenalien. *Arch Fr Pediatr.* 1973;30:997.

59. FLUGE G, STOA KD, AARSKOG D. Endocrinological aspects at follow-up studies in neonatal hypoglycemia. *Acta Paediatr Scand.* 1975;64:280.

60. ARTAVIA-LORIA E. CHAUSSAIN JL, BOUGNERES PF, JOB JC. Frequency of hypoglycemia in children with adrenal insufficiency. *Acta Endocrinol (Copenh).* 1986;279:275.

61. VERMA M, AHMED N. SOOD SK. Congenital adrenal hyperplasia with hypoglycaemia. *J Assoc Physicians India.* 1984;32:457.

62. VIDNES J, OYASAETER S. Glucagon deficiency causing severe neonatal hypoglycemia in a patient with normal insulin secretion. *Pediatr Res.* 1977;11:943.

63. KOLLEE LA, MONNENS LA, CEJKA V, WILMS RH. Persistent neonatal hypoglycaemia due to glucagon deficiency. *Arch Dis Child.* 1978; 53:422.

64. POSKITT EME, RAYNER PHW. Isolated growth hormone deficiency. Two families with autosomal dominant inheritance. *Arch Dis Child.* 1974; 49:55.

65. CHALEW SA, KOWARSKI AA. The catecholamine response to hypoglycemia in children with isolated growth hormone deficiency syndromes and multiple pituitary hormone defects. *Pediatr Res.* 1986; 20:1097.

66. VOORHESS ML, MacGILLIVRAY MH. Low plasma norepinephrine responses to acute hypoglycemia in children with isolated growth hormone deficiency. *J Clin Endocrinol Metab.* 1984;59:790.

67. MIGEON CJ, KENNY FM, KOWARSKI A, et al. The syndrome of congenital adrenocortical unresponsiveness to ACTH. Report of six cases. *Pediatr Res.* 1968;2:501.

68. MIGEON CJ. Hypoadrenocorticism. In: Rudolph AM, Hoffman JIE, eds. *Pediatrics, 18th ed.* Norwalk: Appleton & Lange, 1987;1484.

69. GEMELLI M, DELUCA F, BARBERIO G. Hypoglycaemia and congenital adrenal hyperplasia. *Acta Paediatr Scand.* 1979;68:285.

70. GUTAI JP, MIGEON CJ. Adrenal insufficiency during the neonatal period. *Clin Perinatol.* 1975;2:163.

71. KAYE R, BAKER L, KUNZMAN EE, PRASAD ALN, DAVIDSON MH. Catecholamine excretion in spontaneously occurring asymptomatic neonatal hypoglycemia. *Pediatr Res.* 1970;4:295.

72. WHITE PC, NEW MI, DUPONT B. Congenital adrenal hyperplasia. *N Engl J Med.* 1987;316:1519, 1580.

73. MULLIS P, PATEL M, BRICKELL PM, BROOK CGD. Isolated growth hormone deficiency: analysis of the growth hormone (GH)-releasing hormone gene and the GH gene cluster. *J Clin Endocrinol Metab.* 1990;70:187.

74. McQUARRIE I, BELL ET, ZIMMERMAN B, WRIGHT WA. Deficiency of alpha cells of pancreas as possible etiological factor in familial hypoglycemosis. *Fed Proc.* 1950;9:337. (Abstract.)

75. GOTLIN RW, SILVER HK. Neonatal hypoglycaemia, hyperinsulinism and absence of pancreatic alpha cells. *Lancet* 1970;1:1346 (Letter to the Editor), and personal communication, 1975.

76. GRAHAM EA, HARTMANN AF. Subtotal resection of the pancreas for hypoglycemia. *Surg Gynecol Obstet.* 1934;59:474.

77. TALBOT NB, CRAWFORD JD, BAILEY CC. Use of mesoxalyl urea (alloxan) in treatment of an infant with convulsions due to idiopathic hypoglycemia. *Pediatrics.* 1948;1:337.

78. BRODER LE, CARTER SK. Pancreatic islet cell carcinoma. II. Results of therapy with streptozotocin in 52 patients. *Ann Intern Med.* 1973; 79:108.

79. YALOW RS, BERSON SA. Immunoassay of endogenous plasma insulin in man. *J Clin Invest.* 1960;39:1157.

80. WOLFF FW, PARMELEY WW. Aetiological factors in benzothiadiazine hyperglycaemia. *Lancet.* 1963;2:69.

81. ELLIS EF, SMITH RT. The role of the spleen in immunity. *Pediatrics.* 1966;37:111.

82. HARKEN AH, FILLER RM, AVRUSKIN TW, CRIGLER JF JR. The role of "total" pancreatectomy in the treatment of unremitting hypoglycemia of infancy. *J Pediatr Surg.* 1971;6:284.

83. THOMAS CF JR, CUENCA RE, AZIZKHAN RC, UNDERWOOD LE, CARNEY CN. Changing concepts of islet cell dysplasia in neonatal and infantile hyperinsulinism. *World J Surg.* 1988;12:598.

84. RICH RH, DEHNER LP, OKINAGA K, DEEB LC, ULSTROM RA, LEONARD AS. Surgical management of islet-cell adenoma in infancy. *Surgery.* 1978;84:519.

85. LAIDLAW GF. Nesidioblastoma, the islet tumor of the pancreas. *Am J Path.* 1938;14:125.

86. YAKOVAC WC, BAKER L, HUMMLER K. Beta cell nesidioblastosis in idiopathic hypoglycemia of infancy. *J Pediatr.* 1971;79:226.

87. HEITZ PU, KLOPPEL G, HACKI WH, POLAK JM, PEARSE AGE. Nesidioblastosis: the pathologic basis of persistent hyperinsulinemic hypoglycemia in infants. *Diabetes.* 1977;26:632.

88. SOLTESZ G, JENKINS PA, AYNSLEY-GREEN A. Hyperinsulinaemic hypoglycaemia in infancy and childhood: a practical approach to diagnosis and medical treatment based on experience of 18 cases. *Acta Paediatr Acad Scien Hungaricac.* 1984;25:319.

89. AMENDT P, KOHNERT KD, KUNZ J. The hyperinsulinemic hypoglycaemias in infancy: a study of six cases. *Eur J Pediatr.* 1988;148:107.

90. ANTUNES JD, GEFFNER ME, LIPPE BM, LANDAW EM. Childhood hypoglycemia: differentiating hyperinsulinemic from nonhyperinsulinemic causes. *J Pediatr.* 1990;116:105.

91. GORDEN P, SHERMAN B, ROTH J. Proinsulin-like component of circulating insulin in the basal state and in patients and hamsters with islet cell tumors. *J Clin Invest.* 1971;50:2113.

92. AYNSLEY-GREEN A, JENKINS P, TRONIER B, HEDING LG. Plasma proinsulin and c-peptide concentrations in children with hyperinsulinaemic hypoglycaemia. *Acta Paediatr Scand.* 1984;73:359.

93. DERSHEWITZ R, VESTAL B, MacLAREN NK, CORNBLATH M. Transient hepatomegaly and hypoglycemia—a consequence of malicious insulin administration. *Am J Dis Child.* 1976;130:998.

94. STANLEY CA, BAKER L. Hyperinsulinism in infancy: diagnosis by demonstration of abnormal response to fasting hypoglycemia. *Pediatrics.* 1976;57:702.

95. KIRKLAND J, BEN-MENACHEM Y, AVSHTAR M, MARSHALL R, DUDRICK S. Islet cell tumor in a neonate: diagnosis by selective angiography and histological findings. *Pediatrics.* 1978;61:790.

96. INGEMANSSON S, KUHL C, LARSSON L-L, LUNDERQUIST A, LUNDQUIST I. Localization of insulinomas and islet cell hyperplasias by pancreatic vein catheterization and insulin assay. *Surg Gynecol Obstetr.* 1978; 146:725.

97. TEICHMANN RK, SPELSBERG F, HEBERER G. Intraoperative biochemical localization of insulinomas by quick radioimmunoassay. *Am J Surg.* 1982;143:113.

98. SHERWIN RS, FELIG P. Hypoglycemia. In: Felig P, Baxter JD, Broadus AE, Frohman LA, eds. *Endocrinology and Metabolism.* 2nd ed. New York: McGraw-Hill Book Co., 1987;1186.

99. HIRSCH HJ, LOO S, EVANS N, CRIGLER JF JR, FILLER RM, GABBAY KH. Hypoglycemia of infancy and nesidioblastosis: studies with somatostatin. *N Engl J Med.* 1977;296:1323.

100. BLOOMGARDEN ZT, SUNDELL H, ROGERS LW, O'NEILL JA, LILJENQUIST JE. Treatment of intractable neonatal hypoglycemia with somatostatin plus glucagon. *J Pediatr.* 1980;96:148.

101. POLLAK A, LISCHKA A, GHERARDINI R, et al. Persistent hyperinsulinemic hypoglycemia in infants: diagnosis and preoperative management. In: Stern L, Oh W, Friis-Hansen B, eds. *Physiologic Foundations of Perinatal Care.* New York: Elsevier, 1987; Chpt 11.

102. WUTHRICH CL, SCHUBIGER G, ZUPPINGER K. Persistent neonatal hyperinsulinemic hypoglycemia in two siblings successfully treated with diazoxide. *Helv Paediat Acta.* 1986;41:455.

103. BONEH A, LANDAU H. ABRAMOVITCH N. Raw cornstarch as an additional therapy in nesidioblastosis. *Am J Clin Nutr.* 1988;47:1001.

104. THOMAS CG JR, UNDERWOOD LE, CARNEY CN, DOLCOURT JL, WHITT JJ. Neonatal and infantile hypoglycemia due to insulin excess. *Ann Surg.* 1977;185:505.

105. GAUDERER M, STANLEY CA, BAKER L, BISHOP HC. Pancreatic adenomas in infants and children: current surgical management. *J Pediatr Surg.* 1978;13:591.

106. KRAMER JL, BELL MJ, DESCHRYVER K, BOWER RJ, TERNBERG JL, WHITE NH. Clinical and histological indications for extensive pancreatic resection in nesidioblastosis. *Am J Surg.* 1982;143:116.

107. MOAZAM F, RODGERS BM, TALBERT JL, ROSENBLOOM AL. Near-total pancreatectomy in persistent infantile hypoglycemia. *Arch Surg.* 1982; 117:1151.

108. CARCASSONE M, DELARUE A, LETOURNEAU JN. Surgical treatment of organic pancreatic hypoglycemia in the pediatric age. *J Pediatr Surg.* 1983;18:75.

109. GREENE SA, AYNSLEY-GREEN A, SOLTESZ G, BAUM JD. Management of secondary diabetes mellitus after total pancreatectomy in infancy. *Arch Dis Child.* 1984;59:356.

110. GRUPPUSO PA, DELUCA F, O'SHEA PA, SCHWARTZ R. Near-total pancreatectomy for hyperinsulinism. Spontaneous remission of resultant diabetes. *Acta Paediatr Scand.* 1985;74:311.

111. JAFFE R, HASHIDA Y, YUNIS EJ. Pancreatic pathology in hyperinsulinemic hypoglycemia of infancy. *Lab Invest.* 1980;43:356.

112. JAFFE R. The pancreas. In: Wigglesworth JSW, Singer DB, eds. *Fetal and Perinatal Pathology.* Oxford: Blackwell Scientific Publ, Inc., 1991.

113. GOULD VE, MEMOLI VA. Nesidiodysplasia and nesidioblastosis in infancy. *Pediatr Pathol.* 1983;1:7.

114. WITTE DP, GREIDER MH, DESCHRYVER-KECSKEMETI K, KISSANE JM, WHITE NH. The juvenile human endocrine pancreas: normal v. idiopathic hyperinsulinemic hypoglycemia. *Semin Diag Pathol.* 1984;1:30.

115. BECKWITH JB. Extreme cytomegaly of the adrenal fetal cortex, omphalocele, hyperplasia of kidneys and pancreas, and Leydig-cell hyperplasia: Another syndrome? Presented at Annual Meeting of Western Society for Pediatric Research, Los Angeles, California, Nov. 11, 1963.

116. BECKWITH JB, WANG C, DONNELL GN, GWINN JL. Hyperplastic fetal vis-

ceromegaly, with macroglossia, omphalocele, cytomegaly of the adrenal fetal cortex, postnatal somatic gigantism and other abnormalities: A newly recognized syndrome. Abstract read by title, at Annual Meeting of American Pediatric Society, Seattle, Washington, June 16–18, 1964.

117. WIEDEMANN HR. Complexe malformatif familial avec hernie ombilicale et macroglossie. Un "syndrome nouveau"? *J Genet Hum.* 1964;13:223.

118. PETTENATI MJ, HAINES JL, HIGGINS RR, WAPPNER RS, PALMER CG, WEAVER DD. Wiedemann-Beckwith syndrome: presentation of clinical and cytogenetic data on 22 new cases and review of the literature. *Human Genet.* 1986;74:143.

119. WIEDEMANN HR. Tumor and hemihypertrophy associated with Wiedemann-Beckwith's syndrome. *Eur J Pediatr.* 1983;141:129.

120. ENGSTROM W, LINDHAM S, SCHOFIELD P. Wiedemann-Beckwith syndrome. *Eur J Pediatr.* 1988;147:450.

121. COMBS JT, GRUNT JA, BRANDT IK. New syndrome of neonatal hypoglycemia. *N Engl J Med.* 1966;275:236.

122. STEFAN Y, BONDI C, GRASSO S, ORCI L. Beckwith-Wiedemann syndrome: a quantitative, immunohistochemical study of pancreatic islet cell populations. *Diabetologia.* 1985;28:914.

123. SCHIFF D, COLLE E, WELLS D, STERN L. Metabolic aspects of the Beckwith-Wiedemann syndrome. *J Pediatr.* 1973;82:258.

124. GRUNT JA, ENRIQUEZ AR. Further studies of the hypoglycemia in children with the exomphalos-macroglossia-gigantism syndrome. *Yale J Biol Med.* 1972;45:15.

125. KOH THHG, COOPER JE, NEWMAN CL, WALKER TM, KIELY EM, HOFFMANN EB. Pancreatoblastoma in a neonate with Wiedemann-Beckwith syndrome. *Eur J Pediatr.* 1986;145:435.

126. SOTELO-AVILA C, SINGER D. Syndrome of hyperplastic fetal visceromegaly and neonatal hypoglycemia (Beckwith's Syndrome). A report of seven cases. *Pediatrics.* 1970;46:240.

127. WAZIRI M, PATIL SR, HANSON JW, BARTLEY JA. Abnormality of chromosome 11 in patients with features of Beckwith-Wiedemann syndrome. *J Pediatr.* 1983;102:873.

128. SPENCER GSG, SCHABEL F, FRISCH H. Raised somatomedin associated with normal growth hormone. A cause of Beckwith-Wiedemann syndrome? *Arch Dis Child.* 1980;55:151.

129. ROBINOW M, SCHAFER AD. Somatomedin-C in the Beckwith-Wiedemann syndrome. *Arch Dis Child.* 1981;56:77. (Letter.)

130. WENINGER M, LISCHKA A, POLLAK A, VERGEBLICH C, OGRIS E, FRISCH H. Somatomedin aktivitat bei Wiedemann-Beckwith syndrome. *Monatsschr Kinderheilkd.* 1984;132:900.

131. SPRITZ RA, MAGER D, PAULI RM, LAXOVA R. Normal dosage of the insulin and insulin-like growth factor II genes in patients with the Beckwith-Wiedemann syndrome. *Am J Hum Genet.* 1986;39:265.

132. GOTLIN RW. Diazoxide therapy in the syndrome of Beckwith-Wiedemann-Coombs. *J Pediatr.* 1973;83:342. (Letter to the Editor.)

133. ROE TF, KERSHNAR AK, WEITZMAN JJ, MADRIGAL LS. Beckwith's syndrome with extreme organ hyperplasia. *Pediatrics.* 1973;52:372.

134. FILIPPI G. MCKUSICK VA. The Beckwith-Wiedemann syndrome. *Medicine.* 1970;49:279.

135. DONOHUE WL. Clinicopathologic conference at the Hospital for Sick Children: dysendocrinism. *J Pediatr.* 1948;32:739.

136. DAVID TJ, WEBB BW, GORDON IRS. The Patterson syndrome, leprechaunism, and pseudoleprechaunism. *J Med Genet.* 1981;18:294.

137. ROSENBERG AM, HAWORTH JC, DEGROOT W, TREVENEN CL, RECHLER MM. A case of leprechaunism with severe hyperinsulinemia. *Am J Dis Child.* 1980;134:170.

138. CANTANI A, ZIRVOLO MG, TACCONI ML. Un syndrome polydysmorphique rare: le leprechaunisme. *Ann Genet.* 1987;30:221.

139. KAPLOWITZ PB, D'ERCOLE AJ. Fibroblasts from a patient with leprechaunism are resistant to insulin, epidermal growth factor and somatomedin C. *J Clin Endocrinol Metab.* 1982;55:741.

140. ELSAS LJ, ENDO F, STRUMLAUF E, ELDERS J, PREIST JH. Leprechaunism: an inherited defect in a high-affinity insulin receptor. *Am J Hum Genet.* 1985;37:73.

141. KADOWAKI T, BEVINS CL, CAMA A, et al. Two mutant alleles of the insulin receptor gene in a patient with extreme insulin resistance. *Science.* 1988;240:787.

142. MOLLER DE, FLIER JS. Detection of an alteration in the insulin-receptor gene in a patient with insulin resistance, acanthosis nigricans and the polycystic ovary syndrome (type A insulin resistance). *N Engl J Med.* 1988;319:1526.

143. ROSE SR, CHROUSOS G, CORNBLATH M, SIDBURY J. Management of postoperative nesidioblastosis with zinc protamine glucagon and oral starch. *J Pediatr.* 1986;108:97.

HYPERGLYCEMIA

IN THE

NEONATE

During the past 30 years, the major focus has been on hypoglycemia in the neonate, and relatively little attention has been given to hyperglycemia. When reported, the emphasis has been on infants with transient diabetes mellitus [1,2] or the rare neonate with permanent diabetes [3,4].

Over the past two decades, however, the survival of very low birth weight (VLBW) and stressed, small, premature infants [5–7] and the use of supplemental and total parenteral nutrition [8–10] have resulted in a number of reports emphasizing the problems of hyperglycemia and the ensuing glycosuria, dehydration, and hyperosmolality [11]. These complications have included an increased mortality [12,13] and frequency of ventricular hemorrhage [12], as well as major handicaps [14]. Unfortunately, these reports contained a number of confounding variables and did not permit evaluation of the hyperglycemia alone as an independent variable [11].

More recently, both Pildes and Raivio [15] presented preliminary data that showed a positive statistical correlation between hyperglycemia and neurodevelopmental and behavioral outcomes in very low birth weight infants after correcting for a number of confounding variables.

The definition of hyperglycemia in the neonate is a plasma glucose concentration over 125 mg/dl (6.9 mM) obtained preprandially (see Chapter 2). Transient hyperglycemia in the high-risk neonate of low birth weight and short gestational age is often associated with low Apgar scores, respiratory distress [13], intravenous glucose therapy [16], supplemental or total parenteral nutrition [5,9], medications [17] and/or anesthetic and surgical stress [18]. The plasma values often exceed 180 mg/dl (10 mM) and may be as high as 300 mg/dl (16.7 mM) or more and are usually associated with glucosuria as well [19]. In both permanent and transient neonatal diabetes mellitus, the plasma glucose levels usually exceed 250 mg/dl (13.9 mM) and can be over 2,000 mg/dl (111 mM).

Neonatal hyperglycemia, transient diabetes mellitus and permanent diabetes mellitus are discussed here.

• Transient Neonatal Hyperglycemia

This past 15 years has seen the survival of many infants between 500 and 1000 gm birth weight and between 25 and 30 weeks gestation—the "micropremie" [20]. All VLBW, the majority of preterm, low birth weight, and sick newborns are given parenteral therapy. This includes glucose, alone or in combination with amino acids, lipids, and electrolytes in order to provide as adequate nutrition as possible and to support the metabolic milieu of these precarious neonates until adequate oral feedings can be tolerated. This has not been without untoward consequences since hyperglycemia appears to be a common, albeit, probably preventable complication in the care of these high-risk babies.

The frequency of hyperglycemia, as summarized by Dweck and Miranda [5], varied between 20 and 83 percent of low birth weight infants (mean weights = 890 to 1,376 gm) of short gestation (mean gestational ages = 27 to 31 weeks) in both prospective and retrospective studies [13,21–24]. Highest glucose values in some 186 infants ranged between 192 mg/dl (10.7 mM) [22] and 2,000 mg/dl (111 mM) [21]. Most of the infants were being given parenteral glucose. With glucose rates exceeding 6 mg/kg/min (0.36 gm/kg/hr) in one study, 72 percent (36 of 50) of infants with a mean birth weight of 890 gm and a mean gestational age of 27 weeks had glucose values greater than 300 mg/dl (16.7 mM) [24].

In a more recent study, Louik et al. [16] emphasized the problems that can ensue with the administration of parenteral glucose alone. The risk for hyperglycemia is 18 times greater in infants weighing under 1,000 gm than in those weighing over 2,000 gm.

Clinical manifestations depended upon the severity and duration of the hyperglycemia. While no specific acute problems were associated with plasma glucose values between 125 and 200 mg/dl (6.9 and 11.1 mM), higher plasma glucose concentrations caused significant osmotic diuresis, dehydration, and weight loss. Secondary effects included metabolic disturbances such as hyponatremia, hypernatremia, hyperosmolality, and acidosis. The consequences of these developments include cerebral fluid shifts and hemorrhage, with CNS manifestations, including seizures. While none of these are specific, the correction of the hyperglycemia is important to establish whether or not it alone is responsible.

Early studies have also implicated hyperglycemia in long-term consequences such as an increase in both mortality and morbidity [12–15]. Unfortunately, these studies were not adequately controlled, and further study will be required before definitive conclusions are justified. One current hypothesis indicates that the hyperglycemia, itself, is secondary to high-stress diseases such as sepsis, underlying CNS or neurologic disorders, or cardiorespiratory distress syndromes in these high-risk neonates. Thus, hyperglycemia may be a consequence rather than a cause of both the acute and long-term clinical problems.

Clinical Management

Clinical management of the infants at risk involves anticipating the problem by carefully controlling the amounts of parenteral glucose being given. Glucose infusion rates between 3 and 4 mg/kg/min have been recommended because they do not produce hyperglycemia in very low birth weight infants and are adequate to prevent hypoglycemia [11]. However, since this is not invariably true, it is important to monitor plasma and urine glucose concentrations in all of these high-risk newborns when they are being given parenteral glucose either alone or in conjunction with supplemental or total parenteral feedings. This is especially true during the first 24 to 48 hours of parenteral glucose [13,24] and in babies of low birth weight [<1,250 gm] and short gestation (<31 weeks) [13,25].

These low rates of glucose administration, unfortunately, are often inadequate to promote weight gain and growth. Recent studies suggest that the careful administration of regular insulin, either as an IV infusion [26–28] or intermittently [11], can support the utilization of increasing quantities of glucose without hyperglycemia or glycosuria [28,29] and allow weight gains equivalent to those of euglycemic low birth weight neonates [28].

Binder et al. [28], in an inadequately controlled, nonrandomized, retrospective analysis of 112 infants with birth weight ≤1000 gm born between November 1983 and November 1986, reported positive results from giving insulin to 34 infants with significant hyperglycemia, defined as the blood glucose concentration associated with glucosuria $\geq$0.5 percent as determined by Clinitest tablets. No specific blood glucose concentrations were provided in this report. These values were likely to have been highly variable, in part due to the immaturity of renal glucose reabsorption in these VLBW infants.

Thirty-six infants were excluded from the study, 34 were given insulin for 1–58 days, and 42 never received insulin (i.e., no glycosuria). In this study, glycosuria occurred in 45 percent of VLBW infants and in 80 percent of those with a birth weight <750 gm.

Rapidly changing insulin tolerance in some patients required careful monitoring to modify insulin therapy. Blood glucose concentrations were monitored every 1–2 hours during insulin administration. If they were less than 40 mg/dl (2.2 mM), hypoglycemia was suspected, and a laboratory glucose oxidase determination of plasma glucose was obtained. Insulin dose was titrated as necessary to maintain blood glucose concentrations between 100 and 150 mg/dl (5.6 and 8.3 mM).

While the treated infants were significantly smaller and more immature and required ventilation longer than the untreated group, they achieved an intake of 100 kcal/kg/day at 15 $\pm$ 8 days versus 17 $\pm$ 11 days for the untreated group and regained birth weight at 12 $\pm$ 6 days versus 13 $\pm$ 6 days of life with this regimen. The authors concluded that ". . . insulin infusion improves glucose tolerance in extremely low birth weight infants and allows hyperglycemic infants to achieve adequate energy intake similar to that of infants who do not become hyperglycemic" [28].

A prospective controlled randomized intervention study will be necessary to confirm these results before any definitive recommendations regarding insulin infusion therapy for general clinical use can be made.

Monitoring Plasma Glucose Values

Monitoring plasma glucose values should be done frequently during the first 24–48 hours of parenteral glucose administration and then less often as long as glucose is being given either alone or in conjunction with other substrates (lipid or amino acid supplements). This may be done every 4–8 hours during the first 48 hours, daily thereafter, or whenever there is *glucosuria over 0.25 percent, a diuresis, or weight loss.*

With insulin therapy, more frequent monitoring is necessary. Samples should be obtained at 1–2-hour intervals during insulin infusions. If insulin is given intermittently, monitoring is recommended at 3–4-hour intervals. Monitoring should be continued at these frequent intervals for another 24 hours after insulin is discontinued.

Ostertag et al. [27] have suggested the following practical steps for such frequent sampling in these VLBW infants:

1. A 25-gauge needle is used instead of a lancet to obtain blood samples to avoid soft tissue damage [29].
2. Hexokinase or glucose oxidase laboratory glucose determinations should be done when glucose values are 40 mg/dl (2.2 mM) or less.

Infants should also be monitored regularly after exchange transfusions; after surgical procedures; if stress of any sort is present (e.g., intraventricular hemorrhage, respiratory distress syndrome, patent ductus arteriosus); or with infections or hypoxia [6,11]. Intermittent monitoring is indicated during theophylline therapy [11,17].

While inadequate to establish a diagnosis, bedside glucose oxidase stick methods, if done precisely as directed, appear to be more reliable between 100 and 300 mg/dl (5.6 and 16.7 mM) than below 50 mg/dl (2.8 mM). However, values above 300 mg/dl (16.7 mM) become less reliable and require frequent confirmation with a laboratory plasma glucose determination.

Any abnormal glucose value (>125 mg/dl [6.9 mM]) should be confirmed by a reliable laboratory plasma glucose analysis to establish the diagnosis of hyperglycemia.

Therapy

Therapy is probably not necessary for plasma glucose concentrations less than 200 mg/dl (11.1 mM) unless an osmotic diuresis occurs. Careful monitoring of blood glucose values and reducing the rate of the glucose infusion, alone, should be sufficient to prevent further hyperglycemia.

In symptomatic infants, a reduction in the rate or concentration of the glucose infusion is indicated. This should be done in a gradual manner by 2 mg/kg/min every 4–6 hours until plasma glucose levels are less than 125 mg/dl (6.9 mM).

Caution must be exercised in using hypotonic as well as non-glucose-containing solutions.

In infants with plasma glucose concentrations over 250–300 mg/dl (13.9–16.7 mM), insulin therapy has been utilized cautiously to both reduce the plasma glucose levels as well as allow greater caloric input [27–30]. Insulin has been given as an infusion utilizing a pump, inserted "piggyback" as close as possible to the parenteral nutrition solution [27,28], or intermittently as regular insulin [11,26].

Intermittent insulin may be given at a dose of 0.1–0.2 U/kg every

6–12 hours until glucose levels are stable. Plasma glucose concentrations should be measured at regular intervals, with the goal of keeping the blood glucose values between 100–150 mg/dl (5.6–8.3 mM).

The duration of insulin therapy has been highly variable in all infants and may be necessary for 1–2 doses only or for as long as several days to weeks, depending upon the purpose of therapy.

With conflicting reports of efficacy and safety and the lack of a prospective controlled randomized intervention trial, the use of insulin in these very low birth weight infants must still be considered under investigation and experimental [26,31].

Prognosis

Prognosis for hyperglycemia alone is difficult to evaluate in view of the multiplicity of problems presented by these VLBW immature infants. Hyperglycemia alone, if sufficiently severe, may be responsible for cerebral hemorrhage in VLBW infants by increasing serum osmolality, resulting in shifts of water from the intracellular to the extracellular compartments of the brain. Since each 18-mg/dl (1.0 mM) increment in glucose concentration increases serum osmolality by 1 mOsm/L, a plasma glucose concentration of 270 mg/dl (15 mM) would increase total serum osmolality by about 10 mOsm/l and could produce shifts in intracellular fluid. Furthermore, it should be noted that transient hyperglycemia has been described in two infants with severe hypernatremia and hyperosmolality following improper preparation of formula [32].

In the presence of hypoxia-ischemia, which is so common in these infants, hyperglycemia has been postulated to produce cellular damage by yet another mechanism. The increased glucose levels result in excessive lactic acidosis in the brain which, in turn, produces brain damage. While this sequence of events has been shown to be true in adult animals and man, studies in immature rats [33] and in vitro brain glial cell cultures [34] suggest either no effect [33] or a protective one [34] for hyperglycemia in the neonate.

Why specific infants develop hyperglycemia and others do not has not been adequately explained. Studies of hormone assays, hepatic glucose output, stress, and glucose infusion rates have all been suggestive of causation in specific infants. No generalizations are indicated, and each infant must be evaluated for the best approach to prevention, therapy, and maintenance of adequate growth and development.

The goal of therapy in all infants, including the VLBW, is to provide sufficient nutrients to meet energy requirements and establish growth [35]. Under fasting conditions, catabolism results in loss of tissue nitrogen (protein), while glucogenic amino acids may provide glucose via gluconeogenesis. The provision of exogenous glucose alone or with insulin may reduce catabolism, but cannot, in itself, result in real growth. For insulin to produce growth, even in the presence of hyperglycemia, all other essential nutrients (including nonessential and essential amino acids and fatty acids) must be available as well, in addition to adequate energy sources. This must all be achieved, while avoiding both hyperglycemia and hypoglycemia.

· Transient Diabetes Mellitus

A discrete clinical entity that simulates diabetes mellitus has been described in small-for-gestational-age infants during the first 6 weeks of life. Characteristically, in this temporary or transient diabetes mellitus, ketonuria is minimal or absent, but hyperglycemia, glycosuria, and dehydration may be severe [1,2]. However, these infants are insulin sensitive. This syndrome has also been referred to as congenital neonatal pseudodiabetes, paradiabetes mellitus infantum, or congenital temporary diabetes [36–39].

Probably the first patient identified as having this syndrome was the son of a physician who presented with "honeyed napkins," polyuria, polydipsia, polyphagia, dry skin, and emaciation a few days after birth. Glycosuria was identified at 14 days of age, and the infant died of a urinary tract infection after 6 months (Kitselle, 1852) as described by Lawrence and McCance [40]. Ramsey [41] reported the first neonate with this syndrome whose hyperglycemia and glycosuria was well documented. After a 25-year follow-up, the patient remained healthy and was accepted for military service [36]. Subsequently, reports of over 45 patients with variations of this condition have been published [1,36–70], and others are known to the authors.

At least two patients have now been reported to develop permanent insulin-dependent diabetes mellitus, one at 18 years [71] and one at 15 years of age [65]. The latter was one of three half-siblings (one brother and two sisters) who developed transient diabetes mellitus in early infancy [60,65], and who represent a unique genetic pattern in having the same father, but three different mothers. Another report of successive siblings having this transient syndrome included three boys born of the same mother [50,51]. In addition, first cousins, one with transient and one with permanent neonatal diabetes mellitus [69], and a set of twins [70] have been reported as well. The frequency of this syndrome is relatively rare and sporadic in occurrence.

Clinical Manifestations

Characteristically, the infants were small for gestational age. The sexes were equally represented (Table 6-1). There was a positive family history of diabetes mellitus in 34 percent of the patients. The most striking presenting signs and symptoms were marked dehydration and wasting, often in the presence of an adequate food intake and in the absence of vomiting or diarrhea. These infants had a "peculiar pallor and lined, aged appearance which was associated with remarkably 'open-eyed' alert facies," according to Hutchison et al. [39] (Fig. 6-1). Subcutaneous fat was minimal. Occasionally, there was evidence of infection and vomiting; sudden weight loss, polyuria and fever were also recorded. Three patients have been reported to have macroglossia as well [37,47,62].

The diagnosis was made as early as one day of age [51] or as late

TABLE 6-1. Summary of data of 46 patients with transient diabetes mellitus

LOW BIRTH WEIGHT/GESTATION (small for gestational age)	MAJORITY	%
Sex		
Male	25	54
Female	21	46
Positive diabetic family history	12(35)*	34
Age of detection		
Mean	12 days	
Range	1–42 days	
Moderate to severe dehydration	32(44)	73
Complicating infection	10(40)	25
Highest blood sugar level		
Mean	792 mg/dl	
Range	245–2,472 mg/dl	
Metabolic acidosis	12(16)	75
Ketonuria	15(41)	37
Insulin therapy	36(44)	82
Mean	7.4 units/day	
Range	0.5–60 units/day	
Duration of insulin therapy		
Mean	72 days	
Range	0 to 540 days	
Follow-up		
Mean	25 months	
Range	1 to 300 months	

*Number in parentheses represents numbers of infants about whom information was known.

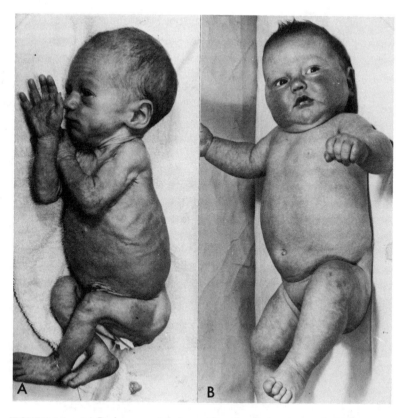

FIGURE 6-1.   (a) Patient was 14 days old and emaciated, yet alert after 48 hours of therapy. (b) Picture taken at 3½ months of age. (From Hutchison et al. *Br Med J.* 1962; 2:435, with permission.)

as six weeks, with a mean age of 12 days. All the clinical manifestations may be present at birth or shortly thereafter. While a number have had low Apgar scores at birth, others have been normal.

The diagnosis is based on glycosuria, present in all, and hyperglycemia, ranging between 245 and 2,470 mg/dl (13.6 and 137 mM). Glucose tolerance tests are not necessary for diagnosis. Ketosis has not been reported. However, ketonuria has definitely been reported as a transient phenomenon in 15 of 41 patients.

Lumbar punctures have been done on several infants, and the cerebrospinal fluid sugar was elevated to levels exceeding 400 mg/dl (22.2 mM) [50,70]. Thus, the sugar content of the CNS can be diagnostic in transient diabetes mellitus, in contrast to hypoglycemia.

Only limited laboratory data are available for the patients reported. The information given suggests that acid-base derangements may be common, since 12 of 16 infants had a metabolic acidosis (pH 7.05–7.20, $HCO_3 < 15$ mEq/L). Serum electrolytes, reported at the time of diagnosis, indicated normal or minimal elevations of serum sodium concentrations in most, although hypernatremia [32] and hyponatremia have occurred as well. Serum potassium values were usually within normal limits but may be elevated. Studies of steroid metabolism have been normal in some ten infants.

In one infant, umbilical serum radioimmunoassayable insulin and insulinlike growth factor I (IGF-I) were low, but insulinlike growth factor II (IGF-II), measured by a specific radioreceptor assay, was normal. At 2.5 months of age, after insulin treatment was discontinued, endogenous insulin secretion was documented by increased urinary C-peptide concentrations [64]. This study concluded that growth failure in these infants may be related not only to a lack of insulin but also to IGF-I deficiency.

Serum insulin concentrations have been reported in at least ten infants [1,51–53,55,61,64,66,71] and urine insulin values in two [51,64]. Low serum proinsulin and plasma C-peptide values were reported in three patients [67,70]. While low initially, repeated measurements of C-peptide in urine suggest that recovery of beta cell function occurs. However, low values may persist for as long as 5 months and still be transient [68]. Insulin antibodies were negative in two infants [70].

Clinical Course

Clinical course is characterized by insulin sensitivity and a dramatic clinical improvement in appearance and behavior (see Fig. 6-1). In view of the profound and repeated hypoglycemic episodes reported in two of the early patients treated with 30–60 units of regular insulin daily (extremely high doses), the majority of infants have subsequently been treated with significantly less insulin, from 0.5–3 units per kilogram body weight or 1.6–4, maximum 8 units/day. Some have not even required insulin therapy [70] and responded to hydration alone.

In many instances, the infants could be maintained on oral feedings and were not given intravenous fluids. In contrast, some were severely dehydrated and acidotic and required parenteral fluids for 24–72 hours. Dehydration was rapidly corrected, weight gain ensued, and the clinical manifestations were quickly reversed. Glycosuria persisted for as long as 18 months or subsided within 1–2 weeks. The duration of hyperglycemia was also variable.

Currently, such patients should have repeated studies of serum insulin, C-peptide, electrolytes, and acid-base status. Such studies, done both fasting and postprandially over time (months), may be necessary to differentiate the transient syndrome from permanent diabetes mellitus. Permanent diabetes has been reported to occur as early as nine days of age [72].

These infants have also been mistaken for patients with the salt-losing type of congenital adrenal hyperplasia and galactosemia. An acute onset of weight loss, vomiting, and dehydration can occur in both of these conditions. It is important to test the urine specifically for glucose (glucose oxidase). The urine should be tested for both total reducing substances and glucose, and the plasma for glucose concentration and, if high, for insulin and C-peptide levels as well. All of these are especially important in the neonate to diagnose diabetes mellitus and to differentiate between the permanent and transient types.

Therapy

Therapy in these infants should be directed toward control of the hyperglycemia and its associated hypertonicity and dehydration. Insulin therapy must be individualized; small, intermittent, subcutaneous doses of regular insulin ("human" insulins) and frequent measurements of plasma glucose concentrations are essential to avoid hypoglycemia. Total doses varying between 0.5 to 3.0 U/kg/day have been found to be effective. Plasma glucose values between 100 and 180 mg/dl (5.6 and 10 mM) can be achieved and appear to be adequate to relieve the clinical manifestations. With adequate feedings, this level of control is associated with appropriate weight gain and growth. When glycosuria and hyperglycemia have been controlled, the dose of insulin must be tapered slowly (days to weeks) before stopping completely. Since the condition is transient, there have not been any reports, to our knowledge, on the use of glycosylated hemoglobin in monitoring control in these infants.

In the presence of marked hyperglycemia (>400 mg/dl [22.2 mM]) and dehydration, parenteral fluids are necessary. Physiologic management can be achieved, provided repeated mircroblood analyses are available for sugar, blood gases, and electrolytes, and are used. Under these conditions, the hypertonicity and the osmotic diuresis, which are responsible for the dehydration, are best corrected by the use, initially, of non-glucose-containing fluids. Solutions of hypotonic electrolytes (75 mEq/liter sodium, e.g., 1/2 Ringer's, 1/2 water) in quantities of 60 to 80 ml/kg are given in the first 12 hours or until the plasma glucose concentration has fallen to 300 mg/dl (16.7 mM). Thereafter, additional fluids containing 40 mEq/liter sodium (as 1/4 Ringer's solution) and 2.5 or 5 percent dextrose in quantities up to 150 to 200 ml/kg/day are recommended.

In view of the variable and changing sensitivity to insulin in these infants and the dangers of prolonged or recurrent hypoglycemic reactions, dextrose (2.5 percent) can be included in the initial fluids if careful monitoring of the plasma glucose is not possible and the initial plasma glucose concentration is less than 500 mg/dl (27.8 mM).

Chlorpropamide was reported to be useful in weaning one patient from insulin after some 40 days [62]. However, others [69,70] have tried Chlorpropamide, even in a set of twins in which only one was treated, and have not found it useful.

Etiology and Pathogenesis

A variety of etiologic factors have been suggested in this syndrome, including a transient hypothalamic imbalance, infection, adrenocortical abnormalities, insulin resistance, or relative or absolute hypoinsulinism due to hypoplasia of the beta cells [51–53,55,58,64,67,70]. A number of glucose tolerance tests during pregnancy have been reported in the mothers of these infants. These have varied from flat [47,50,62] to normal [44,50] to diabetic curves [59,60].

Many studies support the concept that a temporary delay in the maturation of beta cell function may occur in these infants. Urinary insulin [55] or C-peptide [64] secretion, as well as insulin and glucose responses to glucose [1,44,51,52,55,61,64,67], tolbutamide [44,52,53,55,61], and caffeine benzoate [55,61], support this hypothesis. The deficient or delayed pancreatic insulin release could be related to a number of steps in the process of insulin synthesis, storage, or release. Whether receptors on the beta cell, transport mechanisms, or enzymatic activating systems, such as those involving adenylyl cyclase or others, may be involved in this delay is still not known.

On the basis of the growth pattern in one affected infant, Schiff et al. [52] suggested that insulin may act as a stimulus to growth in early life. More recently, in another such infant, Blethen et al. [64] found that both insulin and IGF-I were low, but IGF-II was normal in umbilical blood. After 2.5 months, endogenous insulin secretion was documented by urinary C-peptide measurements. Normal growth and IGF-I levels persisted. More studies of this type will be necessary to understand fully the various factors involved in both the growth failure and the transient diabetes mellitus in these infants.

Case Report (Patient 6-1): Hypoglycemia Followed by Transient Diabetes Mellitus [1]

A full-term female infant was born by vaginal delivery to a 21-year-old primipara after a midforceps rotation under caudal anesthesia. Apgars were 2 and 4 at 1 and 5 minutes. The infant was intubated, given oxygen, glucose, and sodium bicarbonate via an umbilical catheter.

The pregnancy had been uneventful except for maternal acute trauma resulting in a fractured mandible on the day of delivery. There was no family history of diabetes mellitus.

Birth weight was 2,780 gm (10–25th percentiles), length 49 cm (50th percentile), head circumference 34 cm (50th percentile) (see Fig. 6-2 for clinical course).

At 5 hours of age, she had a generalized convulsion, and the blood sugar concentration was <10 mg/dl (0.6 mM). She responded promptly to continuous intravenous 10 percent glucose in water. The lumbar puncture (LP) at that time and those done subsequently were all within normal limits. At 7 hours of age, seizures recurred, with the blood sugar at 10 mg/dl (0.6 mM) with the glucose infusion in place. At that time, a modified intravenous glucose tolerance test was done by giving 1.0 gm/kg of 50 percent glucose and measuring plasma glucose and insulin concentrations at regular intervals (see Fig. 6-3a). The test was terminated after 44 minutes when the glucose concentration fell to 25 mg/dl (1.4 mM) and a third seizure occurred. The clearance rate for glucose was abnormally rapid (Kt = 4.5 percent/min; normal = <1.0 percent/min). The infant was given 15 mg hydrocortisone twice daily, and the concentration of the dextrose infusion was increased to 15 percent.

With blood glucose concentrations between 40 and 50 mg/dl (2.2 and 2.8 mM), she continued to have seizures that gradually subsided over the next three days. Phenobarbital, dilantin, paraldehyde, and pyridoxine had

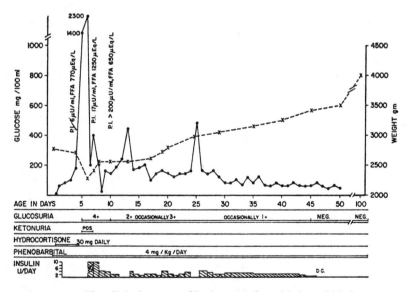

FIGURE 6-2. The clinical course of Patient 6.1 from birth to 100 days of age, showing blood sugar (solid line) and body weight (broken line). Recurrence of marked hyperglycemia occurred on days 13 and 25 when insulin was temporarily omitted. (PI = plasma insulin.) (From Gentz and Cornblath. *Adv Pediatr.* 1969; 16:345, with permission.)

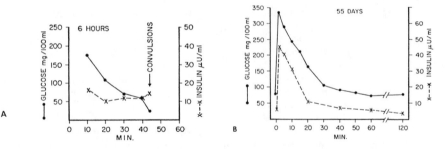

FIGURE 6-3. Blood glucose and serum insulin levels in an infant with transient diabetes studied by intravenous glucose tolerance tests at (a) 6 hours and (b) 55 days. (From Gentz and Cornblath. *Adv Pediatr.* 1969; 16:345, with permission.)

been given without any effect. A repeat LP was within normal limits. Seizures stopped on day 4.

At 5 days of age, blood glucose concentration was >250 mg/dl (13.9 mM) by Dextrostix. Hydrocortisone was discontinued and intravenous fluid changed to half-isotonic saline. Within the next 12 hours, she became severely dehydrated, was lethargic, and had polyuria with marked glucosuria and moderate ketonuria. Capillary pH was 7.25; serum acetone positive; sodium was 143, potassium 5.0, chloride 105 mEq/l. The blood glucose concentration reached a maximum of 2,300 mg/dl (127.8 mM), at which time a plasma insulin concentration was 17 μU/ml (102 pM) and FFA 1,250 uEq/l. At a blood glucose value of 1,280 mg/dl (71.1 mM), the plasma insulin concentration was 6 μU/ml (36 pM) and FFA, 770 uEq/l.

On day 6, the infant was given a total of 20 units of regular insulin in divided doses during the first 24 hours of therapy, and the blood glucose was 170 mg/dl (9.4 mM) (see Fig. 6-2). Glycosuria and polyuria diminished and hydration improved. Ketonuria was no longer present. She was subsequently maintained on 4–8 units of insulin (2–4 U/kg/day), and blood glucose values remained between 100 and 200 mg/dl (5.6 and 11.1 mM). On the second day of insulin therapy, one blood glucose value was below 20 mg/dl (1.1 mM) without symptoms. Within a few days, she began to gain weight and continued to do so.

Abrupt cessation of regular insulin therapy resulted in a recurrence of hyperglycemia and glycosuria within 6 hours at 7, 14, and 25 days of life. The dose of insulin was gradually reduced to 2 units/day; blood glucose values approximated 100 mg/dl (5.6 mM). Insulin therapy was discontinued at 44 days of age.

At 55 days of age, another IV glucose tolerance test was done. The clearance rate (Kt = 5.7 percent/min) remained rapid, with a prompt normal insulin response (Fig. 6-3b).

When last seen at 13 months of age, the infant had shown normal growth and development. There was no glycosuria.

Comment

First reported by Chance and Bower [56], the sequence of symptomatic hypoglycemia followed by transient diabetes mellitus requiring insulin therapy demonstrates the profound disturbance in carbohydrate homeostasis that can occur during the neonatal period. This patient illustrates the caution necessary in treating symptomatic hypoglycemia and the necessity of carefully monitoring plasma glucose concentrations during therapy. Excessive hyperglycemia occurred due to the failure to recognize hyperglycemia as a result of utilizing only glucose oxidase strips for follow-up.

The intravenous glucose tolerance test at 55 days of age shows a normal insulin response, indicating the transient nature of the diabetes.

This case clearly illustrates the importance of tapering the therapy slowly and not discontinuing the insulin abruptly once glucose control has been attained.

• Permanent Diabetes Mellitus (IDDM)

In young infants, permanent insulin-dependent diabetes mellitus (IDDM) occurs less often than the transient type. In fact, by 1975, Dorchy, Ooms, and Loeb reported only the eleventh case of persistent IDDM appearing during the first month of life [73]. In addition to the fact that their patient still required insulin after 30 months, tests that stimulate insulin secretion indicated nearly total failure of beta-cell responses with only one exception. Large pharmacological doses of glucagon produced a moderate increase in plasma insulin concentration. Their patient did not have ketonuria.

Subsequently, permanent IDDM has been reported in at least seven additional patients [4,68,69,74–76], often in unique family situations. One [4] was the infant of a diabetic mother; neither infant nor mother had HLA phenotypes associated with IDDM. Two siblings [76], also diagnosed during the first week of life, were HLA DW 3/DW 4 positive and had a "novel autoantibody" to acinar non-islet cells. However, none of the three had islet cell antibodies. Another patient [69] had a first cousin with transient diabetes mellitus.

Low values have been reported for immunoreactive insulin (IRI) and C-peptide [4,68,74] either measured in serum or in urine [4,74] following various stimuli. These low C-peptide values may also develop over time and provide the basis for the diagnosis of permanent IDDM.

It is now clear that the clinical presentation and initial laboratory findings, including IRI, C-peptide, islet cell, and insulin antibodies, may be identical in transient and permanent neonatal diabetes mellitus [1,68,69]. *Therefore, one should be cautious in making a definitive diagnosis too soon.* It is important to monitor beta-cell responsiveness (plasma C-peptide concentrations) to stimulation, e.g., mixed meal, glucagon, or tolbutamide, over time as well as the clinical requirements for insulin therapy to distinguish between these two conditions. The patient described in detail below will illustrate how this can be done effectively.

Certainly, the implications and prognosis for permanent IDDM beginning in the neonatal period differ from those for transient diabetes mellitus. The former requires a lifetime of exogenous insulin therapy, whether provided by injection, pump, or transplant, whereas the latter rarely develops into IDDM.

While the etiology of permanent IDDM in the neonate remains obscure, as is true for any age group with IDDM, the approach to therapy is similar to that in any child with diabetes mellitus. Caution in the amounts of insulin given, as well as the value of monitoring both blood glucose and urine ketone measurements, should be stressed. Glycosylated hemoglobin measurements have been made in these infants and can be as useful as in the older patient.

In summary, both transient and permanent IDDM must be considered in the differential diagnosis of a neonate or young infant who presents with glycosuria, persistent hyperglycemia, dehydration, acidosis, with or without ketonuria, in the absence of vomiting, diarrhea, or poor food intake [1].

Case Report (Patient 6-2): Permanent Neonatal Diabetes in an Infant of an Insulin-Dependent Mother

A male infant was born after 36 weeks gestation to a 27-year-old, insulin-dependent diabetic mother who required a cesarean delivery because of an exacerbation of proliferative retinopathy (White Class F). Delivery was complicated by an incision through the anterior placenta. The placenta weighed 461 gm, had two grossly evident infarcts (<2.5 cm in diameter), and microscopic features consistent with prematurity.

The infant had Apgar scores of 3 and 5 at 1 and 5 minutes. Weight was 2,100 gm (10th to 25th percentile), length 43 cm (>10th percentile), and head circumference 32 cm (>25th percentile). Dubowitz score confirmed the 36 weeks gestation. A venous hematocrit was 31 percent. He improved rapidly after intravenous therapy with volume expanders, including packed red blood cells. A mild respiratory distress subsided after 2 days.

No hypoglycemia was evident in the first days of life. However, Dextrostix determinations were elevated to more than 200 mg/dl (11.1 mM). This was confirmed by a plasma glucose value of 242 mg/dl (13.4 mM) on the fifth day of life during a dextrose infusion of 6 mg/kg/min. With the reduction of intravenous fluids and increase in oral intake, hyperglycemia persisted in the range of 250–350 mg/dl (13.9–19.4 mM). Glycosuria was noted but without ketonuria or polyuria. Insulin treatment was not given since the infant was gaining weight and there was no evidence of dehydration or acidosis.

The infant was carefully observed and a number of diagnostic studies were done to determine the etiology of the persistent hyperglycemia and glycosuria during 8 weeks of hospitalization. These included the following:

1. Umbilical cord serum insulin antibodies were 3–4 U/L (presumably due to maternal-fetal transfer).

2. Islet cell surface antibodies were undetectable.
3. At 2 weeks of age, glucose turnover rate using stable D-[U-^{13}C]-glucose was 5.8 mg, glucose/kg/min (normal = 3.0–4.0).
4. At 35 days of age, IV tolbutamide tolerance test (20 mg/kg) after a 4-hour fast yielded the following:

TIME (min)	GLUCOSE (mg/dl)	[mM]	C-PEPTIDE (pmol/ml)	GH (ng/ml)	CORTISOL (µg/dl)	GLUCAGON (pg/ml)
0	375	[20.8]	0.36	19	5.6	125
15	312	[17.3]	—	—	—	—
40	207	[11.5]	1.76	25	11.8	340
90	103	[5.7]	0.92	—	—	—

5. At 42 days, after a 3-hour fast, plasma glucose values fell from 400 to 250 mg/dl (22.2 to 13.9 mM) and plasma beta-hydroxybutyrate concentrations were normal at basal (0.06 mM) and at the end of a 4.5-hour fast (0.09 mM).
6. Tolbutamide tolerance tests were repeated at 4 and 16 months, of age, with the following results:

Time (min)	4 MONTHS Glucose (mg/dl)	[mM]	C-Peptide (pmol/ml)	16 MONTHS Glucose (mg/dl)	[mM]	C-Peptide (pmol/ml)
0	260	[14.4]	0.07	425	[23.6]	0.00
15	230	[12.8]	—	388	[21.6]	0.72
40	185	[10.3]	0.35	335	[18.6]	—
90	185	[10.3]	0.14	273	[15.2]	—

7. Tissue antigens DR$_3$ and DR$_4$ were not found in HLA typing, and BF*F1 and C2*B were not found in complement typing.
8. Erythrocyte, cultured B lymphocytes, and fibroblasts from a skin biopsy in mother and child were measured for specific insulin receptor binding and were found to be normal.
9. Serum autoantibodies against islet cell cytoplasmic antibodies, thyroglobulin, thyroid microsomes, gastric parietal cell, and other antinuclear, antimitochondrial and antismooth muscle antibodies were all negative.

At 13 weeks of age, he developed an upper respiratory infection and ketonuria. At that time, his weight was 3,600 gm, length 55 cm, and head circumference 37 cm. He responded promptly to insulin therapy and has been managed with twice-daily insulin injections at a dose of 8–10 U/day. He continued to have hyperglycemia, with glycosylated hemoglobin values fluctuating between 9.4 and 11.75 percent of total hemoglobin (normal range = 4.6 to 6.4 percent). His weight and length have progressed well and at 20 months of age were close to the 50th percentile. There have been no episodes of ketoacidosis or hyperosmolar coma. Except for a delay in language development, his neurologic and psychologic development have been normal.

Family History. The mother developed insulin-dependent diabetes mellitus at 12 weeks of age, at which time she had fever, poor weight gain, polydipsia, and polyphagia. The course of the mother's IDDM has been a difficult one, with multiple hospitalizations for ketoacidosis, the development of proliferative retinopathy, and proteinuria at 24 years of age. In addition, a maternal great-grandmother had maturity onset diabetes (NIDDM), and a paternal grandmother had been treated with insulin for 10 years before her death at age 42 [4].

Comment

While it is rare to have the infant of an IDDM mother develop diabetes mellitus as a neonate, this patient illustrates how well a neonate can gain weight, grow, and develop with significant persisting hyperglycemia as long as he remains well. In contrast to the patients with transient neonatal diabetes mellitus, beta cell function continued to fail rather than improve in this boy. He is also an example of the difficulty in maintaining normoglycemic blood glucose levels in an infant with IDDM even when the mother has IDDM herself.

• Summary

In recent years, hyperglycemia in the neonate has become a more common problem, requiring careful evaluation and management. With increased numbers and survival rates of VLBW infants and other high-risk, stressed premature infants, the frequency of significant hyperglycemia with its associated diuresis, dehydration, hyperosmolality, and failure to thrive has increased. This has been especially evident since total or supplemental parenteral nutrition has been given early in life.

Three different clinical entities have now evolved. The most common is transient glucose intolerance related to immaturity, stress, or disease. Hyperglycemia may be minimal and asymptomatic, but often exceeds 200 mg/dl (11.1 mM) and is acutely symptomatic. These infants require careful surveillance and skillful management, usually without, but sometimes with, exogenous insulin.

Much less frequent is transient diabetes mellitus associated with the SGA infant, who is wasted, looks alert, becomes quickly dehydrated (in the absence of vomiting or diarrhea), and has marked glycosuria, often without ketonuria. Hyperglycemia is usually striking, often as high as 700 mg/dl (38.9 mM) or more. The infants are insulin-sensitive, respond dramatically, and only require insulin for periods of days, weeks, or months. A rare patient may become an IDDM years later.

Even rarer is permanent insulin-dependent diabetes mellitus beginning in the neonatal period or in the first months of infancy. Clinically, the infants may be SGA or AGA and have an identical presentation, both clinically and by laboratory study, as the neonate with transient diabetes mellitus. However, the need for insulin therapy persists.

In order to distinguish between the two latter syndromes, repeated stimulation tests to measure beta-cell function as reflected in changes in plasma C-peptide concentrations are necessary.

REFERENCES

1. GENTZ JCH, CORNBLATH M. Transient diabetes of the newborn. *Adv Pediatr.* 1969;16:345.
2. CORNBLATH M, SCHWARTZ R. *Disorders of Carbohydrate Metabolism in Infancy.* 2nd ed. Philadelphia: W.B. Saunders Co., 1976;218.
3. GREENWOOD RD, TRAISMAN HS. Permanent diabetes mellitus in a neonate. *J Pediatr.* 1971;79:296.
4. WIDNESS JA, COWETT RM, ZELLER WP, SUSA JB, RUBENSTEIN AH, SCHWARTZ R. Permanent neonatal diabetes in an infant of an insulin-dependent mother. *J Pediatr.* 1982;100:926.
5. DWECK HS, MIRANDA LEV. Perinatal glucose homeostasis: The unique character of hyperglycemia and hypoglycemia in infants of very low birth weight. *Clin Perinatol.* 1977;4:351.
6. LILIEN LD, ROSENFIELD RL, BACCARO MM, PILDES RS. Hyperglycemia in stressed small premature neonates. *J Pediatr.* 1979;94:454.
7. BRANS YW. Parenteral nutrition of the very low birth weight neonate. A critical review. *Clin Perinatol.* 1977;4:367.
8. FILLER RM, ERAKLIS AJ, RUBIN VG, DAS JB. Long-term total parenteral nutrition in infants. *N Engl J Med.* 1969;281:589.
9. HEIRD WC, DRISCOLL JM, WINTERS RW. Total parenteral nutrition in infants of very low birth weight. In: Elliott K, Knight J, eds. *Size at Birth.* Amsterdam: Associated Scientific Publishers, 1974;329.
10. GHADIMI H. Newly devised amino acid solutions for intravenous administration. In: Ghadimi H, ed. *Total Parenteral Nutrition: Premises and Promises.* New York: J. Wiley and Sons, 1975;393.
11. PILDES RS. Current literature and clinical issues: neonatal hyperglycemia. *J Pediatr.* 1986;109:905. (Editorial.)
12. DWECK HS, CASSADY G. Glucose intolerance in infants of very low birth weight: incidence of hyperglycemia in birth weights 1100 gms or less. *Pediatrics.* 1974;53:189.
13. ZARIF M, PILDES RS, VIDYASAGAR D. Insulin and growth hormone responses in neonatal hyperglycemia. *Diabetes.* 1976;25:428.
14. RAVAL D, BAGNUOLO L, HENEK T, et al. Follow-up of very low birth weight (VLBW) infants of very low socioeconomic families. *Pediatr Res.* 1986;20:363A.
15. CORNBLATH M, SCHWARTZ R, AYNSLEY-GREEN A, LLOYD JK. Hypoglycemia in infancy: the need for a rational definition. *Pediatrics.*

1990;85:834. (Personal communication.) Presented at the Ciba Foundation Discussion Meeting, Oct. 17, 1989, London.

16. LOUIK C, MITCHELL AA, EPSTEIN MF, SHAPIRO S. Risk factors for neonatal hyperglycemia associated with 10 percent dextrose infusion. *Am J Dis Child.* 1985;139:783.

17. SRINIVASAN G, SINGH J, CATTAMANCI G, YEH TF, PILDES RS. Plasma glucose changes in preterm infants during oral theophylline therapy. *J Pediatr.* 1983;103:473.

18. SRINIVASAN G, JAIN R, PILDES RS, KANNAN CR. Glucose homeostasis during anesthesia and surgery in infants. *J Pediatr Surg.* 1986;21:718.

19. DWECK HS, CASSADY G. Glucose intolerance in infants of very low birth weight. *Pediatrics.* 1974;53:189.

20. COWETT RM, HAY WW JR, eds. *The micropremie: the next frontier.* Report of the Ninety-Ninth Ross Conference on Pediatric Research. Columbus, Ohio: Ross Laboratories, 1990.

21. BRYAN MH, WEI P, HAMILTON JR, CHANCE GW, SWYER PR. Supplemental intravenous alimentation in low-birth-weight infants. *J Pediatr.* 1973;82:940.

22. CHAIVORARAT O, DWECK HS. Effects of prolonged continuous glucose infusion in preterm infants. *Pediatr Res.* 1976;10:406A.

23. DWECK HS, BRANS YW, SUMNERS JE, et al. Glucose intolerance in infants of very low birth weight. II. Intravenous glucose tolerance tests in infants of birth weight 500–1380 grams. *Biol Neonate.* 1976; 63:1492.

24. DWECK HS, CASSADY G. Glucose intolerance in infants of very low birth weight. I. Incidence of hyperglycemia in infants of birth weight 1100 grams or less. *Pediatrics.* 1974;53:189.

25. CSER A, MILNER RDG. Glucose tolerance and insulin secretion in very small babies. *Acta Paediatr Scand.* 1975;64:457.

26. SCHWARTZ R. Should exogenous insulin be given to very low birth weight infants? *J Pediatr Gastroenterol Nutr.* 1982;1:287. (Editorial.)

27. OSTERTAG SG, JOVANOVIC L, LEWIS B, AULD PAM. Insulin pump therapy in the very low birth weight infant. *Pediatrics.* 1986;78:625.

28. BINDER ND, RASCHKO PK, BENDA GI, REYNOLDS JW. Insulin infusion with parenteral nutrition in extremely low birth weight infants with hyperglycemia. *J Pediatr.* 1989;114:273.

29. VAUCHER YE, WALSON PD, MORROW G. Continuous insulin infusion in hyperglycemic very low birth weight infants. *J Pediatr Gastroenterol Nutr.* 1982;1:211.

30. POLLAK A, COWETT RM, SCHWARTZ R, OH W. Glucose disposal of low birth weight infants during steady state hyperglycemia. Effects of exogenous insulin administration. *Pediatrics.* 1978;61:546.

31. OGATA ES. Problems of glucose metabolism in the extremely low-birth-weight infant. In: Cowett RM, Hay WW Jr, eds. *The micropremie: the next frontier.* Report of the Ninety-Ninth Ross Conference on Pediatric Research. Columbus, Ohio: Ross Laboratories, 1990, p 55.

32. JUNG AL, DONE AK. Extreme hyperosmolality and "transient diabetes." *Am J Dis Child.* 1969;118:859.

33. VANNUCCI RC, VASTA F, VANNUCCI SJ. Cerebral metabolic responses of hyperglycemic immature rats to hypoxia-ischemia. *Pediatr Res.* 1987; 21:524.

34. CALLAHAN DJ, ENGLE MJ, VOLPE JJ. Hypoxic injury to developing glial cells: Protective effect of high glucose. *Pediatr Res.* 1990;27:186.
35. Nutritional needs of low-birth-weight infants. Committee on Nutrition. American Academy of Pediatrics. *Pediatrics.* 1985;75:976.
36. AREY SL. Transient diabetes in infancy. *Pediatrics.* 1953;11:140.
37. ENGLESON G, ZETTERQVIST P. Congenital diabetes mellitus and neonatal pseudodiabetes mellitus. *Arch Dis Child.* 1957;32:193.
38. BRUGSCH H. Diabetes mellitus im sauglingsalter. *Z Aerztl Fortbild.* 1962;51:439.
39. HUTCHISON JH, KEAY AJ, KERR MM. Congenital temporary diabetes mellitus. *Br Med J.* 1962;2:436.
40. LAWRENCE RD, MCCANCE RA. Gangrene in an infant associated with temporary diabetes. *Arch Dis Child.* 1931;6:343.
41. RAMSEY WR. Glycosuria in the new-born treated with insulin. *Trans Am Pediatr Soc.* 1926;38:100.
42. STRANDQVIST B. Infantile glucosuria simulating diabetes. *Acta Paediatr.* 1932;13:421.
43. NAWROCKA-KANSKA B. Diabetic syndrome in intracranial haemorrhage in newborn. *Pediatr Pol.* 1952;27:1067.
44. WYLIE MES. A case of congenital diabetes. *Arch Dis Child.* 1953;28:297.
45. KEIDAN SE. Transient diabetes in infancy. *Arch Dis Child.* 1955;30:291.
46. JEUNE M, RIEDWEG M. Syndrome diabetique transitoire chez un nouveau-ne. *Pediatrie.* 1960;15:63.
47. GERRARD JW, CHIN W. The syndrome of transient diabetes. *J Pediatr.* 1962;61:89.
48. BURLAND WL. Diabetes mellitus syndrome in the newborn infant. *J Pediatr.* 1964;65:122.
49. KOUVALAINEN K, VAÄNÄNEN I, HIEKKALA H. Neonatal pseudodiabetes mellitus. *Ann Paediatr Fenniae.* 1961;7:242.
50. FERGUSON AW, MILNER RDG. Transient neonatal diabetes mellitus in sibs. *Arch Dis Child.* 1970;45:80.
51. MILNER RDG, FERGUSON AW, NAIDU SH. Aetiology of transient neonatal diabetes. *Arch Dis Child.* 1971;46:724.
52. SCHIFF D, COLLE E, STERN L. Metabolic and growth patterns in transient neonatal diabetes. *N Engl J Med.* 1972;287:119.
53. FERGUSON IC. Neonatal hyperglycaemia: Case report with plasma insulin studies. *Arch Dis Child.* 1967;42:509.
54. HORNER R, THOMSON AJ, MCDONALD R. Neonatal transient diabetes mellitus. *S Afr Med J.* 1968;42:71.
55. PAGLIARA AS, KARL IE, KIPNIS DM. Transient neonatal diabetes: Delayed maturation of the pancreatic beta cell. *J Pediatr.* 1973;82:97.
56. CHANCE GW, BOWER BD. Hypoglycaemia and temporary hyperglycaemia in infants of low birth weight for maturity. *Arch Dis Child.* 1966; 41:279.
57. OSBORNE GR. Congenital diabetes. *Arch Dis Child.* 1965;40:332.
58. LEWIS SR, MORTIMER PE. Idiopathic neonatal hyperglycaemia. *Arch Dis Child.* 1964;39:618.
59. HAGER H, HERBST R. Das Transitorische Diabetes Mellitus Syndrom des Neugeborenen ein Krankheitsbild Sui Generis. *Z Kinderheilkd.* 1966; 95:234.
60. COFFEY JD, WOMACK NC. Transient neonatal diabetes mellitus in half sisters. *Am J Dis Child.* 1967;113:480.

61. TAKEUCHI T. Insulin as a growth factor of the fetus and newborn—clinical and endocrinological study of two cases with "transient" neonatal diabetes. Presented at Neonatal Society, London, Nov. 13, 1975.

62. DACOU-VOUTETAKIS C, ANAGNOSTAKIS D, XANTHOU M. Macroglossia, transient neonatal diabetes mellitus and intrauterine growth failure: a new distinct entity? *Pediatrics.* 1975;55:127.

63. KUNA P, ADDY DP. Transient neonatal diabetes mellitus. Treatment with chlorpropamide. *Am J Dis Child.* 1979;133:65.

64. BLETHEN SL, WHITE NH, SANTIAGO JV, DAUGHADAY WH. Plasma somatomedins, endogenous insulin secretion and growth in transient neonatal diabetes mellitus. *J Clin Endocrinol Metab.* 1981;52:144.

65. COFFEE JD JR, KILLELEA DE. Transient neonatal diabetes mellitus in half sisters. A sequal. *Am J Dis Child.* 1982;136:626.

66. MCGILL JJ, ROBERTON DM. A new type of transient diabetes mellitus of infancy? *Arch Dis Child.* 1986;61:334.

67. SCHINDLER AM, PLEASURE JR. The diabetic baby who got better. *Hospital Practice.* 1987;22:147.

68. CAVALLO L, MAUTONE A, LAFORGIA N, FIORE R, ZUPPINGER K, SCHETTINI F. Neonatal diabetes mellitus: evaluation of pancreatic beta-cell function in two cases. *Helv Paediatr Acta.* 1987;42:437.

69. MATHEW PM, HANN RW, HAMDAN JA. Neonatal diabetes mellitus in first cousins. *Clin Pediatr.* 1988;27:247.

70. NIELSEN F. Transient neonatal diabetes mellitus in a pair of twins. *Acta Paediatr Scand.* 1989;78:469.

71. CAMPBELL IW, FRASER DM, DUNCAN LJP. Permanent insulin-dependent diabetes mellitus after congenital temporary diabetes mellitus. *Br Med J.* 1978;276:174.

72. GUEST GM. Infantile diabetes mellitus: 3 cases in successive siblings, 2 with onset at 3 months of age and 1 at 9 days of age. (Abstract). *Am J Dis Child.* 1948;75:461.

73. DORCHY H, OOMS H, LOEB H. Permanent neonatal diabetes mellitus: a case report with plasma insulin studies. *Z Kinderheilkd.* 1975; 118:271.

74. KNIP M, KOIVISTO M, KAAR ML, PUUKKA R, KOUVALAINEN K. Pancreatic islet cell function and metabolic control in an infant with permanent diabetes mellitus. *Acta Paediatr Scand.* 1983;72:303.

75. BARBOTTE E, SIMONIN G, UNAL D, COIGNET J. Le diabete neonatal. A propos de deux observations. *Pediatrie.* 1986;41:553.

76. IVARSSON SA, MARNER B, LERNMARK A, NILSSON KO. Nonislet pancreatic autoantibodies in sibship with permanent neonatal insulin dependent diabetes mellitus. *Diabetes.* 1988;37:347.

C H A P T E R 7

DISORDERS
OF GLYCOGEN
METABOLISM

A variety of types of disturbances of glycogen metabolism have been described over the past 60 years. The first patient was reported by Snapper and van Creveld in 1928 [1], who attributed the hepatomegaly, hypoglycemia, and ketonuria in a young boy to a defect in glycogen mobilization. This hepatic form of glycogen storage disease was further elucidated by pathologic studies (von Gierke [2]) and by biochemical studies (Schönheimer [3]). Von Gierke's patient also had renal involvement, hence, the designation "hepatonephromegalia glycogenica." An apparently unrelated syndrome of glycogen accumulation in the heart of a 7-month-old infant was noted by Pompe in 1932 [4] and subsequently in skeletal muscle as well by van Creveld [5,6]. Van Creveld [5] reviewed the glycogen storage syndromes in detail in 1939 and emphasized the variations in the clinical and pathologic observations. Mason and Andersen [7] in 1941 reported a patient with hepatomegaly, hypoglycemia, and acidosis in the newborn period who died from infection at 2 months of age. The accumulation of excessive fat in the livers of these patients was emphasized by Debré [8].

Initially, two categories of disease were apparent: the hepatorenal group and the cardiomuscular group. Two other distinct syndromes were described subsequently: Andersen's [9], with an increased concentration of an abnormal glycogen in the liver and a progressive course that terminated in cirrhosis with hepatic failure, and McArdle's [10], with skeletal muscle involvement only and an onset in childhood but not usually diagnosed until adulthood. The classification based on clinical manifestations was then expanded to hepato-renal, cardiomuscular, hepatic cirrhotic, or muscular types of glycogen storage disease.

Biochemical classification was not possible until the details of the pathways of glycogen metabolism were elucidated by the Coris, Leloir, Kalckar, Colowick, the Stettens, Sutherland, Larner, Illingworth, and Hers [11–13]. Initially, the biochemical classification of the five glycogen storage diseases was presented by G.T. Cori [11] in 1954. Subsequently, this schema included six distinct biochemical and clinical types (Fig. 7-1) [11]. In addition, a number of specific enzymatic defects related to glycogen metabolism have been described and found to be associated with variable clinical manifestations. Various investigators have designated these types, ranging from type VII to type XI [14,15].

Recent reviews have summarized the clinical findings as well as biochemical abnormalities in all of the glycogen storage diseases [13,16,17].

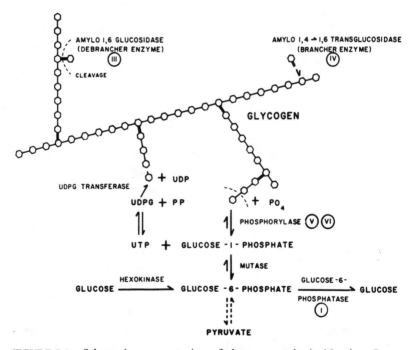

FIGURE 7-1. Schematic representation of glycogen synthesis. Numbers I to VI refer to sites of enzymatic defect in the various types of glycogen storage disease. Type II (alpha acid maltase) and type 0 (synthase or UDPG transferase) are not indicated specifically.

• Classification of Disorders of Glycogen Metabolism

Defects in glycogen metabolism could appear at any of the enzymatic steps described in Figure 1-13 in Chapter 1. The absence of glucose-6-phosphatase in liver was the first proven enzyme defect in the glycogen diseases [18]. The most intensely studied defects involve glucose-6-phosphatase, phosphorylase, and debrancher enzymes. Hers [19] has described a lysosomal system that hydrolyzes glycogen at an acid pH (acid alpha glucosidase) which is important in regulating cytoplasmic glycogen accumulation. He first reported the absence of this enzyme in type II, the musculocardiac form of glycogen storage disease.

A classification based on the organs involved has been combined with that based on the biochemical defects to provide a useful clinical and physiologic approach to these inborn errors of metabolism (see Table 7-1).

The hepatorenal glycogen diseases may result from deficiencies of four different enzymes: glucose-6-phosphatase (type Ia), glucose-6-phosphate translocase (type Ib), amylo-1,6-glucosidase (type III), and phosphorylase (type VI). The other, rarer hepatic type (IV) involves the deficiency or absence of amylo-1,4-1,6-transglucosidase. The muscular types include the cardiomuscular, with a general deficiency of acid maltase or α-glucosidase (type II), the skeletomuscular, with absence of phosphorylase (type V), or absence of phosphofructokinase (type VII) in muscle. A defect in hepatic glycogen synthase (type 0) has also been reported [20]. Abnormalities of the phosphorylase-activating (kinase) systems have been included as variants of type VI [13].

• Hepatic (Renal) Syndromes

Glucose-6-Phosphatase Defect (Type I)

The classical disease is manifested early in infancy by hepatomegaly without splenomegaly, with or without symptoms associated with hypoglycemia [21]. The liver is firm and smooth and may extend to the iliac crest, filling a major portion of the protuberant abdomen. There are no signs of cirrhosis or portal hypertension. Although the kidneys are often enlarged, they may not be palpable because of the massive hepatomegaly. Cardiomegaly does not occur. The infant or child is short in stature but appears well-nourished. The cheeks and extremities have excessive adipose tissue ("doll-like facies") (Fig. 7-2), but the musculature is diminished and flabby. The face appears

TABLE 7-1. Classification of major glycogen diseases

TYPE	ORGANS INVOLVED	GLYCOGEN CONTENT (g/100 g)	BIOCHEMICAL EFFECTS		PHYSIOLOGIC EFFECTS		
			Glycogen Structure	Enzyme Activity Decreased	Blood Glucose	Blood Lactate	OTHERS
Ia (von Gierke)	Liver	> 8.0	N†	Glucose-6-phosphatase	Very low	High	Pyruvate ↑
	Kidney	Increased	N	Glucose-6-phosphatase			Urate ↑
	Intestine	Increased		Glucose-6-phosphatase			FFA ↑
							Lipids ↑
Ib	Liver			Glucose-6-phosphatase‡			
III* (Cori)	Generalized	Increased	Abnormal	Amylo-1,6-glucosidase	Very low or low	Normal	Lipids ↑ sl.
	Esp. liver	Increased	Abnormal				
	RBC	N or H	Abnormal				
	WBC	?	Abnormal	Amylo-1,6-glucosidase (±)			
VI* (Hers)	Liver	Increased	N?	Phosphorylase	Low	Normal– high	Lipids ↑
	Kidney	?	N				
	RBC	N or H	N				
	WBC	?		Phosphorylase			
V (McArdle)	Muscle	Increased	N	Phosphorylase	Normal	Low	Myopathy
	RBC	?		Normal			
	WBC			Normal			
	Liver						

II (Pompe)	Generalized Liver Heart Muscle RBC WBC Amniotic cells	Increased Increased Increased Increased N† ?	Normal	α1,4-glucosidase α1,4-glucosidase α1,4-glucosidase α1,4-glucosidase α1,4-glucosidase α1,4-glucosidase	Normal	Normal	Cardiomegaly Myopathy CNS
IV (Andersen)	Generalized Liver R-E system RBC WBC	Normal Normal	Abnormal Abnormal Abnormal	Amylo-1,4→ 1,6-transglucosidase Amylo-1,4→ 1,6-transglucosidase	Normal	Normal	Cirrhosis
0 (Lewis)	Liver Kidney RBC	Decreased	Normal	Glycogen synthase ? Normal	Very low	High§	Fatty liver

*See text for variants.

†N = normal, H = high.

‡Assayed on fresh liver; normal on frozen liver.

§Postgalactose.

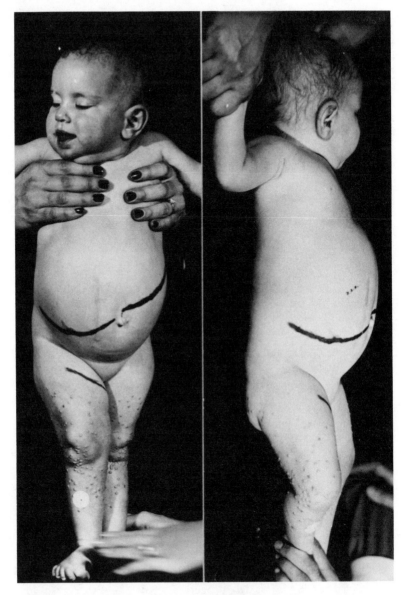

FIGURE 7-2. Infant with proven glycogen storage disease, glucose-6-phosphatase deficiency, showing the doll-like facies, hepatomegaly, and xanthomata on the lower extremities.

plethoric and may be moist with perspiration. If the patient is starved, agitated, or ill, respirations may be rapid and deep owing to acidosis. Easy bruising and a hemorrhagic tendency are common. Nose bleeds occur frequently. Some untreated patients have xanthomata, which appear as orange-colored papules over the upper and lower extremities. Lipemia retinalis may also be noted. Ophthalmoscopic examination may reveal multiple bilateral, symmetrical, yellowish, nonelevated, discrete paramacular lesions [22]. The neurologic examination is unremarkable. Mental development varies: some children have been reported to be mentally retarded; others are normal. This appears to be unrelated to the hypoglycemia.

In the neonate, this syndrome may present as severe respiratory distress in the absence of pulmonary disease which is due to profound metabolic lactic acidosis. The liver is markedly enlarged. Ketonuria [23] occurs in contrast to the older infant and child [24], and symptomatic hypoglycemia can be present as well. If undiagnosed, there may be rapid progression to death [23].

Alternatively, the infant may be asymptomatic and only later in infancy or early childhood fail to thrive or grow and show a protuberant abdomen that is due to hepatomegaly.

Laboratory Tests

Lactic acidosis with a low pH is often present after a brief fast, although the routine urine and blood studies are usually within normal limits. Ketonuria has been observed transiently in very young infants [23] but not in older patients [24]. Thrombocytemia has been reported. The bleeding disorder includes prolonged bleeding time, low values for platelet adhesiveness, increased numbers of platelets, and high values for prothrombin and fibrinogen [25]. Routine chemical analyses usually reveal low or unmeasurable fasting blood glucose concentrations, depending on the duration of the fast. Glycohemoglobin (Hb A_{1c}) is normal, but Hb A_{1a+b} is elevated [26]. The carbon dioxide content is low. Serum concentrations of sodium, potassium, chloride, urea, and bilirubin are usually normal. Serum protein concentrations may be slightly elevated, with a normal electrophoretic pattern. The levels of glutamic oxalacetic transaminase (SGOT), glutamic pyruvic transaminase (SGPT), fructose 1,6-diphosphate aldolase (ALD), and ornithine carbamoyl transferase (OCT) may be elevated, but lactic dehydrogenase (LDH) is normal [27]. Concentrations of lactate and pyruvate in blood are elevated, as may be those of urate and free fatty acids in plasma [28]. The plasma may be lactescent as a result of a generalized increase in lipids, including triglycerides, phospholipids, and cholesterol (Fig. 7-3) [29]. Plasma lipoprotein analyses have indicated that the concentrations of very low-density lipoprotein (VLDL) cholesterol and triglycerides are elevated, high-density lipoprotein (HDL) cholesterol is low, and low-density lipoprotein (LDL) cholesterol is within normal limits.

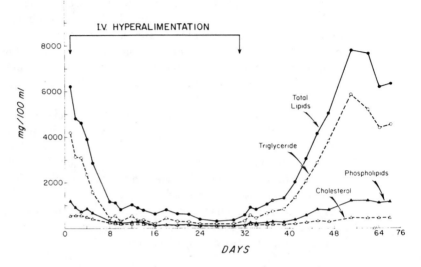

FIGURE 7-3. Correction of hyperlipidemia by total parenteral alimentation and continuous normoglycemia in a patient with type Ia glycogen storage disease. (From Folkmann. *Surgery.* 1972;72:306, with permission.)

Ultrasound demonstrates the abdomen to be filled with a large liver mass and bilateral symmetrical enlargement of the kidneys.

Special Studies

Neither erythrocyte nor leukocyte analysis for glycogen content or structure [30] or enzyme activity [31,32] are diagnostic in Type Ia glycogen storage disease (GSD).

The diagnosis may be inferred from the results of tolerance tests that measure the breakdown of glycogen to glucose and lactate, and the conversion of hexoses (galactose or fructose) and other substrates (glycerol or dihydroxy-acetone) to glucose. Glucagon, which acutely stimulates glycogenolysis and release of glucose from the liver [33,34], is given following a short fast of 4–6 hours. It is given (100 μg/kg– 1 mg maximum) intravenously or intramuscularly. Serial blood samples are obtained for 2 hours at 15-minute intervals for measuring both blood glucose and lactate concentrations. The response is shown in Figure 7-4. Blood glucose concentrations may decline to unmeasurable levels, remain unchanged, or increase slightly. Rarely, patients with undetectable hepatic glucose-6-phosphatase activity have responded to glucagon with a prompt, significant (but subnormal) hyperglycemia. The explanation for this unexpected reaction remains obscure. Blood lactate concentrations increase rapidly and markedly

GLUCAGON TOLERANCE
IN GLYCOGEN STORAGE (Type I a)
(K.Y. 7 mos., white male)

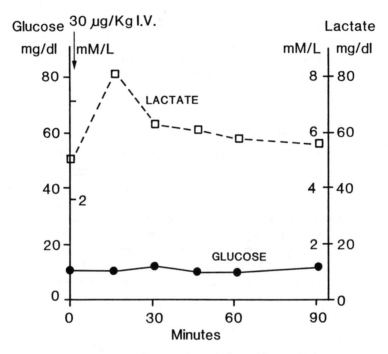

FIGURE 7-4. Response to glucagon in an infant with type I glycogen storage disease. Note the lactic acidosis, hypoglycemia, and failure to increase plasma glucose concentration.

(occasionally to values over 150 mg/100 ml) within 30–60 minutes, in contrast to little or no rise in the normal individual.

In contrast to GSD I, failure of a rise in blood glucose with a normal lactate response can be caused by a defect in amylo-1,6-glucosidase (III), phosphorylase (VI), phosphorylase kinase (VI), or deficient liver glycogen. Thus, the blood glucose response alone in the glucagon test is neither specific nor sufficient.

Another tolerance test to evaluate glucose-6-phosphatase activity indirectly and to bypass glycogenolysis is the intravenous galactose tolerance test described by Schwartz et al. [35]. After a short fast of 4–6 hours, galactose (1 g/kg body weight) is given rapidly intravenously as a 25 percent solution. Blood samples are taken to determine total hexose or galactose, glucose (glucose oxidase or hexokinase technique), and lactate at 10-minute intervals for 1 hour. Galactose disappears rapidly from the circulation. The absence of a rise in blood glucose (glucose oxidase) concentration with a significant increase in lactate is presumptive evidence of a defect in glucose-6-phosphatase (Fig. 7-5).

These tolerance tests can result in sufficient increases in lactic acid to produce reciprocal effects on buffer bicarbonate with decreased pH and carbon dioxide (CO_2) contents. If the patient is tachypneic and hyperpneic (acidotic) at the conclusion of the test, feedings should be supplemented with sodium bicarbonate in a dose of 2 mEq/kg body weight.

Biochemical Diagnosis

The diagnosis is established by biochemical analysis of a liver biopsy. Prior to the biopsy, consultation and arrangements must be made with an experienced metabolic-biochemical laboratory to assure proper handling and analysis of the specimen. The laboratory will provide details for collecting and transporting the tissue.

Hers [14] has developed a technique for analysis of micro quantities of tissue, which can safely be obtained from an infant by punch biopsy. Open biopsy at laparotomy carries the advantage of availability of larger tissue samples for multiple analyses as well as control

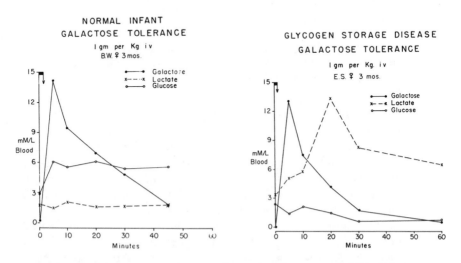

FIGURE 7-5. (a) Intravenous galactose tolerance test in a normal child. Galactose disappeared rapidly, glucose rose, while lactate remained low. (b) Intravenous galactose tolerance test in an infant with absence of glucose-6-phosphatase. Galactose disappeared rapidly, glucose decreased, while lactate rose markedly. (From Schwartz et al. *Pediatrics.* 1957;19:585, with permission.)

of bleeding. The patient must be carefully evaluated for bleeding disorders and for the ability to withstand anesthesia. Lactic acidosis, hypoglycemia, and infection must be corrected prior to surgery (vide infra). The child is given a continuous infusion of glucose at 8–10 mg/kg/min on the night before surgery and during exploration. An adequate biopsy sample must be immediately divided and one-half analyzed fresh for the diagnosis of type Ib GSD. The other half is frozen on solid carbon dioxide or in liquid nitrogen (*not in alcohol or acetone—dry ice*) for further biochemical and enzymatic analyses. Separate specimens should be placed in alcohol to allow for glycogen staining, as well as in Zenker's acetic acid and in formalin for routine histologic examination. At the time of laparotomy, muscle samples should also be obtained for biochemical and histologic examination, as described for the liver.

In every child who has an exploratory laparotomy for hepatomegaly of any cause, an adequate portion of the specimen should be frozen on solid carbon dioxide (dry ice) or in liquid nitrogen for possible future biochemical and enzymatic analyses.

The fresh and frozen biopsy material should be analyzed for glycogen content and structure and for activities of the enzymes of the glycogen cycle [14,36]. The liver specimen has a high glycogen content, greater than 5 percent of wet weight, and a high fat content, greater than 4–8 percent of wet weight. The presence of excessive fat results in a falsely low glycogen content per unit total tissue.

A lack of glucose-6-phosphatase activity is evidence for the diagnosis of type Ia glycogen storage disease. Levels of 10 percent or less of normal glucose-6-phosphatase activity may represent nonspecific "alkaline" phosphatases or incomplete defects. Other enzyme activities, including those of glycogenolysis and glycolysis (phosphorylase, amylo-1,6-glucosidase, phosphoglucomutase, and phosphofructokinase) and glycogen synthesis (UDPG pyrophosphorylase and UDPG transglucosylase or synthase) have been found to be normal.

Glucose-6-phosphatase is bound inside the endoplasmic reticulum. A specific glucose-6-phosphate transporter is required to carry this substrate to the active site. Thus, at least two defects have been described. In type Ia, there is absence of the specific glucose-6-phosphatase. In type Ib, this enzyme is intact, but the transporter (glucose-6-phosphate translocase) is defective. This accounts for the differences observed between analyses performed on fresh versus frozen (disrupted) tissue [37].

Pathology

At laparotomy, the liver is large and smooth, with a gleaming capsule. It has a definite yellow, fatty appearance. There is no nodularity or irregularity in its surface. Microscopically, the hepatic cells are large and swollen with centrally placed nuclei (Fig. 7-6). Staining with a standard hematoxylin and eosin preparation indicates normal preservation of lobular architecture without any inflammation, cirrhosis, or tumor. There are many vacuolated areas, both within and apparently outside the hepatic cells. Examination of the alcohol-fixed specimens with Best's stain or with the Schiff's periodic acid (PAS) technique indicates numerous red- or purple-staining granules of carbohydrate in the hepatic cells. Vacuoles often persist, however, and are identified as fat by Sudan stain on Zenker's or formalin-fixed

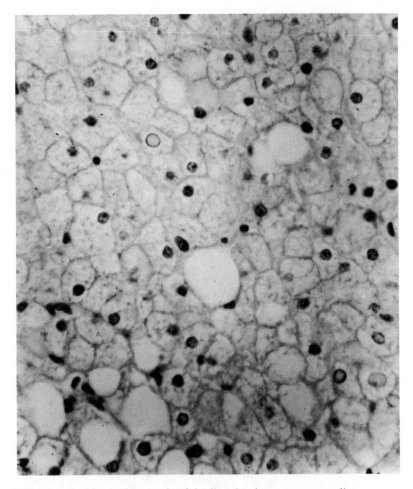

FIGURE 7-6. Photomicrograph of the liver in glycogen storage disease associated with an absence of glucose-6-phosphatase. The cells are swollen, and the nuclei are centrally placed. The large clear areas reflect loss of fat.

material. In some instances, the amount of fat exceeds that of glycogen. Examination of skeletal muscle in type I disease shows no particular abnormalities. The kidney is grossly enlarged and has normal architecture: microscopic examination indicates glycogen-laden proximal tubular cells.

Pathophysiology

The pathophysiology of this type I defect is best considered developmentally, beginning in utero. While the human fetus has been shown to have glucose-6-phosphatase activity as early as 10 weeks' gestation [38], the primary energy source in utero is glucose derived transplacentally from the mother, relegating the fetal liver to a minor role in glucose homeostasis. Furthermore, the fetal circulation uniquely provides for a bypass of the liver via the ductus venosus so that only a fraction of the glucose supplied by the mother passes through the liver. The constant infusion of glucose from the mother maintains intact peripheral glucose metabolism, prevents hypoglycemia, and results in relatively normal intrauterine growth. The variable manifestations of type I disease in the newborn period may be related to differences in intrauterine hepatic blood flow.

Following delivery, the infant with complete absence of glucose-6-phosphatase is unable to sustain a normal blood glucose level, and hypoglycemia supervenes unless frequent glucose feedings are provided. Fortunately, feeding the infant by breast or formula every 3–4 hours may prevent hypoglycemia. Hepatic glycogen synthesis derives not only from excess glucose, but also from galactose and fructose. As the interval between feedings is extended, hypoglycemia occurs just prior to the next feed.

During the period of starvation, the liver is unable to sustain a normal glucose level, resulting in a variety of secondary effects on hormone and substrate concentrations. The hormonal response to hypoglycemia includes an initial release of epinephrine, glucagon, and growth hormone, and later glucocorticoid. Phosphorylase is activated and hepatic glycogenolysis is increased, but glucose release from the liver only occurs by hydrolysis of branch points by amylo-1,6-glucosidase. This can result in approximately 8 percent free glucose release. Studies with stable isotopes, ^{13}C-glucose, have indicated a persistent hepatic glucose output of 2.0 mg/kg/min with fasting [39,40]. This explains why hypoglycemia does not always accompany starvation and why a minor rise in blood glucose sometimes occurs with administration of glucagon.

Normally, lactate produced in the peripheral tissues, especially in erythrocytes and muscle, is removed from the circulation by the liver and either metabolized via the Krebs cycle or converted to glucose via the gluconeogenetic pathway. Mason and Sly [41] first reported the presence of excessive lactate in the blood of patients with glycogen storage disease. Several studies have confirmed this important observation and elucidated the origin of the lactate [33,34]. Intrahepatic changes of sugar phosphates and inorganic phosphate have been observed in patients with type Ia glycogen storage disease by P-31 magnetic resonance spectroscopy [42].

The increased intrahepatic metabolism of glucose results in overactivity of all pathways from glucose-6-phosphate so that production of DPNH and TPNH is presumably increased [28]. These key cofactors are necessary for a variety of biochemical reactions, including the conversion of pyruvate to lactate and the synthesis of fatty acids, ketones, and cholesterol. Thus, the reason for hepatic fat accumulation and lactate formation may be secondary to the single defect, a failure to convert glucose-6-phosphate to glucose [28]. Decreased ketone formation may be due to increased malonyl CoA which inhibits carnitine acyl-transferase I [43].

In addition to secondary effects, at least one tertiary effect has been noted, that being the rise in plasma urate concentration. This has been attributed to either an increase in purine metabolism or an increased tubular reabsorption. The latter appears most likely since it is related to the elevation in blood lactate concentration, which inhibits urate secretion in the renal tubule [44]. Roe and Kogut [45] inferred enhanced nucleotide catabolism from studies of responses to fructose or glucagon. Gout has been reported [21].

Previously, growth retardation in inadequately treated patients could not be satisfactorily explained on a biochemical or endocrinologic basis. However, the catch-up growth observed with intragastric continuous feedings or with administration of raw, uncooked cornstarch make chronic hypoglycemia a major factor (vide infra).

Hypoglycemia

Previously, hypoglycemia without symptoms occurred frequently in this disease. Unmeasurable blood glucose levels (well under 10 mg/dl [0.56 mM]) have been documented for several hours, without seizures or any symptoms of hypoglycemia. The implication is that, under these circumstances, the brain metabolizes a substrate or substrates other than glucose. Lactate is the likely substrate for brain in these children [46].

Schulman [23] reported electroencephalographic studies in two biochemically proven patients and could perceive no differences in electrical activity whether blood glucose concentrations were high or low. Both EEGs were interpreted as normal at very low blood sugar levels.

Now, with current management maintaining normoglycemia throughout the 24 hours, these patients manifest all of the clinical signs and symptoms of hypoglycemia when their blood glucose concentrations are low [47]. The full spectrum of neuroglycopenia, including death, has occurred in the treated patients.

Other problems can occur: (1) An intermittent diarrhea without intolerance to mono-· or disaccharides or to fat remains unexplained [48]. (2) In older subjects, malignant changes may occur in the liver [49]. Both radionuclide scintiscan and ultrasonography have been used to define these hepatic tumors [50–52]. Solitary and multiple lesions have been reported in adults. While most lesions are benign hepatomas, occasional transformation to carcinoma has been found. Cirrhosis does not precede this change. (3) Renal abnormalities have been reviewed by Moses [16] and include the Fanconi syndrome and uric acid nephropathy. Chen et al. [53] observed significant renal dysfunction in older patients. In some subjects, initial microalbuminuria progressed to gross proteinuria and renal failure. Recently, hyperfiltration and hypercalcinuria, hypocitraturia, and nephrocalcinosis have also been reported [54]. Patients over 10 years of age should be assessed for renal dysfunction.

Therapy

The major objective of therapy, namely, maintenance of normoglycemia, anteceded the discovery of the specific enzyme defect. However, diet therapy was refined when hepatic glucose-6-phosphatase was found to be absent. A high-protein diet was no longer recommended. Since neither gluconeogenesis nor the conversion of the monosaccharides (fructose and galactose) to glucose would support blood glucose concentrations, fruits and milk were to be avoided.

While diet therapy has improved over the past 40 years, the observations of Folkmann et al. [29] placed renewed emphasis on maintenance of normoglycemia. In preparation for portocaval shunt surgery, they used continuous total parenteral nutrition with a central catheter for over 30 days. They observed regression in size of the liver and correction of the lactic acidemia and hyperuricemia. In addition, hyperlipidemia (triglyceridemia and hypercholesterolemia) reverted to normal, as did the platelet dysfunction. This remarkable demonstration of the effects of prolonged normoglycemia is shown in Figure 7-3 (see p. 256).

The next major advance occurred in the 1970s when Greene et al. [55] proposed continuous nighttime feedings. Several regimens evolved, including nasogastric administration of a high-dextrose (with or without amino acids), pump-controlled continuous feeding or the installation of a permanent gastric button device for intermittent gastric insertion of the enteral feeding tube without reflux. These regimens markedly increased growth in both height and weight and adolescent maturation but were not without risk. At least one fatality was reported from accidental malfunction of a pump during the night in a previously "hypoglycemic-resistant" child [47]. The maintenance of normoglycemia appears to restore brain glucose sensitivity (i.e., primary dependence on glucose substrate), in contrast to the ability of the poorly controlled subject to utilize an alternate substrate, presumably lactate.

Another technique was intermittent nighttime feedings by the clock, every 3 hours. A 16-year-old patient of ours has grown normally and achieved male adolescence with this regimen (see Case Report on Patient 7.1).

The next significant advance in diet therapy occurred in the 1980s when Chen et al. [56] described the ability of raw, uncooked cornstarch to maintain normal plasma glucose concentrations for 4 to 6 hours. The underlying nutritional biochemistry has not yet been clarified. It is noteworthy that cooked starches (corn, potato, and rice) were rapidly hydrolyzed and absorbed and have no prolonged effects on blood glucose levels; these do not differ from dextrose (glucose monohydrate) or Polycose (medium-length polymers). Uncooked cornstarch is absorbed more slowly than raw potato or rice starch. The recommended dose is 1.75–2.5 gm/kg per feeding in cool, chilled diet soda or Kool-Aid or water. The exact dose and time interval should be evaluated by hourly monitoring of plasma glucose concentrations and initiated in the hospital. Infants must be tested to determine their ability to digest and absorb the raw cornstarch before this therapy is instituted. After the initial evaluation, home blood glucose monitoring is used to evaluate dosage and effectiveness. In addition to safety, a major advantage of raw cornstarch therapy is in preventing and treating obesity induced by continuous or frequent night feeding. Cornstarch has also been effective in maintaining euglycemia in pregnancy [57]. Consensus recommendations for treatment of the glycogen storage diseases were reported by representatives of the European communities [58] in 1988.

Diet therapy should include a caloric intake appropriate for age, ideal weight, and expected height and an adequate protein intake according to National Research Council age-dependent standards. Carbohydrate sources should only be glucose or its polymers. Fructose and galactose and their disaccharides and polymers are to be avoided. Practically, this means no fruits or honey or milk of any type. Appropriate sugar substitutes may be used. Stanley et al. have suggested an average glucose rate of 10 mg/kg/min to avoid lactic acidosis [43]. This is equivalent to approximately 58 kcal/kg/day, an inordinately high carbohydrate intake for the older child. This recommendation has recently been questioned by Kalhan and Rossi from stable isotope studies during nasogastric infusion [59]. A recent European workshop suggested graded doses of glucose intake according to age [58]. These varied from 8–9 mg/kg/min in infancy to 5–7 mg/kg/min in the older child. The actual intake is best assessed with frequent blood glucose monitoring preprandially, day and night, for intake adjustment. Excessive caloric intake may contribute to abnormal weight gain and obesity.

Another important aspect of management is lactic acidosis which can occur promptly with a decrease in blood glucose concentration or with infection. Under stable conditions, normoglycemia prevents excessive lactic acid production. However, all children are vulnerable to this complication with intercurrent infections, especially those manifest by vomiting and diarrhea. We recommend the prophylactic administration of sodium bicarbonate (baking soda) at 2 mEq/kg/day. This is easily achieved by adding a single solution (1 tsp dry powder, i.e., 56 mEq/tsp, to 90 ml (3 oz) or 100 ml water) to a milk substitute or any liquid (e.g., Kool-Aid). All GSD patients are given a note with specific instructions to emergency room physicians to evaluate and treat with parenteral dextrose at 10 mg/kg/min plus 75 mEq/L of sodium bicarbonate (*not sodium lactate or lactate Ringers*) until they are stable (no vomiting) and feeding is resumed.

Patients may have hyperuricemia and benefit from allopurinol therapy at 150–300 mg/day, depending on age.

Several surgical procedures to bypass the liver have been utilized in the past [29,60], but none are recommended currently. Platelet dysfunction and abnormal bleeding, especially epistaxis, may occur. Even minor surgery, such as removal of a verruca, may result in uncontrolled bleeding. Elective surgery should be deferred until normoglycemia and reversal of the bleeding diathesis have been achieved.

Prognosis

Until the 1950s, infants with glycogen storage disease type I were usually diagnosed postmorten following minor illnesses which were fatal because of the associated metabolic lactic acidosis. Now, if the diagnosis is made and appropriate treatment instituted, early mortality associated with infections or hypoglycemia should be preventable.

Optimal management results in near-normal growth and development. In particular, adolescent maturation is appropriate in well-stabilized subjects. Interestingly, no significant adverse neurobehavioral effects of early onset hypoglycemia have been reported in these patients.

Late complications associated with hyperuricemia have included pseudogout. Management with allopurinol has been effective. Maintenance of normoglycemia should minimize its occurrence.

A more significant late complication is the presence of hepatomata [50–52]. These tumors may be identified by ultrasound, CT scan, or MRI. There is inadequate data to indicate that malignant transformation does occur. No specific therapy is known to prevent this complication at this time.

Female patients have not only achieved successful physical and sexual maturation, but have also completed successful normal pregnancies and fetal outcomes. No untoward events have been reported for well-controlled pregnant individuals.

Genetics

Based on family history and frequency of this disorder (type Ia) in siblings, it is considered a simple Mendelian recessive that may affect either sex. There are less data to characterize the genetics of the type Ib defect. The frequency has not been estimated. The chromosome locus of the enzyme defect has not been identified, and molecular genetic techniques have not yet been applied to the identification of homozygotes or heterozygotes. Enzyme activity of glucose-6-phosphatase has been studied in liver, kidney, and small intestine. The latter has the potential for genetic studies [61], but no follow-up reports have been made.

Variants of Type I

A subset (about 10 percent) of phenotypically similar patients have significant neutropenia and bacterial infections. Described in 1968, liver glucose-6-phosphatase activity was initially normal in frozen liver [62]. With the recognition of microsomal membrane transport systems for glucose-6-phosphate (T1) and for inorganic phosphate, pyrophosphate, and carbamyl phosphate (T2), subsequent studies on fresh liver demonstrated a deficiency of the glucose-6-phosphate translocase (type Ib) [37]. Shin et al. [63] have developed a sensitive radioisotope method for glucose-6-phosphatase in polymorphonuclear leukocytes for the diagnosis of type Ib. Recent interest has focussed on the impaired leukocyte function. Defects in glucose transport

[64,65], chemotaxis, and neutrophil function [66,67] have been reported. Except for the infections and impaired neutrophil function, these patients appear and are managed similarly to the classic Von Gierke's, type Ia.

Summary

Hepatomegaly in a neonate, infant, or young child with a "doll-like" facies may be associated with epistaxis, hypoglycemia, lactic acidosis, and transient ketonuria. The basic problem is an inability to release glucose from the liver because of an absence of glucose-6-phosphatase activity. The diagnosis is dependent upon an adequate biochemical analysis of liver tissue taken by biopsy, but it may be inferred from glucagon and galactose tolerance tests. Complications associated with plasma lipid elevations, lactic acidemia, and hyperuricemia may be minimized by maintaining normoglycemia by frequent feedings with raw cornstarch or by continuous nighttime nasogastric glucose administration.

Debrancher, Amylo-1,6-Glucosidase Deficiency (Type III)

Although the first documented case with an abnormal glycogen structure due to an absence of the enzyme amylo-1,6-glucosidase was studied by Illingworth and Cori [68] and reported by Forbes [69], the original two cases described by van Creveld have been reevaluated and reclassified into this group [21,70]. The latter cases represent an experience extending over more than 30 years of careful clinical observation.

This disorder has clinical and physiologic abnormalities similar to those of type I disease. In the absence of biochemical analyses of liver tissue, distinction may be difficult. However, certain differences that are generally present lead the clinician to suspect this type of defect. The type III patients tend to have a milder disease and are not as seriously affected by minor infections. While hepatomegaly and hypoglycemia are present, the latter is usually not as severe as in type I disease. In addition, lactic acidosis, an important complication of type I disease, is less frequent and less severe. Ketonuria after fasting does occur [24], but ketoacidosis is not a problem.

Diagnosis

The disease is often unsuspected until a protuberant abdomen and enlarged liver are found. Evaluation shows no evidence of liver dysfunction or splenomegaly. Laboratory studies may reveal nothing more than low fasting blood glucose values. Mild elevation of plasma cholesterol concentration has been noted, but marked hyperlipemia is unusual. The blood sugar is not well-sustained during fasting. A glucagon stimulation test may give variable results. When performed after a brief period of starvation (4–6 hours), a prompt, significant elevation of blood sugar may be found; however, when performed after a 12–14-hour fast, there is usually no rise in blood glucose or lactic acid concentrations [71]. Both the galactose and fructose tolerance tests show normal disappearance of hexose, with prompt elevation of blood glucose (glucose oxidase). Types I, III, and VI have been differentiated by blood lactate response to oral hexoses or glucose [72]. The results of these tolerance tests may be used to make a presumptive diagnosis of type III disease.

The diagnosis may be further established by analysis of erythrocytes [30,73] or of leukocytes [32,74]. The erythrocytes may contain an excessive content of glycogen, which can be isolated and characterized to be a limit dextrin. The leukocytes have been shown to have a deficiency in debrancher enzyme activity. Definitive proof of the diagnosis is obtained by analysis of muscle and liver obtained at biopsy. The studies of Illingworth [75] and Hers [14] have indicated the nature of the defect to be an absence of amylo-1,6-glucosidase, which results in a multibranched glycogen with short outer chains. Recently, immunoblot analyses of glycogen debranching enzyme have been reported for different subtypes of glycogen storage disease type III [76].

Histologically, the liver may be indistinguishable from that found in type I disease, including the accumulations of fat and glycogen in hepatic cells. Skeletal muscle from type III disease cannot be distinguished from type V since glycogen accumulation is found beneath the sarcolemmal membrane in both [77]. Selective glycogenesis of Schwann cells in unmyelinated nerve fibres from intramuscular nerves has been reported [78].

Course

The course of this disease appears to be milder than that of type I, as evidenced by the survival to adulthood of van Creveld's patients [21] and many others [12]. With adolescence, the hepatomegaly becomes less prominent, and ketonuria is less severe. Growth is no longer impaired, and maturation, while delayed, does occur [16]. Although the underlying defect persists, no adverse consequences have been reported. The two patients of van Creveld had normal motor and intellectual development, were married, and had normal sons. Mental retardation does not appear to be a complication.

Recently, transient acute cortical blindness has been associated with hypoglycemia in a 7-year-old boy on two occasions [79]. High-voltage slowing on the electroencephalogram was observed over both occipital areas in both instances.

In a study of 16 patients with type III disease, Moses et al. [80] found widespread evidence of myopathy with heterogeneous expression. They [81] also found a high incidence of cardiomyopathy by echocardiography and x-ray.

Management

Management is directed toward maintenance of normoglycemia and prevention of progressive hepatic enlargement. Since blood sugar cannot be sustained during prolonged starvation, the long overnight fast should be avoided and a feeding taken in the middle of the night. Excessive calories from any source should also be avoided. While galactose and fructose may be converted to glucose (since glucose-6-phosphatase activity is intact), any excessive hexose would be converted to glycogen and stored in the liver. Protein and amino acids should be able to sustain blood glucose through gluconeogenesis since glucose-6-phosphatase activity is normal; therefore, the suggestion of Bridge and Holt [82] for a night feeding high in protein is worthwhile. Hepatic fat accumulation can best be limited by maintenance of normoglycemia. A diet rich in proteins and containing starch as a major source of carbohydrate has been recommended [83]. As in type I disease, raw cornstarch is beneficial and prolongs the interval between feedings.

Prognosis

Prognosis in this disorder is good for attaining adulthood. Some patients may manifest a progressive myopathy in adult life, whereas others do not. All have elevated creatine phosphokinase activity. This myopathy is most evident in North African patients, in contrast to European and North American patients [80].

Genetics

While the genetics of this disorder have not been clearly established, the occurrence in both sexes suggests simple autosomal recessive inheritance. In Israel, where there is a predominance of type III disease, a frequency of 1/5,420 has been reported [84].

It is interesting that eight of the nine patients reported by van Creveld and Huijing were female [85]. Huijing was unable to detect heterozygotes by leukocyte enzyme studies [86]. Prenatal diagnosis may be made from analysis of cultured fibroblasts obtained by amniocentesis [87]. Recently, Ding et al. [88] reported marked molecular heterogeneity of mRNA. They had sequenced the cDNA of the debrancher enzyme.

Summary

Asymptomatic hepatomegaly in childhood may be associated with hypoglycemia and ketonuria, which are more apparent during a period of fasting. Absence of debrancher enzyme amylo-1,6-glucosidase may be noted in leukocytes and an excess quantity of an abnormal glycogen in erythrocytes. Normal growth and development, with diminution in hepatic size at adolescence, is usual. Prolonged fasting and excessive caloric intake should be avoided. Skeletal neuromyopathy and cardiomyopathy are frequently found later in the disease.

Liver Phosphorylase Defect (Type VI)

This disease, which is similar to types I and III clinically and therefore considered a form of hepatic glycogen storage disease, was identified biochemically in 1959 by Hers [89]. He has observed that one third of 1118 Europeans with GSD have this disorder [13].

The disease has been described in siblings and usually has an early onset with hepatomegaly. Fasting blood sugar values and carbohydrate tolerance are variable; low or normal blood glucose values are reported with fasting. The hyperglycemic responses to glucagon may be absent, subnormal, or normal. The blood lactic acid level is not usually elevated, but ketonuria may be present. Galactose given intravenously produces a prompt elevation of blood glucose concentration [90]. Erythrocyte glycogen may be normal or elevated.

Biochemical Studies

Histologically, the liver is similar to that in type I and has a high glycogen content with a normal structure. Enzyme analyses have shown normal activities of glucose-6-phosphatase and amylo-1,6-glucosidase, but depressed levels of phosphorylase (as low as one-seventh normal activity) [89]. Complete absence of the enzyme has not been reported [36]. Activators of the phosphorylase system appear intact, and inhibitors have not been found. Hers emphasized the variability in this enzyme's activity in liver specimens obtained at biopsy and cautioned against overinterpretation of the biochemical data. Muscle phosphorylase activity in these patients is normal.

In normal individuals, phosphorylase activity is present in the leukocytes [31,91,92]. Low total phosphorylase but normal debrancher enzyme [32] activity levels have been reported in patients with type VI disease, proved by biopsy of the liver.

The variability in responsiveness to tolerance tests (glucagon, galactose), in fasting hypoglycemia, and in ketonuria may be due to the variations in the enzymatic defect. Even low levels of activity of this enzyme are apparently sufficient in some patients to produce adequate blood glucose elevations after administration of glucagon.

Course and Prognosis

The course and prognosis in this disease have not yet been adequately defined. Physiologically, greater similarity would be expected to type III, glycogen debrancher defect, than to type I, glucose-6-phosphatase deficiency. In contrast to type III disease, skeletal muscle is rarely involved. However, hepatic adenomata occur, as in type I disease. In view of the site of the enzymatic defect, gluconeogenesis should be unimpaired, and gluconeogenic substrates should be able to sustain the blood glucose. Therefore, a high-protein diet with frequent feedings should be beneficial. In addition, glucocorticoids, which increase gluconeogenesis, may also be of value. It is not known to what extent the glucose formed will be released or synthesized to glycogen.

Variants

The group considered to have a phosphorylase deficiency has been further characterized with reference to the adenylyl cyclase cascade. Christiansen et al. reported a 2½-month-old infant with hepatomegaly and normoglycemia. A hepatoma removed surgically had a defect in dephosphophosphorylase kinase [93]. Hug first reported a similar defect in a girl with increased hepatic glycogen in 1966 [94]. He later reported five children with asymptomatic hepatomegaly without biochemical or clinical evidence of hypoglycemia who had less than 10 percent activation of liver phosphorylase in vitro [95]. The defect was overcome by addition of kinase in vitro, indicating the integrity of the phosphorylase enzyme. This deficiency in dephosphophosphorylase kinase was associated with glycogen accumulation, both intercellularly and within the hepatocytes. Surprisingly, all five patients responded to glucagon acutely, but its effectiveness therapeutically was not clearly shown. Short stature occurred, and mental development was normal. The long-term prognosis is unknown, and therapy is supportive only. Huijing has observed different leukocyte responses in heterozygotes compared to Hug [96]. They characterized phosphorylase kinase deficiency as an X-chromosomal defect. Hemolysate analysis has been used to distinguish two subgroups based on phosphorylase kinase activity, endogenous phosphorylase b, and amylo-1,6-glucosidase activity [97].

Willems and associates [98] have reported both the initial findings and the longitudinal outcome of 41 patients with kinase deficiency. Most adult patients are asymptomatic. Shin and associates [99] have classified patients in four groups based on erythrocyte activities of phosphorylase kinase, phosphorylase, and amyloglucosidase. Tuchman and associates [100] studied a young child who did not have hypoglycemia and who did not respond to a high-protein diet, but did to a high-carbohydrate diet.

The phosphorylase system may be associated with defects [101] resulting in (1) the X-linked phosphorylase b kinase deficiency, in which the muscle enzyme is unaffected; (2) the autosomal phosphorylase b kinase deficiency, which affects both liver and muscle; and (3) the deficiency of liver phosphorylase, which may be complete or partial. The gene coding for liver phosphorylase has been assigned to chromosome 14 [102]. The alpha subunit of phosphorylase kinase has been assigned to the proximal long arm of the X chromosome, but the beta subunit to chromosome 16 [103].

Summary

A decrease in hepatic and leukocytic phosphorylase activity has been found to be associated with hepatomegaly and hypoglycemia in early childhood. This entity is difficult to differentiate from the other two types of hepatic glycogen storage disease on clinical and physiologic observations alone. Multiple forms of this type of glycogen storage disease have been described, depending upon the mechanism of the reduction in phosphorylase activity.

• Glycogen Disease of Skeletal Muscle

Muscle Phosphorylase Deficiency (Type V), McArdle's Syndrome

This rare myopathy, first recognized in 1951 [10], is of particular significance because it represents the first discovery of a genetic disease of muscle caused by the absence of a single, specific enzyme.

Clinical Considerations

The disease is characterized by a late onset. In early childhood, the patient is relatively free of symptoms, although one noted muscle fatigue and inability to keep up with his playmates by 7 years of age. Generally, symptoms are absent or minimal in the first decade. During the teens, muscle fatigue, particularly with strenuous exercise, may be evident. Transient episodes of dark urine due to myoglobinuria may occur. Hepatomegaly is also absent, and the cardiopulmonary system is not remarkable.

Laboratory Studies

Laboratory studies, including blood and urine, are singularly unrewarding, except for the rare, postexercise episode of transient myoglobinuria. Serum enzyme and carbohydrate studies are particularly unremarkable. Electrolytes, including potassium and calcium, and concentrations of glucose, phosphate, lactate, and pyruvate are normal in the resting state.

Carbohydrate tests, including glucose tolerance, glucose and insulin tolerance, epinephrine and glucagon tolerances, are all normal. The latter two tests indicate that liver phosphorylase is normal.

Physiologic Studies

McArdle [10] studied his 30-year-old male patient extensively and noted particularly a failure of ischemic exercise to produce an elevation in venous blood lactate. Normally, prolonged exercise produces a significant elevation of the lactate concentration in venous blood, and ischemic exercise, depending upon duration, similarly produces a characteristic elevation of from 25–30 mg/dl above the basal level.

Biochemical Studies

Biochemical studies of biopsied muscle have indicated an absence of phosphorylase a and b, but the presence of UDPG-glycogen synthase, phosphorylase kinase, and phosphoglucomutase [104,105]. Glycogen content in muscle in the three original cases was excessive at 2.4–4g/100 gm (normal is less than 1 percent wet weight). The glycogen has been found to be structurally normal.

Pathology

Histologic examination of muscle has indicated variable tissue structure. In younger individuals, muscle appears normal, while in the older person with muscle atrophy, hypertrophied fibers with blebs of raised sarcolemma are found [106,107]. The damaged fibers appear necrotic and may disappear altogether.

Pathogenesis

Resting muscle derives its energy mainly from oxidation of noncarbohydrate substances, although glucose uptake and degradation to lactate do occur [108]. Glycogen is not an important source of energy for resting muscle. In contrast, contracting muscle has an enormous demand for high-energy phosphates, which cannot be supplied adequately by substrates from the blood, even though blood flow increases with exercise. Under these conditions, glycogenolysis and the anaerobic metabolism of glucose with lactate production are important sources of energy to sustain muscle activity. The limitation of the individual with phosphorylase myopathy to sustain muscle during exercise is directly related to the inability to degrade glycogen.

Differential Diagnosis

Differential diagnosis is confined to other muscular disorders, including muscular dystrophy and congenital myotonia (Thomsen's disease). Defects in a variety of glycogenolytic and glycolytic enzymes of muscle must be considered, including phosphorylase b kinase, amylo-1,6-glucosidase, glucose phosphate isomerase, and type VII muscle phosphofructokinase.

Course

The course of the disease is variably benign; longevity does not appear to be affected. Improvement in work and exercise tolerance has been reported following either glucagon injections and glucose or fructose ingestion (30–45 g by mouth, 3 or 4 times daily) [109]. Avoidance of strenuous activity is important.

Genetics

The genetics of this rare disease have been clarified in a detailed family study in which 3 cases (two proven) were found in a sibship of 13 individuals [110]. These findings suggest a single, completely recessive, rare, autosomal gene. Molecular genetic techniques have been used to assign this gene to chromosome 11 [111].

Summary

Myopathy due to the absence of muscle phosphorylase is a rare genetic disease manifest by intolerance to exercise. The abnormal response to ischemic exercise is characterized by a fall in venous lactate concentration. Muscle biopsy is necessary to demonstrate the biochemical defect. Other phosphorylases (liver, leukocyte, etc.) are not affected.

Muscle Phosphofructokinase Deficiency: Type VII

Glycogen storage in muscle from patients with a similar clinical picture to that of McArdle's disease has been reported by Tarui and associates [112,113]. In addition to the muscular disorder, the three young Japanese adult siblings also had a nonspherocytic hemolytic anemia. Myoglobinuria was observed in one subject. As in phosphorylase deficiency, ischemic exercise failed to increase venous blood lactate. The low muscle phosphofructokinase activity was associated with increased concentrations of glucose-6-phosphate and fructose-6-phosphate in muscle, while fructose-1,6-diphosphate was low.

Muscle phosphofructokinase was found to be a different isozyme from that in liver, while erythrocytes normally have approximately half of each form. Tarui and associates [114] noted that total erythrocyte enzyme levels of phosphofructokinase were about 50 percent of normal, with absence of the muscle isozyme and persistence of the hepatic form. They related the reduced erythrocyte life span and hemolysis to the deficient red cell enzyme. Layzer et al. [115] have studied a similar patient from the United States. They were unable to demonstrate any material in a muscle biopsy that would react with an antibody prepared against purified human muscle phosphofructokinase.

While only a few patients have been reported, the disorder is presumably inherited as an autosomal recessive, since it has been observed in both sexes and has been associated with reduced erythrocyte enzyme levels in parents.

• Generalized Glycogen Storage Disease

Deficiency of α-Acid Glucosidase (Acid Maltase) (Type II) (Pompe's Disease)

Although this type of glycogen storage disease was one of the first to be described in terms of pathology [4], the biochemical origin was unknown until the report of Hers in 1963 [19]. This group of glycogen storage diseases represents a clinical spectrum including idiopathic cardiomegaly of infancy, a neuromuscular disorder simulating amyotonia congenita, and a diffuse cardioneuromuscular disease [116,117]. This disease is characterized by an early onset, with a rapidly progressing deterioration to death, often within the first year of life and generally by the second year. The adult onset type may be benign in its course, as noted in survivors.

In a review in 1950 [116], the criteria for a diagnosis of glycogen storage disease of the heart were: (1) marked enlargement of the heart, (2) death within the first year of life, (3) typical "lacework" appearance of histologic sections of myocardium, resulting from the massive deposition of stored material in all cardiac fibers, and (4) chemical or histochemical demonstration of the material as glycogen. These were based on the original observations of Pompe [4] and van Creveld [5,6].

However, these criteria are too rigid, since cases have been reported without cardiomegaly but with predominantly muscular involvement; also, the child may live beyond the first year of life [117].

Clinical Considerations

Onset can be at any time within the first year of life, from the first day to a few months of age. In the generalized type, the clinical manifestations often include diffuse muscular weakness, respiratory difficulty, and progressive cardiac failure. Undernutrition due to difficult feeding, with failure to thrive and loss of subcutaneous fat, may be early manifestations. The muscles feel firm, although hypotonia may be present. Reflexes are sometimes totally absent. The heart is enlarged on percussion, but auscultation reveals no murmurs. The liver is normal or only minimally enlarged. The tongue may be large and protuberant, giving the infant the appearance of a cretin or of a baby with 21 trisomy. Progressive muscle weakness may involve the respiratory muscles, thus simulating amyotonia congenita. Cardiac enlargement progresses to failure, with dyspnea and cyanosis. Respiratory infection with fever is common and is often the precipitating terminal event.

In contrast to the fatal infantile form of this disease, there is a milder, adult form in which muscular weakness is most evident. Survival into middle decades is not unusual.

Laboratory Studies

Laboratory studies are remarkable in that they afford no clues pointing toward an abnormality of glycogen metabolism. Routine blood and urine analyses are merely consistent with the infant's nutritional and infection status. Low blood glucose concentrations, when reported, have been due to inadequate nutrition; blood glucose levels are usually normal. Glucose, epinephrine, glucagon, and galactose tolerance tests have been normal. Blood lactic acid concentration is normal and rises normally after administration of epinephrine. Ketosis, ketonuria, and acidosis are not features of this disorder. Neostigmine responses and electromyography have not been diagnostic.

X-Ray Findings

Roentgen examination may reveal a large, globular heart that is diffusely involved and fills both sides of the thorax. Consolidation of the lungs may be present. The kidneys are not enlarged.

Cardiac Studies

The electrocardiogram is abnormal in those patients with involvement of the heart [118]. Supraventricular tachycardia has been reported as an initial presentation. The P-R interval is short, while the QRS complex may be high. Echocardiography indicates a diffusely, symmetrically enlarged heart. Dincsoy observed endocardial fibroelastosis in two siblings [119].

Differential Diagnosis

The diagnosis, which can only be suspected from clinical evidence, depends upon pathologic and biochemical studies. The patients with cardiac enlargement must be differentiated from the group of infants with primary endomyocardial disease, such as primary endocardial sclerosis, anomalous origin of a coronary artery, myocarditis, calcification of the coronary arteries, and idiopathic myocardial hypertrophy. Skeletal muscle involvement is a distinguishing feature. The latter must be differentiated from amyotonia congenita, a more common entity [120]. The general appearance of the infant with protuberant, large tongue and umbilical hernia may suggest Down's syndrome or congenital hypothyroidism.

Diagnosis

The glycogen content of tissues, especially the heart and skeletal muscle, is high and can exceed 10 percent by wet weight. Glycogen structure is normal. The activity in liver of the enzymes phosphorylase, debrancher, and glucose-6-phosphatase have been normal. Erythrocyte glycogen is not elevated [121]. Acid maltase activity was low in the leukocytes of some patients with type II disease [122].

Pathology

Tissues taken for histochemical analysis must be handled carefully, as the glycogen is highly soluble in water. The changes in cardiac, skeletal, and smooth muscle are similar: a honeycombed or lacework appearance due to extensive vacuolization is characteristic. Alcoholic PAS stains reveal heavy deposits of glycogen with intensively stained, closely packed granules of different sizes. Glycogen deposition granules may be found in a variety of tissues, including the central nervous system. This may occur diffusely and include brain, spinal cord, and peripheral nervous system, or be localized to specific areas such as the spinal cord and the autonomic nervous system.

Pathogenesis

Although an enzymic defect has been demonstrated, the pathogenesis is not entirely clear. Lejeune, Thines-Sempoux, and Hers [123] have localized α-acid glucosidase in the lysosomes in rat liver. These subcellular fractions contain a variety of hydrolases, which are capable of breakdown and digestion of localized areas within the cell. Apparently, there is a continual breakdown and synthesis of local cell constituents. Glycogen, which is synthesized normally and usually degraded by glycogenolytic enzymes (phosphorylase and debrancher), may also be degraded locally within the lysosome by α-acid glucosidase to maltose and glucose. In the absence of this enzyme, other lysosomal hydrolases might destroy the enzymes that usually break down glycogen, allowing normal glycogen to accumulate in the vacuoles. In other cellular sites, containing glycogen and the enzymes of synthesis and degradation, no physiologic defect in glucose metabolism is apparent. The accumulation of glycogen in localized vacuolated areas within the cell would be progressive, impair cellular function, and disrupt muscle fibers.

The enzyme α-acid glucosidase has been identified in a variety of tissues, including leukocytes, liver, and muscle. Skin fibroblasts and amniotic fluid cells have been cultured and assayed for α-glucosidase activity [124,125], allowing in utero diagnosis [126,127]. Shin et al. [128] made a diagnosis in the first trimester by chorionic villus biopsy.

Genetics

The disease is familial, with as many as three affected siblings having been reported in a single family. Over 200 cases of this apparently genetically determined, autosomal recessive disorder have been cited

[128,129]. Parents of affected children have decreased enzyme activity in cultured fibroblasts. Differences in enzyme activities between the infantile and late onset form have been attributed to different allelic mutations [130]. The human gene for α-acid glucosidase has been cloned and assigned to chromosome 17 [131].

Therapy

As with other inherited molecular disorders, therapy has been unsuccessful and primarily supportive. Digitalization and surgical intervention have been notably without benefit. Exogenous enzyme administration has not been beneficial. Recombinant DNA biosynthesis or targeted gene therapy may be effective in the future.

Summary

Generalized glycogenosis is a progressive disorder of young infants in whom cardiac hypertrophy, skeletal muscle dysfunction, and central nervous system deterioration usually result in a fatal outcome in the first year of life. Abnormalities of carbohydrate physiology are not found, although excessive glycogen accumulation in a variety of tissues is characteristic. Diagnosis is established by muscle biopsy and the biochemical demonstration of an absence of α-acid glucosidase. The enzymatic defect may also be shown in the leukocyte and liver. There is no satisfactory therapy.

• Abnormal Glycogen

Storage of Abnormal Glycogen: Amylopectinosis Brancher Deficiency (Type IV) (α-1,4 Glucan:α-1,4 Glucan 6-Glycosyl Transferase)

This disorder was first described clinically by Andersen [9], and the structure of the glycogen was characterized biochemically by Cori [13]. Absence of the enzyme in liver and leukocytes was reported by Brown and Brown [132]. The clinical course was uniform in the group in that the affected infant appeared normal at birth, grew well in the initial months, but failed to thrive early in infancy. By the sixth month of life, abdominal distention, hepatomegaly, and splenomegaly appeared. Dilated superficial veins were present over the upper abdomen. Minimal icterus was present in Andersen's case.

Laboratory Findings and Diagnosis

The hemogram indicated a mild anemia. Carbohydrate studies revealed a normal fasting blood sugar level, rarely as low as 30 mg/100 ml (1.7 mM). Oral and intravenous glucose, galactose, and fructose tolerance tests were not remarkable. Response to administration of epinephrine and glucagon was variable, with a flat or delayed rise in blood glucose levels. In contrast to other forms of glycogen storage disease, no abnormalities in blood concentrations of pyruvate, lactate, or urate were observed either in the fasting state or during the tolerance tests [133].

The major laboratory abnormalities were in liver function tests. SGOT rose as high as 240 units (normal <30), while SGPT reached levels of 114 units (normal <30). In addition to transaminase, elevations of aldolase and lactate dehydrogenase, especially its isoenzyme V form, occur [133]. Values for cholesterol and total lipids were not elevated. Serum electrolyte concentrations were not remarkable. A severe metabolic acidosis has been reported and is thought to be of renal origin [134].

Initial diagnosis, as determined by biopsy in early cases, was glycogen storage disease with diffuse early portal cirrhosis.

Course

The patients reported have had a similar course, with progressive liver or cardiac failure; most patients succumbed between 6 and 24 months, although survival until four years of age has been noted [135]. The complications of portal hypertension and cirrhosis predominated. Ascites, esophageal varices with hemorrhage, jaundice, and malnutrition were present. Hypoproteinemia occurred late in the course of the disease, while hypoprothrombinemia occurred early. Intercurrent infections were frequent.

Pathology

At postmortem, the livers were large and firm, with golden-yellow nodules. The spleen was large. The kidneys were enlarged but otherwise grossly normal on inspection. Histologically, the liver contained fibrous tissue and bile duct proliferation. Best's stain indicated the liver cells to be packed with red granules. On iodine stain, this material gave a purplish-brown color instead of the usual reddish-brown characteristic of normal glycogen. Excess polysaccharide was identified histologically in many tissues, including liver, spleen, lymph nodes, and intestinal mucosa, as well as kidneys, heart, muscle, reticuloendothelial system, and nervous system.

Andersen noted difficulty in chemically isolating glycogen and submitted tissue to Cori for further biochemical analysis, who isolated the polysaccharide and characterized it as an amylopectin with abnormal inner and outer straight chains. On this basis, she postulated a deficiency of brancher enzyme. Sidbury studied a variety of enzymes in liver and muscle and noted a general depression, without absence of a specific enzyme. He isolated and characterized the polysaccharide also as an amylopectin. It is of interest that the liver did not contain an excessive content of this glycogenlike material (0.18–2.86 percent) or of fat.

The diagnosis was suspected, in one case, from an analysis of red blood cell glycogen [136]. While the amount of material (polysaccharide) was not increased in content, the iodine spectrum was similar to that found with amylopectin and different from that of normal glycogen. Shin et al. [133] have measured the enzyme activity in erythrocytes in controls and in three affected children.

The diagnosis of type IV can be established by liver biopsy and accompanying histochemical and biochemical studies [135,137]. The liver glycogen content is usually below normal (<5 g/100 g liver), although a high value (10.7 g/100 g) may occur [135]. One hypothesis suggested that the polysaccharide acts as a foreign body to produce a reaction in the reticuloendothelial system and in liver parenchymal cells.

Genetics

Although few cases have been reported, a familial incidence is evident. In one family, skin fibroblast studies from the propositus established the diagnosis, while those from the parents had enzyme values below those of controls. The disorder appears to be inherited as a simple autosomal recessive.

Therapy

Until recently, management has been nonspecific and supportive. Dietary therapy has been unsuccessful (high protein, low carbohydrate with corn oil). Portocaval transposition was attempted late in one patient without success [135]. Glucagon, both short and long acting, has not modified the course. Another patient survived with steroid therapy until 4 years of age.

A highly purified α-glucosidase from Aspergillus niger has been administered intravenously without success. No unfavorable reactions were observed. The liver did not diminish in size. This therapy did not modify the patient's course.

As noted earlier, the implications of substitution enzyme therapy in inherited molecular diseases may be great. Liver transplants have already begun to influence management in selected acquired (e.g., biliary atresia) and genetic diseases (hereditary tyrosinemia) [138,139]. The possibility of intervention with liver transplant early in life may offer a mechanism for modifying this rapidly progressive disease.

Summary

The accumulation of an abnormal polysaccharide due to a deficiency of brancher enzyme results in pathologic changes in the reticuloen-dothelial system. In particular, cirrhosis occurs with progressive signs of hepatic dysfunction and, ultimately, death due to liver failure. The clinical and chemical picture cannot be distinguished from other causes of cirrhosis in infancy but is readily differentiated from hepatorenal forms of glycogen storage diseases. Identification of the abnormal glycogen in red blood cells, leukocytes, or liver, or an analysis for the specific enzyme in fibroblasts or liver establishes the diagnosis. Liver transplant may be beneficial.

• Glycogen Deficiency Disease

Glycogen Synthase Defect

The absence of glycogen synthase in the liver is the second clinical condition that may result from a defect in glycogen synthesis (see above). This is the first example of a defect in the synthetic pathway leading to inadequate glycogen formation.

First reported in 1963 [20], a set of twins was found to be apneic at 46 and 40 hours of age prior to the initiation of feeding at 48 hours. After 7 months of age, withdrawal of the night feeding was associated with pallor, transient strabismus, and then early morning convulsions prior to morning feeding. Another 9-year-old girl had early morning hypoglycemia with onset after discontinuance of night-time feeds as an infant [140].

In another family [141] in which three prior siblings died in infancy with central nervous system signs, an infant did poorly with feedings during the first days of life but then thrived until 3½ months of age. At 4 months, she had an acute illness with 12 hours of marked lethargy and poor feeding, followed by a "stiffening out spell" and unresponsiveness. She had a "doll-like facies" and an enlarged liver. Her blood sugar concentration was 4 mg/dl (0.2 mM), although spinal fluid sugar was 40 mg/dl (2.2 mM). Glucagon 3 hours after a meal produced a prompt and significant elevation of the blood glucose concentration but had no effect after an overnight fast.

Diagnosis

Liver biopsy is necessary for enzyme analyses to establish the diagnosis. Although glycogen synthase activity has been demonstrated in the erythrocyte by Cornblath et al. [142], this tissue does not serve as a possible source for verification of the diagnosis. Erythrocytes from patients and other family members were found to contain normal glycogen synthase activity [143]. Thus, erythrocyte glycogen synthase appears to be unrelated to hepatic glycogen synthase.

A liver biopsy taken from one twin while the patient was maintained by intravenous glucose contained 0.45 percent glycogen and 9.8 percent total lipid. Histologically, there was glycogen depletion and pronounced fatty change of the liver. Enzyme studies revealed undetectable glycogen synthase activity, but normal activities of UDPG-pyrophosphorylase, phosphorylase, and glucose-6-phosphatase. Gitzelmann et al. found that the defect is not expressed in skin fibroblasts [144] nor in erythrocytes [145].

Genetics

The data are insufficient to establish the genetic aspects of this familial disease.

Pathogenesis

These three studies may represent a variant of the same basic defect, an absence of glycogen synthase. The pathophysiology and the precise biochemical defect remain to be defined. How glycogen synthesis occurs in the absence of this enzyme activity is unknown. Glycogen is apparently formed after meals, since there was a hyperglycemic response to glucagon at that time. This could result from the reversible phosphorylase action [20]. The failure of glycogen synthesis alone is inadequate to explain the hypoglycemia with fasting, since increased gluconeogenesis should compensate for this. It would appear that the inability to synthesize glycogen effectively may lead to secondary inhibition of gluconeogenesis.

Management

The management of these patients must be individualized. Dietary control with high-protein feedings appears to be effective in the mildly affected patient. When hypoglycemia is persistent and severe, raw cornstarch and/or glucocorticoid therapy may be indicated. Aynsley-Green et al. [146] were successful with frequent feedings of a high-protein diet.

Prognosis

Dykes et al. [147] restudied the original family seven years later. The twins had an improved ability to maintain a normal blood glucose concentration but still had episodes of hypoglycemia. Glucagon responses at 3 and 20 hours after a meal were inadequate and interpreted to indicate diminished liver glycogen production. Galactose tolerance tests produced a rise in both blood glucose and blood lactate concentrations.

Summary

A new familial disease characterized by hypoglycemia with starvation in early infancy has been associated with an absence of glycogen synthase in the liver and decreased glycogen stores. Signs of hypoglycemia may be severe, including convulsions before a feeding. Diagnosis may be suspected from a failure of glucagon response after overnight fast but requires enzyme studies of liver for its establishment.

Case Report (Patient 7.1): Type I GSD Treated with Frequent Feeds and then Cornstarch

A 6-lb, 15-oz white male infant was delivered vaginally after a normal pregnancy to a healthy 27-year-old primiparous female who was a first cousin of the father. The neonatal course was complicated by transient episodes of apnea and focal seizures, mild jaundice and minimal hepatomegaly.

At 5 months, he was admitted for poor appetite, nasal congestion, and fever (102°F). The mother reported "breath-holding spells" similar to earlier episodes and associated with duskiness. In the interval at home, he fed vigorously, taking 4 oz of formula, cereals, fruits, vegetables every 4 hours. Neurodevelopment delay was noted. His weight was at the 50th percentile and length at the 60th. He had a "puffy" facies and protuberant abdomen. The liver was palpated 6 cm below the right costal margin. Shortly after admission, he developed Kussmaul respirations and had a pH of 7.14 and TCO$_2$ mM/L. A blood glucose determination was not done, and therapy was directed toward acidosis and possible sepsis. Shortly thereafter, a blood glucose concentration of 5 mg/dl (0.28 mM) was found. In addition, the blood lactic acid level was 13.2 mEq/L, serum acetone moderate, serum cholesterol 503 mg/dl, triglycerides 2,970 mg/dl, and uric acid 14.4 mg/dl. A glucagon stimulation test was done 3 hours after a feed when the plasma glucose value was 65 mg/dl (3.6 mM). There was not only no rise but a fall in the glucose concentration to 50 mg/dl (2.8 mM) after 20 minutes. A presumptive diagnosis of type I glycogen storage disease was made. A fresh liver biopsy contained 12.8 percent glycogen (w/w) and absent glucose-6-phosphatase activity but normal phosphorylase and debrancher activity. Diet instruction initially included high dextrose, low fat, low protein feeds.

Because the mother was reluctant to use nasogastric feeding, she opted to feed him every 3 hours day and night (by the alarm clock). His regimen included feedings of a carbohydrate free formula (RCF; Ross Laboratories, Columbus, OH) supplemented with glucose polymers (Polycose) (26 gm) with and between meals. Polycose in water (40 gm, 1.2 gm/kg) was given throughout the night at 3-hour intervals. Sodium bicarbonate (baking soda 2 mEq/kg/day) was added to the formula. He also was given allopurinol to control hyperuricemia, and calcium carbonate because of suspected demineralization noted at the time of a femoral fracture in early childhood.

His course required brief hospitalizations for parenteral fluid therapy with sodium bicarbonate (75 mEq/L) and dextrose (10 percent) at 10 mg/kg/min to correct lactic acidosis and hypoglycemia associated with intercurrent infections.

On this regimen, his growth in height was delayed (Fig. 7-7); however, weight was always in the 50–75th percentiles.

At age 10½ years, he was admitted for evaluation and had "around-the-clock" blood sampling for glucose, lactate, and related metabolic studies. For the first day, his mother fed his home regimen of Polycose or RCF with Polycose. The left panel of Figure 7-8 shows the rapid rise and fall in plasma glucose concentration to hypoglycemic levels on two occasions. At 18 and 32 hours, he received raw uncooked cornstarch, as recommended by Chen et al. [56]. He initially received 50 gm cornstarch (1.5 gm/kg), but later this was increased to 60 gm (1.8 gm/kg). The effect on his blood glucose concentration is shown in the right panel of Figure 7-8. Subsequently, the patient was controlled on 1.6–1.8 gm/kg dose every 6 hours. His height improved so that he achieved the 25th percentile by 16 years of age. He has also developed normal secondary sex characteristics.

During the study period, plasma insulin concentration ranged from 5–78 μU/ml (30–468 pM) and correlated with the level of glycemia. Lactic acidosis, which was prominent, initially improved with cornstarch therapy. Many of the secondary and tertiary metabolic abnormalities have corrected with avoidance of intermittent and/or persistent hypoglycemia.

Comment

The complex metabolic interrelationships, growth failure, and tolerance to profound hypoglycemia can all be modified by continuous provision of glucose. This may be accomplished in a variety of ways. Glucose polymers have been given as a continuous nocturnal nasogastric infusion. Raw, uncooked cornstarch by mouth has become a practical, safe, nutritionally satisfactory way to achieve normoglycemia in these patients. The patients must be old enough to digest raw starch.

DISORDERS OF GLYCOGEN METABOLISM

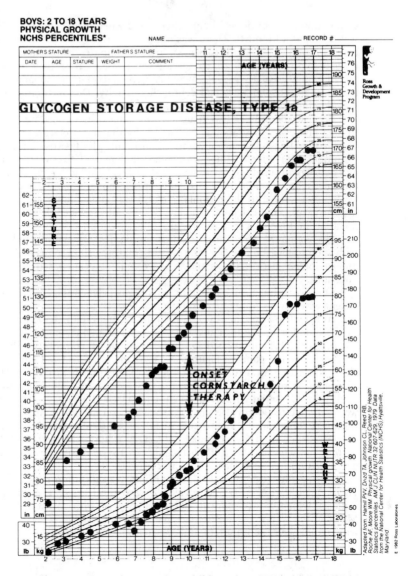

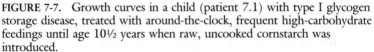

FIGURE 7-7. Growth curves in a child (patient 7.1) with type I glycogen storage disease, treated with around-the-clock, frequent high-carbohydrate feedings until age 10½ years when raw, uncooked cornstarch was introduced.

BLOOD GLUCOSE (MG/DL) VS. MINUTES POSTPRANDIAL

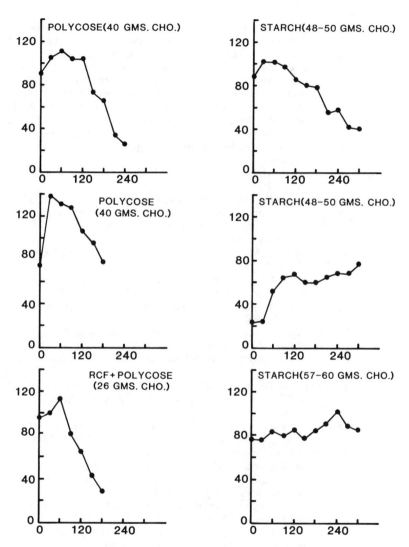

FIGURE 7-8. Comparison of plasma glucose responses in patient 7.1 to high-carbohydrate feedings (Polycose supplemented) compared to raw, uncooked cornstarch. Note the difference in sustaining normoglycemia between the two regimens.

REFERENCES

1. SNAPPER I, VAN CREVELD S. Un cas d'hypoglycémie avec acétonémie chez un enfant. *Bull Mem Soc Med Hop.* (Paris) 1928;52:1315.
2. VON GIERKE E. Hepato-Nephromegalia glykogenica (Glykogenspeich-erkrankheit der Leber und Nieren). *Beitr Pathol.* 1929;82:497.
3. SCHÖNHEIMER R. Über eine eigenartige Storung des Kohlehydrat-Stoff-wechsels. Hoppe Seylers *Z Physiol Chem.* 1929;182:148.
4. POMPE JC. Over idiopatische hypertrophie van het hart. *Ned Tijdschr Geneeskd.* 1932;76:304. (Abstract.)
5. VAN CREVELD S. Glycogen disease. *Medicine.* 1939;18:1.
6. VAN CREVELD S. Investigations on glycogen disease. *Arch Dis Child.* 1934;9:9.
7. MASON HH, ANDERSEN DH. Glycogen disease. *Am J Dis Child.* 1941;61:795.
8. DEBRÉ R. *Les Polyconles.* Paris: Gaston Doin & Cie., 1947.
9. ANDERSEN DH. Studies on glycogen disease with report of a case in which the glycogen was abnormal. In: Najjar VA, ed. *Carbohydrate Metabolism.* Baltimore: Johns Hopkins University Press, 1952;28.
10. MCARDLE B. Myopathy due to a defect in muscle glycogen breakdown. *Clin Sci.* 1951;10:13.
11. CORI GT. Glycogen structure and enzyme deficiencies in glycogen storage disease. *Harvey Lect.* (1952–53) 1954;48:145.
12. STETTEN D JR, STETTEN MR. Glycogen metabolism. *Physiol Rev.* 1960;40:505.
13. HERS H-G, VAN HOOF F, DE BARSY T. Glycogen storage diseases. In: Scriver CR, Beaudet AL, Sly WS, Valle D, eds. *The Metabolic Basis of Inherited Disease, 6th ed.* New York: McGraw-Hill, Inc., 1989; 425.
14. HERS HG. Glycogen storage disease. In: LEVINE R, LUFT R, eds. *Advances in Metabolic Disorders.* Vol. 1. New York: Academic Press, Inc., 1964;1–44.
15. SPENCER-PEET J, NORMAN ME, LAKE BD, MCNAMARA J, PATRICK AD. Hepatic glycogen storage disease. *Q J Med.* 1971;157:95.
16. MOSES SW. Pathophysiology and dietary treatment of the glycogen storage diseases. *J Pediatr Gastroenterol.* 1990;11:155.
17. BROWN DH, BROWN BI. Some inborn errors of carbohydrate metabolism. In Whelan WJ, ed. *M. T. P. International Review of Science vol. 5.* Biochemistry of Carbohydrates. London: Butterworth & Co. and Baltimore: Park Press, 1975;391.
18. CORI GT, CORI CF. Glucose-6-phosphatase of the liver in glycogen storage disease. *J Biol Chem.* 1952;199:661.
19. HERS HG. α-Glucosidase deficiency in generalized glycogen-storage disease (Pompe's disease). *Biochem J.* 1963;86:11.
20. LEWIS GM, SPENCER-PEET J, STEWART KM. Infantile hypoglycemia due to inherited deficiency of glycogen synthetase in liver. *Arch Dis Child.* 1963;38:40.
21. VAN CREVELD S. The Blackader lecture, 1962: the clinical course of glycogen disease. *Can Med Assoc J.* 1963;88:1.
22. FINE RN, WILSON WA, DONNELL GN. Retinal changes in glycogen storage disease type I. *Am J Dis Child.* 1968;115:328.

23. SCHULMAN JL, SATUREN P. Glycogen storage disease of the liver. I. Clinical studies during the early neonatal period. *Pediatrics.* 1954;14:632.

24. FERNANDES J, PIKAAR NA. Ketosis in hepatic glycogenosis. *Arch Dis Child.* 1972;47:41.

25. NILSSON IM, OCKERMAN PA. Bleeding disorder in hepatomegalic forms of glycogen storage disease. *Acta Paediatr Scand.* 1970;59:127.

26. ZELLER WP, CORNBLATH M, SCHWARTZ HC, SCHWARTZ R. Minor hemoglobins in disorders of carbohydrate metabolism. *J. Pediatr.* 1981;98:936.

27. BRANTE G, KAIJSER K, OCKERMAN PA. Glycogenosis type I (lack of glucose-6-phosphatase) in four siblings. *Acta Paediatr.* (suppl.) 1964;157:1.

28. HOWELL RR, ASHTON DM, WYNGAARDEN JB. Glucose-6-phosphatase deficiency glycogen storage disease. Studies on the interrelationships of carbohydrate, lipid and purine abnormalities. *Pediatrics.* 1962;29:553.

29. FOLKMAN J, PHILIPPART A, TZE WJ, CRIGLER J JR. Portocaval shunt for glycogen storage disease: Value of prolonged intravenous hyperalimentation before surgery. *Surgery.* 1972;72:306.

30. SIDBURY JB, CORNBLATH M, FISHER J, HOUSE E. Glycogen in erythrocytes of patient with glycogen storage disease. *Pedatrics.* 1961;27:103.

31. WILLIAMS HE, FIELD JB. Further studies on leukocyte phosphorylase in glycogen storage disease. *Metabolism.* 1963;12:464.

32. WILLIAMS HE, KENDIG EM, FIELD JB. Leukocyte debranching enzyme in glycogen storage disease. *J Clin Invest.* 1963;42:656.

33. SOKAL JE, LOWE CU, SARCIONE EJ, MOSOVICH LL, DORAY BH. Studies of glycogen metabolism in liver glycogen disease (von Gierke's disease): six cases with similar metabolic abnormalities and responses to glucagon. *J Clin Invest.* 1961;40:364.

34. PERKOFF GT, PARKER VJ, HAHN RF. The effects of glucagon in three forms of glycogen storage disease. *J Clin Invest.* 1962;41:1099.

35. SCHWARTZ R, ASHMORE J, RENOLD AE. Galactose tolerance in glycogen storage disease. *Pediatrics.* 1957;19:585.

36. ILLINGWORTH B. Glycogen storage disease. *Am J Clin Nutr.* 1961;9:683.

37. TADA K, NARISAWA K, IGARASHI Y, KATO S. Glycogen storage disease type IB: a new model of genetic disorders involving the transport system of intracellular membrane. *Biochem Med.* 1985;33:215.

38. VILLEE CA. The intermediary metabolism of human fetal tissues. *Cold Spring Harbor Symp Quant Biol.* 1954;19:186.

39. KALHAN SC, GILFILLAN C, TSERNG K-Y, SAVIN SM. Glucose production in type I glycogen storage disease. *J Pediatr.* 1982;101:159.

40. TSALIKIAN E, SIMMONS P, GERICH JE, HOWARD C, HAYMOND MW. Glucose production and utilization in children with glycogen storage disease type I. *Am J Physiol.* 1984;247:E513. (Letter.)

41. MASON HH, SLY GE. Blood lactic acid in liver glycogen disease. *Proc Soc Exp Biol.* 1943;53:145.

42. OBERHAENSLI RD, RAJAGOPALAN B, TAYLOR DJ, RADDA GK, COLLINS JE, LEONARD JV. Study of liver metabolism in glucose-6-phosphatase deficiency (glycogen storage disease type 1A) by P-31 magnetic resonance spectroscopy. *Pediatr Res.* 1988;23:375.

43. STANLEY CA, MILLS JL, BAKER L. Intragastric feeding in type I glycogen

storage disease: factors affecting the control of lactic acidemia. *Pediatr Res.* 1981;15:1504.

44. FINE RN, STRAUSS J, DONNELL GN. Hyperuricemia in glycogen-storage disease type I. *Am J Dis Child.* 1966;112:572.

45. ROE TF, KOGUT MD. The pathogenesis of hyperuricemia in glycogen storage disease, type I. *Pediatr Res.* 1977;11:664.

46. FERNANDES J, BERGER R, SMITH GPA. Lactate as a cerebral metabolic fuel for glucose-6-phosphatase deficient children. *Pediatr Res.* 1984;18:335.

47. LEONARD JW, DUNGER DB. Hypoglycaemia complicating feeding regimens for glycogen storage disease. *Lancet.* 1978;ii:1203.

48. FINE RN, KOGUT MD, DONNELL GN. Intestinal absorption in type I glycogen storage disease. *J Pediatr.* 1969;75:632.

49. MOSES SW, GUTMAN A. Inborn errors of glycogen metabolism. *Adv Pediatr.* 1972;19:95.

50. ROE T, KOGUT M, BUCKINGHAM B, MILLER J, GATES G, LANDING B. Hepatic tumors in glycogen storage disease type I. *Clin Res.* 1978;26:191A.

51. GROSSMAN H, RAM PC, COLEMAN RA, et al. Hepatic ultrasonography in type I glycogen storage disease (von Gierke Disease). *Radiology.* 1981;141:753.

52. BRUNELLE F, TAMMAM S, ODIERRE M, CHAUMONT P. Liver adenomas in glycogen storage disease in children. *Pediatr Radiol.* 1984;14:94.

53. CHEN YT, COLEMAN RA, SCHEINMAN JI, KOLBECK PC, SIDBURY JB. Renal disease in type 1 glycogen storage disease. *N Engl J Med.* 1988;381:7.

54. RESTAINO I, STANLEY C, BAKER L, WEISS R, KAPLAN BS. Renal tubular abnormalities and nephrocalcinosis in patients with type 1a glycogen storage disease. *Pediatr Res.* 1990;27(4):337A. (Abstract.)

55. GREENE HL, SLONIM AE, O'NEILL JA JR, BURR IM. Continuous nocturnal intragastric feeding for management of type 1 glycogen storage disease. *N Engl J Med.* 1976;294:423.

56. CHEN Y-T, CORNBLATH M, SIDBURY JB. Cornstarch therapy in type I glycogen storage disease. *N Engl J Med.* 1984;310:171.

57. JOHNSON MP, COMPTON A, DRUGAN A, EVANS MI. Metabolic control of von Gierke disease (glycogen storage disease type Ia) in pregnancy: maintenance of euglycemia with cornstarch. *Obstet Gynecol.* 1990;75:507.

58. FERNANDES J, LEONARD JV, MOSES SW, ET AL. Glycogen storage disease: recommendations for treatment. *Eur J Pediatr.* 1988;147:226.

59. KALHAN S, ROSSI K. Glucose kinetics in type I and type III glycogen storage disease. In: Chapman TE, Berger R, Reijngoud DJ, eds. *Stable Isotopes in Pediatrics Nutritional and Metabolic Research.* London: Intercept Ltd., 1990:237.

60. STARZL TE, PUTNAM CW, PORTER KA, HALGRIMSON CG, CORMAN J, BROWN BI, GOTLIN RW, RODGERSON DO, GREENE HL. Portal diversion for the treatment of glycogen storage disease in humans. *Ann Surg.* 1973;178:525.

61. FIELD JB, EPSTEIN S, EGAN T. Studies in glycogen storage diseases. I. Intestinal glucose-6-phosphatase activity in patients with von Gierke's disease and their parents. *J Clin Invest.* 1965;44:1240.

62. SENIOR B, LORIDAN L. Studies of liver glycogenoses, with particular reference to the metabolism of intravenously administered glycerol. *N Engl J Med.* 1968;279:958, and Functional differentiation of gly-

cogenoses of the liver with respect to the use of glycerol. *N Engl J Med.* 1968;279:965.

63. SHIN YS, RIETH M, TANSENDFREUND J, ENDRES W. A sensitive radioisotopic method for glucose-6-phosphatase assay and diagnosis of glycogenosis type 1b using polymorphonuclear leukocytes. Personal communication.

64. BASHAN N, POTASHNIK R, HAGAI Y, MOSES SW. Impaired glucose transport in polymorphonuclear leukocytes in glycogen storage disease Ib. *J Inher Metab Dis.* 1987;10:234.

65. BASHAN N, HAGAI Y, POTASHNIK R, MOSES SW. Impaired carbohydrate metabolism of polymorphonuclear leukocytes in glycogen storage disease Ib. *J Clin Invest.* 1988;81:1317.

66. SEGER R, STEINMANN B, TIEFENAUER L, MATSUNAGA T, GITZELMANN R. Glycogenosis Ib: neutrophil microbicidal defects due to impaired hexose monophosphate shunt. *Pediatr Res.* 1984;18:297. (Short communication.)

67. KOVEN ML, CLARK MM, CODY CS, STANLEY CA, BAKER L, DOUGLAS SD. Impaired chemotaxis and neutrophil (polymorphonuclear leukocyte) function in glycogenosis type IB. *Pediatr Res.* 1986;20:438.

68. ILLINGWORTH B, CORI GT. Structure of glycogens and amylopectins. III. Normal and abnormal human glycogen. *J Biol Chem.* 1952;199:653.

69. FORBES GB. Glycogen storage disease. *J Pediatr.* 1953;42:645.

70. VAN CREVELD S, HUIJING F. Differential diagnosis of the type of glycogen disease in two adult patients with long history of glycogenosis. *Metabolism.* 1964;13:191.

71. HUG G, KRILL CE JR, PERRIN EV, GUEST GM. Cori's disease (amylo-1,6-glucosidase deficiency). *N Engl J Med.* 1963;268:113.

72. FERNANDES J, KOSTER JF, GROSE WF, SORGEDRAGER N. Hepatic phosphorylase deficiency. Its differentiation from other hepatic glycogenoses. *Arch Dis Child.* 1974;49:186.

73. MOSES SW, CHAYOTH R, LEVIN S, LAZAROVITZ E, RUBINSTEIN D. Glucose and glycogen metabolism in erythrocytes from normal and glycogen storage disease type III subjects. *J Clin Invest.* 1968;47:1343.

74. HUIJING F. Enzymes of glycogen metabolism in leukocytes in relation to glycogen-storage disease. In: Control of Glycogen Metabolism. Oslo: Oslo University Press (Universitetsforlaget), 1968:115.

75. ILLINGWORTH B, CORI GT, CORI CF. Amylo-1,6 glucosidase in muscle tissue in generalized glycogen storage disease. *J Biol Chem.* 1956; 218:123.

76. DING SH, De BARSY T, BROWN BI, COLEMAN RA, CHEN Y-T. Immunoblot analyses of glycogen debranching enzyme in different subtypes of glycogen storage disease type III. *J Pediatr.* 1990;116:95.

77. NEUSTEIN HB. Fine structure of skeletal muscle in type III glycogenosis. *Arch Pathol.* 1969;88:130.

78. POWELL HC, HAAS R, HALL CL, WOLFF JA, NYHAN W, BROWN BI. Peripheral nerve in type III glycogenosis: selective involvement of unmyelinated fiber Schwann cells. *Muscle and Nerve.* 1985;8:667.

79. GARTY BZ, DINARI G, NITZAN M. Transient acute cortical blindness associated with hypoglycemia. *Pediatr Neurol.* 1987;3:169.

80. MOSES SW, GADOTH N, BASHAN N, BEN-DAVID E, SLONIM A, WANDERMAN KL. Neuromuscular involvement in glycogen storage disease type III. *Acta Paediatr Scand.* 1986;75:289.

81. MOSES SW, WANDERMAN KL, MYROZ A, FRYDMAN M. Cardiac involvement in glycogen storage disease type III. *Eur J Pediatr.* 1989; 148:764.

82. BRIDGE EM, HOLT LE JR. Glycogen storage disease; observations on the pathologic physiology of two cases of the hepatic form of the disease. *J Pediatr.* 1945;27:299.

83. FERNANDES J, VAN DE KAMER JH. Hexose and protein tolerance tests in children with liver glycogenosis caused by a deficiency of the debranching enzyme system. *Pediatrics.* 1968;41:935.

84. LEVIN S, MOSES SW, CHAYOTH R, JAGODA N, STEINITZ K, LEVINSON G. Glycogen storage disease in Israel. *Isr J Med Sci.* 1967;3:397.

85. VAN CREVELD S, HUIJING F. Glycogen storage disease. Biochemical and clinical data in sixteen cases. *Am J Med.* 1965;38:554.

86. HUIJING F, OBBINK HJK, VAN CREVELD S. Activity of the debranching–enzyme system in leucocytes. *Acta Genet.* (Basel) 1968;18:128.

87. MILUNSKY A, LITTLEFIELD JW, KANFER JN, KOLODNY EH, SHIH VE, ATKINS L. Prenatal genetic diagnosis. *N Engl J Med.* 1970;283:1370.

88. DING JH, HARRIS DA, BING-ZI Y, CHEN YT. Cloning of cDNA for human muscle glycogen debrancher, the enzyme deficient in type III glycogen storage disease. *Pediatr Res.* 1989;25:140A.

89. HERS HG. Etudes enzymatiques sur fragments hépatiques; application à la classification des glycogénoses. *Rev Int Hepatol.* 1959;9:35.

90. LAMY M, DUBOIS R, ROSSIER A, FREZAL J, LOEB H, BLANCHER G. La glycogénose par defici. *Arch F Pediatr.* 1960;17:14.

91. HULSMANN WC, OEI TL, VAN CREVELD S. Phosphorylase activity in leukocytes from patients with glycogen storage disease. *Lancet* 1961;2:581.

92. WILLIAMS HE, FIELD JB. Low leukocyte phosphorylase in hepatic phosphorylase deficient glycogen storage disease. *J Clin Invest.* 1961;40:1841.

93. CHRISTIANSEN RO, PAGE LA, GREENBERG RE. Glycogen storage in a hepatoma: Dephosphophosphorylase kinase defect. *Pediatrics.* 1968; 42:694.

94. HUG G, GARANCIS JC, SCHUBERT WK, KAPLAN S. Glycogen storage disease, types II, III, VIII and IX. *Am J Dis Child.* 1966;111:457.

95. HUG G, SCHUBERT WK, CHUCK G. Deficient activity of dephosphophosphorylase kinase and accumulation of glycogen in the liver. *J Clin Invest.* 1969;48:704.

96. HUIJING F, FERNANDES J. X-Chromosomal inheritance of liver glycogenosis with phosphorylase kinase deficiency. *Am J Hum Genet.* 1969;21:275.

97. BAUSSAN C, MOATTI N, ODIEVRE M, LEMONNIER A. Liver glycogenosis caused by a defective phosphorylase system. Hemolysate analysis. *Pediatrics.* 1981;67:107.

98. WILLEMS PJ, GERVER WJ, BERGER R, FERNANDES J. The natural history of liver glycogenosis due to phosphorylase kinase deficiency: a longitudinal study of 41 patients. *Europ J Pediatr.* 1990;149:268.

99. SHIN YS, RIETH M, TAUSENFREUND J, ET AL. Clinical and biochemical variability of phosphorylase B, kinase deficiency: its differentiation using erythrocyte parameters. (Personal communication.)

100. TUCHMAN M, BROWN BI, BURKE BA, ULSTROM RA. Clinical and laboratory observations in a child with hepatic phosphorylase kinase deficiency. *Metabolism.* 1986;35:627.

101. LEDERER B, VAN HOOF F, VAN DEN BERGHE G, HERS HG. Glycogen phosphorylase and its converter enzymes in haemolysates of normal human subjects and of patients with type VI glycogen storage disease. A study of phosphorylase kinase deficiency. *Biochem J.* 1975;147:23.

102. NEWGARD CB, FLETTERICK RJ, ANDERSON LA, LEBO RV. The polymorphic locus for glycogen storage disease VI (liver glycogen phosphorylase) maps to chromosome 14. *Am J Hum Genet.* 1987;40:351.

103. FRANCKE U, DARRAS BT, ZANDER NF, KILIMAN MW. Assignment of human genes for phosphorylase kinase subunits alpha (PHKA) to Xq12-q13 and beta (PHKB) to 16q12-q13. *Am J Hum Genet.* 1989;45:276.

104. LARNER J, VILLAR-PALASI C. Enzymes in glycogen storage myopathy. *Proc Natl Acad Sci USA.* 1959;45:1234.

105. SCHMID R, ROBBINS PW, TRAUT RR. Glycogen synthesis in human muscle lacking phosphorylase. *Proc Natl Acad Sci USA.* 1959;45:1236.

106. SCHMID R, MAHLER R. Chronic progressive myopathy with myoglobinuria; demonstration of a glycogenolytic defect in the muscle. *J Clin Invest.* 1959;38:2044.

107. PEARSON CM, RIMER DG, MOMMAERTS WFHM. A metabolic myopathy due to absence of muscle phosphorylase. *Am J Med.* 1961;30:502.

108. ANDRES R, CADER G, ZIERLER KL. The quantitatively minor role of carbohydrate in oxidative metabolism by skeletal muscle in intact man in the basal state. Measurements of oxygen and glucose uptake and carbon dioxide and lactate production in the forearm. *J Clin Invest.* 1956;35:671.

109. MAHLER RF, MCARDLE B. Specific enzyme defect in glycogen breakdown causing a myopathy. *Q J Med.* 1960;29:638. (Abstract.)

110. SCHMID R, HAMMAKER L. Hereditary absence of muscle phosphorylase (McArdle's syndrome). *N Engl J Med.* 1961;264:223.

111. LEBO RV, GORIN F, FLETTERICK RJ, ET AL. High resolution chromosome sorting and DNA spot-blot analysis assign McArdle's syndrome to chromosome 11. *Science.* 1984;225:57.

112. TARUI S, OKUNO G, IKARA Y, TANAKA T, SUDA M, NISHIKAWA M. Phosphofructokinase deficiency in skeletal muscle. A new type of glycogenosis. *Biochem Biophys Res Commun.* 1965;19:517.

113. OKUNO G, HIZUKURI S, NISHIKAWA M. Activities of glycogen synthetase and UDPG-pyrophosphorylase in muscle of a patient with a new type of muscle glycogenosis caused by phosphofructokinase deficiency. *Nature* (Lond.) 1966;212:1490.

114. TARUI S, KONO N, NASU T, NISHIKAWA M. Enzymatic basis for the coexistence of myopathy and hemolytic disease in inherited muscle phosphofructokinase deficiency. *Biochem Biophys Res Commun.* 1969;34:77.

115. LAYZER RB, ROWLAND LP, RANNEY HM. Muscle phosphofructokinase deficiency. *Arch Neurol.* 1967;17:512.

116. DI SANT'AGNESE PA, ANDERSEN DH, MASON HH, BAUMAN WA. Glycogen storage disease of the heart. I. Report of two cases in siblings with chemical and pathological studies. *Pediatrics* 1950;6:402.

117. BROWN BI, ZELLWEGER H. α-1,4 glucosidase activity in leucocytes from the family of two brothers who lack this enzyme in muscle. *Biochem J.* 1966;101:16C.

118. NIHILL MR, WILSON DS, HUGH-JONES K. Generalized glycogenosis type II (Pompe's disease). *Arch Dis Child.* 1970;45:122.

119. DINCSOY MY, DINCSOY HP, KESSLER AD, JACKSON MA, SIDBURY JB. Generalized glycogenosis and associated endocardial fibroelastosis. *J Pediatr*. 1965;67:728.

120. CLEMENT DH, GODMAN GC. Glycogen disease resembling mongolism, cretinism and amyotonia congenita. *J Pediatr*. 1950;36:11.

121. KAHANA D, TELEM C, STEINITZ K, SOLOMON M. Generalized glycogenosis. *J Pediatr*. 1964;65:243.

122. HUIJING F, VAN CREVELD S, LOSEKOOT G. Diagnosis of generalized glycogen storage disease (Pompe's disease). *J Pediatr*. 1963;63:984.

123. LEJEUNE N, THINES-SEMPOUX D, HERS HG. Tissue fractionation studies. 16. Intracellular distribution and properties of α-glucosidases in rat liver. *Biochem J*. 1963;86:16.

124. DANCIS J, HUTZLER L, LYNFIELD L, COX RP. Absence of acid maltase in glycogenosis type 2 (Pompe's disease) in tissue culture. *Am J Dis Child*. 1969;117:108.

125. NITOWSKY HM, GOUNEFELD A. Lysosomal α-glucosidase in type II glycogenosis. *J Lab Clin Med*. 1967;69:472.

126. NADLER HG, MESSINA AM. In utero detection of type II glycogenosis (Pompe's disease). *Lancet* 1969;2:1277.

127. COX RP, DOUGLAS G, HUTZLER J, LYNFIELD J, DANCIS J. In utero detection of Pompe's disease. *Lancet*. 1970;1:893.

128. SHIN YS, RIETH M, TAUSENFREUND J, ENDRES W. First trimester diagnosis of glycogenosis type II and type III. Unpublished personal communication.

129. BASHAN N, POTASHNIK R, BARASH V, GUTMAN A, MOSES SW. Glycogen storage disease type II in Israel. *Isr J Med Sci*. 1988;24:224.

130. REUSER AJJ, KOSTER JF, HOOGEVEEN A, et al. Biochemical, immunological and cell genetic studies in glycogenosis type II. *Am J Hum Genet*. 1978;30:132.

131. D'ANCONA GG, WURM J, CROCE CM. Genetics of type II glycogenosis: assignment of the human gene for acid alpha-glucosidase to chromosome 17. *Proc Natl Acad Sci USA*. 1977;76:4526.

132. BROWN BI, BROWN DH. Lack of an α-1,4 glucan: α-1,4-glucan 6 glycosyl transferase in a case of type IV glycogenosis. *Proc Natl Acad Sci USA*. 1966;56:725.

133. SHIN YS, STEIGUBER H, KLEMM P, ENDRES W, SCHWAB O, WOLFF G. Branching enzyme in erythrocytes. Detection of type IV glycogenosis homozygotes and heterozygotes. *J Inher Metab Dis*. 1988;11(2):252.

134. FERNANDES J, HUIJING F. Branching enzyme-deficiency glycogenosis: Studies in therapy. *Arch Dis Child*. 1968;43:347.

135. LEVIN B, BURGESS EA, MORTIMER PE. Glycogen storage disease type IV, amylopectinosis. *Arch Dis Child*. 1968;43:548.

136. SIDBURY JB JR, MASON J, BURNS WB JR, RUEBNER BH. Type IV glycogenosis. Report of a case proven by characterization of glycogen and studied at necropsy. *Bull Johns Hopkins Hosp*. 1962;111:157.

137. REED GB JR, DIXON LFP, NEUSTEIN HB, DONNELL GN, LANDING BH. Type IV glycogenosis. *Lab Invest*. 1968;19:546.

138. STARZL TE, ZIFELLI BJ, SHAW BW, et al. Changing concepts of liver replacement for hereditary tyrosinemia and hepatoma. *J Pediatr*. 1985;106:604.

139. KLEINMAN RE, VACANTI JP. Liver transplantation. In: Walker WA, Durie P, Hamilton JE, Walker-Smith JA, Watkins JB, eds. *Pediatric Gas-*

trointestinal Disease: Pathophysiology, Diagnosis and Management. Ontario: BC Decker, Inc., 1990:1105.

140. AYNSLEY-GREEN A, WILLIAMSON DH, GITZELMANN R. Hepatic glycogen synthetase deficiency. Definition of syndrome from metabolic and enzyme studies on a 9-year-old girl. *Arch Dis Child.* 1977;52:573.

141. PARR J, TEREE TM, LARNER J. Symptomatic hypoglycemia, visceral fatty metamorphosis and aglycogenosis in an infant lacking glycogen synthetase and phosphorylase. *Pediatrics.* 1965;35:770.

142. CORNBLATH M, STEINER DF, BRYAN P, KING J. Uridine-diphosphoglucose glucosyl glucosyltransferase in human erythrocytes. *Clin Chim Acta.* 1965;12:27.

143. SPENCER-PEET J. Erythrocyte glycogen synthetase in glycogen storage deficiency resulting from the absence of this enzyme from liver. *Clin Chim Acta.* 1964;10:481.

144. GITZELMANN R, STEINMANN B, AYNSLEY-GREEN A. Hepatic glycogen synthetase deficiency not expressed in cultured skin fibroblasts. *Clin Chim Acta.* 1983;130:111.

145. GITZELMANN R, AYNSLEY-GREEN A, WILLIAMSON DH. Blood cell glycogen synthetase activity in hepatic glycogen synthetase deficiency. *Clin Chim Acta.* 1977;79:219.

146. AYNSLEY-GREEN A, WILLIAMSON DH, GITZELMANN R. The dietary treatment of hepatic glycogen synthetase deficiency. *Helv Paediatr Acta.* 1977;32:71.

147. DYKES JRW, SPENCER-PEET J. Hepatic glycogen synthetase deficiency. Further studies on a family. *Arch Dis Child.* 1972;47:558.

C H A P T E R 8

DISORDERS
OF GALACTOSE
METABOLISM

Galactosuria is one of the better-defined genetic, molecular diseases. The disease, as first described by Von Reuss [1] in 1908, was associated with failure to thrive, liver disease, and galactosemia, with the assumption that the latter was related to the ingestion of milk. Nine years later, Göppert [2] observed that the ingestion of galactose itself as well as milk resulted in galactosuria. The first patient described in the English literature was reported by Mason and Turner in 1935 [3]. Subsequently, scattered cases and large series of cases have been reported [4–11], including a report of the follow-up of Mason's original case by Townsend et al. in 1951 [12]. Initially, attention was focused on: (1) clinical description and course, (2) pathologic findings, and (3) physiologic disturbances of carbohydrate metabolism. These careful clinical investigations resulted in a plan of effective dietary therapy.

In 1933, Fanconi described the first variant of a defect in galactose metabolism, which he called galactose diabetes, in a child with only cataracts [13]. More recently, a number of modifications of the classical syndrome have been defined, based on enzymatic [14–16], metabolic [15–17], and clinical [8,18] observations. These observations evolved from the classical basic investigations of Leloir [19,20], who clarified the metabolic pathway for galactose and for galactose-to-glucose interconversion.

In the cell, galactose is phosphorylated from ATP to galactose-1-phosphate by a specific galactokinase (Fig. 8-1). The galactose-1-P

(1)
$$\text{Galactose} + \text{ATP} \xrightleftharpoons[\text{Galactokinase}]{\text{Mg++}} \text{Galactose-1-Phosphate} + \text{ADP}$$

(2)
$$\text{Galactose-1-Phosphate} + \text{UDP Glucose} \xrightleftharpoons[\text{Transferase}]{} \text{UPD Galactose} + \text{Glucose-1-Phosphate}$$

(3)
$$\text{UDP Galactose} \xrightleftharpoons[\text{4-Epimerase}]{\text{NAD}} \text{UDP Glucose}$$

(4)
$$\text{UDP Glucose} + \text{PP} \xrightleftharpoons[\text{Pyrophosphorylase}]{} \text{Glucose-1-Phosphate} + \text{UTP}$$

(5)
$$\text{Galactose} \xrightleftharpoons[\text{Aldose Reductase}]{\text{NADPH}} \text{Galactitol}$$

FIGURE 8-1. Galactose diabetes results from a deficiency of galactokinase (reaction 1), whereas classical galactosemia results from a deficiency of galactose-1-phosphate uridyl transferase (reaction 2). The transferase enzyme may occur in different molecular forms, thus accounting for some variants of enzyme activity. Recently, an absence of epimerase (reaction 3) has been reported to produce the classical syndrome.

reacts with uridine-diphosphoglucose (UDPG) in the presence of the specific enzyme P-gal uridyl transferase to form uridine-diphosphogalactose (UDPGal) and glucose-1-phosphate. UDPGal-4-epimerase with diphosphopyridine nucleotide (DPN) is necessary for the conversion of the UDPGal to UDPG. UDPG may be metabolized by several pathways [11,21–24]. It can react with pyrophosphate in the presence of UDPG pyrophosphorylase to form uridine triphosphate (UTP) and glucose-1-phosphate, or in the presence of glycogen synthase to form glycogen. (See Chapter 1, p. 26, glycogen cycle). Galactose may also be reduced directly to galactitol by the enzyme aldose reductase (see Fig. 8-1, reaction 5) [25]. Thus, the explanation for the multiple clinical manifestations and syndromes that involve defects in galactose metabolism are beginning to be elucidated on a molecular basis. In 1989, Segal reviewed the metabolism of galactose and its regulation at both the cellular and organ level [11]. The specific enzymatic reactions and the alternate pathways for metabolism are detailed in his report [11].

• Galactosemia

Galactosemia is inherited as an autosomal recessive and was reported by 1972 to occur worldwide in 1:10,000 to 1:187,000 births [26]. In the United States, routine newborn screening has detected from 1 in 14,500 (Maine) to as few as 1 in 119,000 (Ohio) [27]. From screening 2,677,669 neonates in 8 states, 35 affected infants were found, for an average detection rate of 1 in 76,500 [27]. The detection rate depends on sensitivity and specificity as well as precise confirmation. Improved methodology has been described [28–32]. In 1987, Ng and associates reviewed worldwide frequencies of occurrence of galactosemia based on newborn screening data and reported rates of 1/26,000 in Ireland compared to 1/667,000 in Japan [33]. The U.S. frequency was 1/62,000.

Clinical Manifestations

Prenatal Effects

The newborn infant with galactosemia (P-gal uridyl transferase defect) is usually clinically normal at birth. In utero, the fetus may be exposed to variable amounts of lactose or galactose from the mother. The heterozygote mother may be unable to dispose of a galactose load as rapidly as a normal person can. This relative deficiency may result in increased levels of galactose reaching the fetus even under a normal dietary regimen. The presence of nuclear cataracts, which usually develop in the third fetal month and before lens development takes place, has been considered by Ritter to be a further indication of intrauterine fetal abnormalities related to galactose [34]. Roe [35] reported a Negro homozygous woman who was maintained on a lactose-restricted diet since 1950 and gave birth in 1969 to a heterozygote male infant who developed normally (see p. 311). Although lactose and galactitol were present in maternal urine, none was detected in maternal blood or amniotic fluid.

The Neonate and His Problems

At birth, the affected infant appears normal, both physically and developmentally. But shortly after he begins to ingest milk, he develops a characteristic course that varies only in the severity and rapidity of the clinical manifestations [7,36]. Failure to gain weight in the first few days is common, as is jaundice, which increases and persists beyond the usual period of "physiologic jaundice." Subcutaneous bleeding may occur. Vomiting, diarrhea, and dehydration also occur. The skin appears dry, rough, thick, and scaly. The liver enlarges and is smooth, firm, and nontender. If the disease is unrecognized, the course is one of progressive deterioration associated with liver disease (cirrhosis), cataracts, mental retardation, and even death. The characteristic abdominal distention is the combined result of ascites, hepatomegaly, and splenomegaly. Zonular or lamellar cataracts may be seen as early as one month of age. Mental retardation does not become manifest until later in the initial year of life. Malnutrition, extreme loss of subcutaneous fat tissue, and retarded growth become evident as the untreated disease progresses (Fig. 8-2).

In contrast to these marked abnormalities, the onset in some cases may be subtle and the disease manifested only in a failure to feed well or to gain weight. In these infants, the course progresses to a more characteristic clinical picture as they take more lactose-containing foods. Mental retardation, which is the most serious consequence for

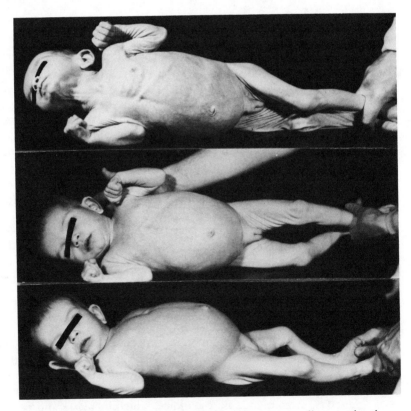

FIGURE 8-2. Infant with chronic diarrhea who was not discovered to have galactose intolerance until 5 months of age. Removal of lactose from the diet resulted in rapid improvement in nutrition.

untreated surviving children with this disorder, varies in severity [37]. The heterozygote does not have clinical manifestations. Furthermore, the disease may be difficult to detect even in the homozygote. Hugh-Jones and associates [38] have reported a family with an affected homozygous grandfather of normal intelligence who had cataracts and hepatomegaly and was not diagnosed until the sixth decade of life.

Laboratory Data

Blood

The galactose concentration in the blood may not be diagnostic since it may be either normal, or elevated postprandially after milk feedings in normal infants. Fasting blood glucose levels as determined with specific glucose oxidase techniques are normal, but may be low following the ingestion of galactose [39,40]. Morphologic studies may show no initial effects on the erythrocytes or leukocytes. No specific abnormalities in blood counts, acid base balance, or electrolyte concentrations are present unless extensive diarrhea or dehydration occur. Under these circumstances, azotemia and metabolic acidosis are found. A normocytic, hypoplastic anemia has been described later in the course of the disease. Liver function tests show variable results. Serum bilirubin and alkaline phosphatase, aspartate, and alanine amino transferases may be elevated. There is no characteristic pattern for other serum enzymes, including SGOT and SGPT.

Urine

Following milk feedings, abnormalities in the urine include generalized proteinuria, positive reducing substances, and a generalized aminoaciduria. The sediment is normal. The reducing substances are positive to Clinitest tablets in the absence of ketonuria. Specific analyses with glucose oxidase chemical reagent strips are negative or show a trace reaction, indicating that the reducing substance is not glucose. Further identification may be made by chromatography, including high-performance liquid chromatography [41], or by the specific enzymatic techniques that utilize galactose oxidase or galactose dehydrogenase [42].

Ultrasound and/or Roentgen Findings

After a variable period of exposure to milk, ultrasonography and roentgen studies may show hepatomegaly, splenomegaly, and ascites.

The kidneys are normal. Late roentgen changes may include generalized osteoporosis.

Diagnosis

A variety of diagnostic tests for this disorder have been devised and have been summarized by Kirkman [43], Hsia [44], and Segal [11]. These include the identification of sugar in urine and specific enzyme tests on red or white blood cells. A variety of enzymatic techniques of variable specificity have been used for the erythrocytes and include a measurement of galactose-1-phosphate, UDPG consumption, and a methylene blue coupled reaction with measurement of $^{14}CO_2$ from 1-^{14}C galactose [11,44]. The diagnostic enzymatic methods may not be available in smaller laboratories. Galactose tolerance tests are contraindicated and carry a risk of central nervous system toxicity.

Prenatal Diagnosis

When galactosemia is suspected from family history, prenatal diagnosis is indicated. The homozygous P-gal uridyl transferase deficiency has been diagnosed successfully in utero early in pregnancy in amnion cells by Nadler and associates [45] and confirmed by others [46]. The diagnosis has also been made successfully by enzyme analysis of chorionic villus biopsy [47]. Several groups have developed techniques, including a stable isotope dilution assay for galactitol in amniotic fluid [48,49]. The activities of galactose-1-phosphate uridyl transferase and of galactokinase have been studied in human fetal organs at various stages of gestation [46,50]. Maximal specific activity for each enzyme was found at 28 weeks' gestation in liver.

Postnatal Diagnosis

If not suspected prenatally, a urinalysis may be done to determine whether reducing substances are present. This determination must be done with Clinitest tablets and not with glucose oxidase reagent strips [42,51]. If reducing substance other than glucose is found, the removal from the diet of lactose-containing foods (milk) should result is disappearance of the sugar (presumably galactose) from the urine within 24–72 hours. If galactosemia is suspected, the infant must be fed a galactose-free diet (see Appendixes II, III) until the results of the enzyme studies in the red blood cells are known. Galactose will not be present in the urine of the newborn before onset of milk feedings. The specific diagnosis is established by the enzymatic methods that utilize red blood cells.

In the newborn infant suspected of having this disorder because of a positive family history or clinical manifestations, the diagnosis should be made by demonstrating the absence of galactose-1-P uridyl transferase in the red blood cells before the initiation of milk feedings, and not upon the presence of reducing sugars in the urine.

Differential Diagnosis

Differential diagnosis in the neonate is concerned principally with mellituria and with hyperbilirubinemia associated with hepatic disease. The latter includes consideration of sepsis, cytomegalic inclusion disease, toxoplasmosis, rubella, syphilis, biliary atresia, neonatal hepatitis, and congenital hypopituitarism with or without congenital optic nerve hypoplasia. A positive blood culture does not rule out galactosemia.

Recent reports have also emphasized the occurrence of gram-negative *(Escherichia coli)* sepsis in infants with undiagnosed galactosemia and have suggested a relationship of substrate (lactose-galactose) requirement to organism [52,53]. In the large U.S. survey noted above, of the 35 infants detected to be deficient in the transferase, 10 had significant neonatal infections. Of these, 9 were fatal and 4 had *E coli* infection [27]. A positive blood culture for *E coli* in the neonate is an indication for a specific diagnostic test for galactosemia. However, the presence of minute amounts of galactose in the urine of the newborn, especially the low birth weight infant, may be a transient physiologic phenomenon [54] related to a decreased tissue uptake of galactose.

Later, the multiple causes for failure of growth, diarrhea, cirrhosis, cataracts, albuminuria, and mental retardation must be considered in the differential diagnosis.

Therapy

In Utero

Once an in utero diagnosis is established, the mother should be provided a galactose-lactose-free diet. Some women who are known heterozygotes or homozygotes are advised to ingest the restricted diet before conception. Irons et al. [55] have observed a woman who maintained her blood concentration of galactose and galactose-1-phosphate at less than 1 mg/dl throughout pregnancy. The affected fetus had a high level of galactose-1-phosphate (4 mg/dl) in cord whole blood. There are over a dozen pregnancies reported with similar findings. Gitzelmann [56] suggested that galactose-1-phosphate in the affected fetus of a mother on a restricted diet is endogenously produced from glucose-1-phosphate via the glucose-4-epimerase and the uridine diphosphogalactose pyrophosphorylase reactions (Fig. 8-1).

Postnatal

The management of patients with this disorder requires meticulous attention to detail. The course changes dramatically when milk sugar (lactose) is removed from the diet. Even an infant with the full-blown disorder that goes unrecognized for many months shows a remarkable response to the simple elimination of lactose from the diet. His appetite increases, vomiting and diarrhea subside within a few days, weight gain ensues promptly, liver function improves, and jaundice subsides. Even the cataracts may disappear on a lactose-free diet. Holzel [36] has indicated that several of the low-galactose formulas are not devoid of oligosaccharides, which contain galactose. However, Gitzelmann and Auricchio [57] have examined critically the ability of a normal and a galactosemic child to metabolize soya α-galactosides. They detected no α-galactosidase activity in the human small intestine, no rise in erythrocyte galactose-1-phosphate after raffinose ingestion, and slow absorption of galactose from the colon of the galactosemic child. They concluded that soybean formulas are generally safe for galactosemic infants, provided that such infants do not have diarrhea. For the infant, several satisfactory proprietary formulas are available [58,59] (see Appendixes II, III). In older children, avoidance of galactose is difficult because many foods contain unlabeled lactose. Thus, candies and compounded foods, especially bread, sausage, frankfurters, and so on, must be rigidly excluded unless the exact composition is known in detail.

Biochemical monitoring of erythrocyte galactose-1-phosphate is necessary to assure compliance with dietary recommendations.

Genetics

A careful family history is essential, as in all inherited disorders. Family counseling regarding further pregnancies can be more specific if enzymatic analysis of erythrocytes from all family members is done to define heterozygotes. Family history has been inadequate in defining the individual heterozygote, but the enzymatic tests have made possible a more precise analysis of the genetic situation. Refinement of the assay system has resulted in the detection of a definite difference in transferase levels in normal adults and in parents of galactosemic children. Donnell [60] studied 278 individuals, including 55 family members from 14 galactosemic families, and clearly identified the heterozygotes (Fig. 8-3).

Molecular Genetics

The galactose-1-phosphate uridyl transferase (GALT) gene has been mapped to human chromosome 9, band p13 [61]. This is transmitted as an autosomal recessive trait with homozygotes estimated to occur in 1 in 50,000 newborns screened. There is no particular ethnic or geographic variation [62].

Reichardt and Berg [63] have utilized a unique technique to clone and characterize the cDNA that encodes human GALT. The cDNA is 1,400 bases in length and encodes a 43,000 M_r protein. The cloning strategy involved the identification of short peptide sequences conserved between the homologous enzymes from *E coli* and yeast, and the construction of oligonucleotide pools corresponding to the conserved patches. These patches of conserved amino acids tend to be present in humans also.

Reichardt [64] has pursued these observations by studies of 15

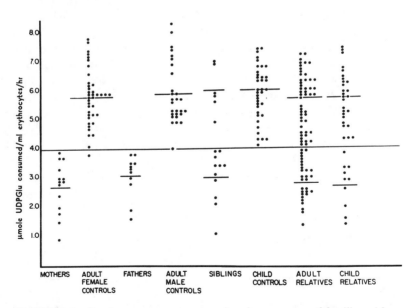

FIGURE 8-3. Erythrocyte enzyme assays in a large survey of families with galactosemia. Observe the difference in the distribution of values between the controls (values above 4 μmoles/ml) and the members of families with affected children. (From Donnell et al. Reproduced by permission of *Pediatrics.* 1960;25:572, copyright 1960.)

galactosemic patients using molecular analysis of DNA, mRNA, and protein by Southern, Northern, and Western blotting techniques. He concluded that galactosemia is caused by missense mutations. He found detectable enzyme activity in all 13 patients studied and speculated that this provided a threshold level of UDPGal which is both the product of the GALT reaction and the substrate for the galactosylation of glycolipids and glycoproteins. He is currently analyzing glycolipids from patients to verify this hypothesis.

Pathology

Pathologic studies indicate that the liver disease is a fatty infiltration with varying degrees of portal fibrosis, resulting in a lobular pattern [12]. The hepatic cells may have a granular appearance. Infiltrates of leukocytes may be seen in the connective tissue. Medline and Medline [65] have described the early histologic changes in liver in twins. One died at 9 days of age of aspiration and the other shortly thereafter of sepsis. The liver was yellow and contained excessively large, fatty droplets in virtually every hepatocyte. Extensive bile ductular proliferation was present in the periportal areas. There was no increase in fibrosis. Bell [66] observed vacuolar changes in the epithelial cells of the proximal tubule of the kidney in one case. Crome [67] reported on the neuropathologic findings in a child with physical and mental retardation who survived to 8 years of age. He found microencephaly with pronounced fibrous gliosis of the white matter; the cerebellum showed marked loss of Purkinje's cells and less conspicuous loss of the granular layer. All the findings were considered nonspecific and could not be differentiated from those seen in other forms of mental retardation. Cataracts are usually lamellar or zonular, although a few nuclear or anterior cortical changes in the lens have been reported [34]. Levy et al. [68] have reported normal follicle development and abundant oocytes in the ovaries of a 5-day-old infant who died (see below).

Pathogenesis

Site of Defect

In galactosemia, Schwarz [69] found that galactose-1-phosphate accumulated in erythrocytes, suggesting that galactokinase was active normally and that the defect was beyond the first phosphorylation step. Kalckar [70] demonstrated the defect to be an absence of the specific transferase, P-gal uridyl transferase, and with Isselbacher [71] showed that the epimerase and UDPG pyrophosphorylase were normal. The latter authors suggested that the reversibility of the epimerase reaction permitted synthesis of UDPGal under circumstances of dietary deprivation. This could account for normal galacto-lipid synthesis and central nervous system development in the absence of exogenous galactose [71].

In contrast, Reichardt [64] proposed that minimal transferase activity is required for survival to produce a threshold level of UDPGal for minimal galactosylation of glycoproteins and glycolipids. He suggested supplemental therapy with uridine in addition to galactose restriction. Kaufman and associates [72] have evaluated UDPGal in erythrocytes. Chronic administration of oral uridine resulted in normalization of erythrocyte UDPGal in two patients. This novel suggestion requires careful, critical evaluation and should be investigated.

Mechanism of Toxicity

The mechanism of toxicity at the biochemical level is not entirely proven. The original suggestion of Mason and Turner that hypoglycemia was responsible for much of the symptomatology is untenable. The toxic effects appear to be more directly related to the accumulation of galactose-1-phosphate. Young rats fed diets high in galactose (up to 80 percent, by weight, of total food) develop cataracts and renal disease [73,74]. The livers, however, do not show histologic changes. Lerman [75] has shown that a tenfold rise in the concentration of galactose-1-P is found in the lens in cataracts in experimental rats. Although little information is available about the metabolism of the human lens in this disease, transferase activity was apparently absent in the lens tissue from one galactosemic infant [76]. Several theories have been proposed to explain the cataracts that develop when there is galactose intolerance. One relates the changes to decreased oxidation of glucose and consequent interference with normal lens metabolism [75]. Another proposes conversion of galactose to its alcohol, galactitol, which accumulates with water to produce vacuoles in the lens [77]. The latter theory suggests that fiber rupture, secondary to the osmotic effects, precedes cataract formation.

The presence of galactose-1-P in erythrocytes impairs oxygen uptake. Tissue damage in liver, kidney, and brain is apparently related to this compound, although the mechanism of action is unknown. In vitro, galactose-1-P has been shown to inhibit phosphoglucomutase, glucose-6-phosphatase or glucose-6-phosphate dehydrogenase, but how this might explain cellular damage is unknown [78]. From a clinical standpoint, both the rate of development and the rate of decline of toxicity suggest the slow accumulation of a toxic metabolite.

This has been demonstrated with respect to aminoaciduria in the study of Cusworth et al. [79]. They showed that a 3 to 5-day interval was necessary after initiation of a galactose diet before renal amino acid excretion increased. Similarly, removal of galactose from the diet resulted in a decrease in aminoaciduria only after a few days had passed. Although extensive liver disease might affect the plasma amino acid levels with overflow aminoaciduria, the studies of Hsia et al. [80] and Cusworth and associates [79] indicate that the primary effect is in the renal tubule, with minimal changes in plasma amino acids. Thus, the aminoaciduria is the result of a reabsorptive alteration in the proximal tubule.

In addition to the well-described biochemical consequences of the transferase defect, there have been two studies indicating nonenzymatic galactosylation of proteins [81,82]. The significance of a more generalized galactosylation of proteins is unknown at this time.

Prognosis

The clinical manifestations are so highly variable that the ultimate course is unpredictable. In undetected severe cases, death occurs in early infancy. In other untreated children, mental retardation and liver disease may be the major complications, with few surviving beyond childhood. Early diagnosis and careful dietary management can result in normal growth and development, both physically and intellectually, without serious complications [36,37] (Fig. 8-4). When the diagnosis has been delayed for several months, there may be some degree of permanent mental retardation, although other signs of galactose toxicity subside with diet therapy.

Recent reviews of experiences with dietary management in large numbers of patients have indicated a significant degree of psychosocial behavioral impairment. Komrower and Lee [83] investigated 60 galactosemic children whose physical health was good under therapy; however, intelligence scores were variable and tended to be low (mean 80, range 30–118). They reported a recurrent pattern of learning difficulties and psychologic upset, which may, in part, have been environmental rather than inherent in the disorder. Similarly, Nadler and associates [45] reported on 55 patients whose mean IQ was lower than that of siblings; 80 percent of the children were one or more grades behind in school; a specific learning disability was characterized by difficulty in mathematics and spatial relationships. Because of a short attention span, behavior problems were observed in school. Both authors concluded that strict diet therapy beyond infancy (above 2 years of age) has not proved additionally beneficial as regards mental development.

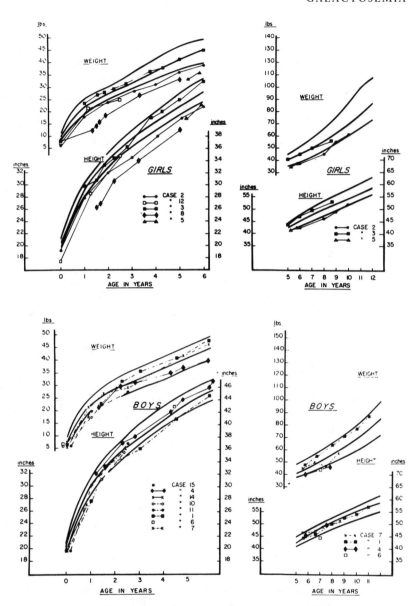

FIGURE 8-4. Growth data in children with galactosemia (GALT). Observe the normal growth patterns in both height and weight of children of both sexes fed galactose-restricted diets. (From Donnell et al. *J Pediatr.* 1962; 58:836, with permission.)

Fishler et al. [84] described the intellectual and personality development of 23 girls and 22 boys treated from infancy and followed up to 23 years. They noted the best developmental progress in the preschool age group. School children aged 6 to 15 years had a mean IQ of 87, and nearly half had poor handwriting and difficulty in visual-perceptual functions. Children who were diagnosed between birth and 1.0 month of age maintained more normal intellectual function as a group than those diagnosed between 4 and 11 months. The authors also assessed the emotional-social aspects of behavior in their patients and concluded that poor self-image was related to their dietary restrictions, which set them apart from their peers. It should be noted that there was no significant difference among the mean IQs of the treated patients, their parents, and their unaffected siblings.

Subsequently, this group [85] reported on the developmental follow-up status of 60 galactosemic infants. Again, the highest level of mental development was in the preschool age group. The lowest level, but still within normal limits, was in the school-age children. Mean IQ was 95 for the entire group, with a range from 50–125. No correlation of IQ with diet compliance was found. One-third of the patients studied by EEG were abnormal. It is unclear how much of the intellectual impairment may be avoided by prompt diagnosis and treatment [86].

Jan and Wilson [87] reported late, unusual neurologic findings in a 19-year-old who had been treated by rigid dietary restrictions since the age of 15 days. The patient showed progressive cerebellar and extrapyramidal disturbances. Although the authors were uncertain as to the cause of the clinical findings, one can speculate that prolonged strict dietary control may not be indicated.

In addition to the long-term mental difficulties, reduced intelligence, and social maladjustment, Packman et al. [88] proposed that a subgroup of galactosemic children may develop a syndrome of mental retardation, tremor, and cerebellar dysfunction. Friedman et al. [89] have reported two adults, a 41-year-old male and a 46-year-old female, one of whom developed complex partial seizures in the fourth decade and the other a severe cerebellar disorder in the fifth decade. They speculated that it seems likely that, as galactosemic adults age, a spectrum of neurologic disorders will occur that will include seizures, cerebellar ataxia, extrapyramidal dysfunction, and apraxia. Whether this is due to the enzymatic defect alone, to other closely linked genetic abnormalities, or to therapy is not yet known. Diagnosis at birth and early intervention with a galactose-free diet does not always assure an optimal outcome. Waisbren et al. [90] reported eight children, diagnosed from 1–15 days of age, treated immediately, and found to have no detectable galactose in the blood or urine and whole blood galactose-1-phosphate concentrations less than 2 mg/dl. At follow-up ages $3^7/_{12}$ and $11^7/_{12}$ years, variable deficits were identified in receptive language (comprehension), short-term memory, expressive language, and articulation. There is speculation that these long-term effects originated in utero.

Tedesco, Morrow, and Mellman [91] have reported a normal pregnancy in a 17-year-old black galactosemic on dietary control, confirming the original report by Roe et al. [35] (see p. 299). The newborn infant was normal and had heterozygote values of transferase and normal values of galactokinase activities in his erythrocytes. The placental tissue was also deficient in transferase activity, which apparently had no deleterious effects on the fetus. Although these two pregnancies suggest that fertility and fetal development can be normal in galactosemic women under dietary control, infertility has emerged as a major problem in these patients.

Kaufman et al. [92] evaluated gonadal function in 18 female and 8 male subjects with galactosemia. The males were normal, but 12 females had hypergonadotropic hypogonadism. All the female patients had a 46,XX karyotype, normal levels of thyroid hormone and prolactin, and no antiovarian antibodies. Urinary gonadotropins were biologically normal. Ovarian tissue was diminished or absent by ultrasonography. They speculated that the abnormality was acquired and related to galactose-1-phosphate toxicity. While there have been other reports substantiating these late findings, the etiology and time of onset have been questioned [68,93–96]. In any event, this is an important observation that merits major attention.

• Variants of Transferase Deficiency

Duarte Variant

In 1966, Beutler and associates [14] reported an extensive survey screening for the incidence of homozygous and heterozygous galactosemia in 1,820 apparently normal individuals and in 352 subjects hospitalized in a mental institution, utilizing a modification of the UDPG consumption technique [97]. Thirty subjects had levels of transferase activity less than those of heterozygote parents of known galactosemic individuals. Nineteen subjects were Caucasian; 11 were unclassified; and none were Negro, Oriental, or native American. In family studies, abnormally low GALT activity suggested two general types of inheritance. In one, present in 15 of 34 subjects, enzyme activity was 50 percent of normal and indicated that a single gene was involved. In the second, enzyme activity was 75 percent of normal or greater than the level associated with the heterozygote carrier state in classical galactosemia. This abnormality has been termed the "Duarte variant." Thus, individuals with red blood cell transferase activities that approximate 50 percent of normal levels could be either heterozygotes for classical galactosemia or homozygotes for the Duarte variant, an allelic gene. Heterozygotes for both the gene for galactosemia and the Duarte variant have approximately one-quarter normal enzyme activity (Table 8-1). In this limited population survey, heterozygotes for galactosemia composed approximately 1.25 percent of the subjects, while those for the Duarte variant, approximately 10 to 13 percent.

By electrophoretic mobility, the transferases for the homozygous Duarte variant have a single band that differs from the normal [98]. Individuals heterozygous for the Duarte variant were found to have both distinct bands.

Gitzelmann [99] has reported two individuals in Switzerland (one infant and one parent of two known galactosemics) in whom family studies have suggested a pattern of enzyme activities similar to that of the Duarte variant. Starch-gel electrophoresis indicated a faster mobility of the patients' enzymes compared to that of normals.

While Levy et al. [100] reported no clinical manifestations for ten individuals with either the homozygous or heterozygous form of the Duarte variant, Kelly [101] reported mild galactose intolerance in the Duarte/classical galactosemia compound. The heterozygous form of classical galactosemia has no clinical abnormalities.

"Negro" Variant

Although relatively rare in the Negro race, classical galactosemia has been reported [15,102]. In studying whole body metabolism of 1-^{14}C-radiogalactose to $^{14}CO_2$ in vivo, Segal [102] noted that 3 of 12 sub-

TABLE 8-1. Distribution of GALT activity in erythrocytes from galactosemic variants

ERYTHROCYTE TRANSFERASE ACTIVITY (percent normal)	GENETIC LOCI REPRESENTED (both chromosomes)	POPULATION	
100	N,N	Normal	
50	D,D	Duarte	Homozygous
0	g,g	Galactosemic	
75	N,D	Normal/Duarte	
50	N,g	Normal/galactosemic	Heterozygous
25	D,g	Duarte/galactosemic	

jects with absent red cell transferase activity had normal net galactose metabolism. The three individuals were Negroes who had had classical galactosemia in infancy, including cataract formation. The investigators suggested that certain Negroes have a capacity to develop alternate pathways for galactose metabolism that circumvent the GALT reaction. This capacity has been designated as the Negro variant.

Similar observations by other investigators have confirmed these differences among affected Negroes. Studies of various tissues have not supported a global enzyme deficiency; thus white blood cell transferase may be present while erythrocytic activity is absent. Molecular techniques should clarify these differences.

Other Variants

In addition to the Duarte and Negro variants, there have been reports [103] of infants (homozygote compounds) with symptoms of vomiting, failure to thrive, hepatomegaly, and cataracts who were found with transferase activity in erythrocytes that varied from 0–35 percent of normal. Electrophoretic mobility patterns were variable. These variants have been named for the place of origin: Indiana, Chicago, Rennes, Los Angeles, etc. Symptomatic infants are managed similarly to those with classical galactosemia.

• Galactose-4-epimerase Deficiency

Gitzelmann [104] has reported on a deficiency of uridine diphosphate galactose-4-epimerase in erythrocytes from a normal infant. Several patients have been reported with the erythrocyte enzyme deficiency without clinical manifestation.

In contrast, in 1981, Holton et al. [105] reported a 5-day-old infant with classical galactosemia. However, the erythrocyte transferase activity was normal, as was galactokinase. There was a lack of activity of epimerase in both erythrocytes and skin fibroblasts. Concentrations of the proximal metabolites, uridine diphosphate galactose, and galactose-1-phosphate were increased in erythrocytes. The erythrocytes from the parents had decreased activity levels of epimerase.

In contrast to the classical transferase abnormality, management included an intake of small amounts of galactose at 1.5 gm daily after 4 months of age. This small intake is essential for the biosynthesis of sphingolipids which are required for brain growth and development as well as for other galactosides. The classical transferase abnormality allows for some endogenous galactose synthesis from glucose via the intact epimerase reaction.

Studies of infants with this defect should permit an estimate of minimal galactose requirements for essential structural compounds.

Chromosomal Alterations and Galactose Metabolism

Transferase activities of either red or white blood cells have been reported to be increased in Down's syndrome (trisomy 21), Cornelia de Lange syndrome, and in other trisomy syndromes [106,107]. The significance of these observations remains obscure.

• Galactokinase Deficiency

In 1933, in Zurich, a nine-year-old boy with von Recklinghausen's neurofibromatosis had an operation for bilaterally recurring cataracts. Fanconi [13] studied the mellituria (2.2–5.8 g/100 ml) in this patient and characterized the disorder as "galactose diabetes" because 50–87 percent of ingested galactose, 80 percent of galactose from ingested lactose, and 60–80 percent of milk lactose were excreted in the urine. The patient metabolized glucose, fructose, and other carbohydrates without mellituria. Gitzelmann [16] restudied this patient at 43 years of age, at which time he appeared to have normal intelligence, no signs of cirrhosis, but was blind. His urine contained 2 gm galactose and 0.04 gm glucose per 100 ml. Studies of the patient's blood indicated that the hemolysate (1) metabolized galactose-1-phosphate normally, (2) had normal GALT activity, and (3) contained minimal concentrations of galactose-1-phosphate. Since these findings were not compatible with classical galactosemia, intact red blood cells were studied for both galactokinase and uridyl transferase activities utilizing ^{14}C-labelled galactose and its conversion to galactose-1-phosphate and uridine diphosphogalactose. In contrast to normal cells, red blood cells of the patient did not produce detectable amounts of either compound, indicating a deficiency of galactokinase (Fig. 8-5). This patient was also studied for the possible relationship of polyol and galactitol to cataract formation [25]. He excreted excessive galactose in concentrations varying from 0.4–1.4 gm and galactitol, from 0.03–0.77 gm per 100 ml urine.

Enzyme Studies

Subsequently, Gitzelmann [18] carried out extensive studies of the family members of the original propositus. An older sister had cataracts and galactokinase deficiency, while another sister with cataracts was suspected to have the defect. Gitzelmann postulated an absence of the enzyme in the liver as well because of the delayed clearance of

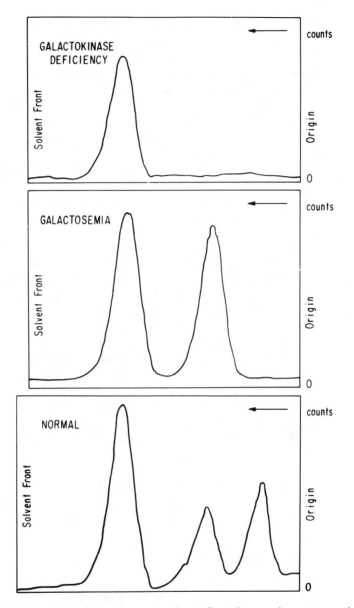

FIGURE 8-5. Radiochromatogram tracings of reaction products separated by paper chromatography following incubation of intact red blood cells with ^{14}C-labelled galactose according to Robinson. In the normal subject (bottom panel), three major fractions (origin to solvent front) are seen: uridine diphosphohexose, galactose-1-phosphate, and galactose. No uridine diphosphohexose is formed by the erythrocytes of a galactosemic individual (middle panel). No phosphorylated intermediates are found on the chromatogram from patient H.K. (top panel). (From Gitzelmann. *Pediatr Res.* 1967;1:14, with permission.)

galactose from the blood after the ingestion of milk. The net clearance of galactose was accomplished by its intact excretion and by its metabolism and excretion as galactitol. Of the approximately two-thirds of dietary galactose accounted for, one-fifth was excreted as galactitol and four-fifths as galactose.

In a patient with hereditary galactokinase deficiency, Gitzelmann, Wells, and Segal [108] studied whole body metabolism by measuring expired $^{14}CO_2$ after the administration of labeled ^{14}C-galactose, ^{14}C-galactitol and ^{14}C-galactonate. The excretion of $^{14}CO_2$ was minimal, suggesting that the defect was extensive and involved all tissues. However, $^{14}CO_2$ was excreted more rapidly after the administration of ^{14}C-1-galactose than after ^{14}C-2-galactose, suggesting the possibility of an alternate oxidative pathway catalyzed by galactose dehydrogenase in this patient.

Galactokinase activity was measured in the red blood cells of 100 control subjects and 18 family members. In the latter, three groups were identified: (1) the two patients had virtually a complete deficiency of enzyme activity, (2) ten relatives had intermediate values, while (3) six members had normal activities. All four of the children of the oldest patient had values clearly in the intermediate group. Additional patients have been reported [109–119].

Ng and associates [116] examined the developmental changes of galactokinase activity in human erythrocytes. Enzyme activities at 24 hours of age were approximately 3 times greater than those of the adult. Leukocyte buffy coats did not significantly affect the assay results. They speculated that a similar developmental pattern existed in the human liver. Dahlqvist [111] also noted higher galactokinase levels in erythrocytes from infants aged 2–4 months as compared to those of children and adults aged 2 to 67 years. Vigneron [117] reported similar control data, but found a transient galactokinase deficiency in a newborn infant. Thus, repeated verification of the defect may be necessary during the first weeks of life.

Clinical Manifestations

The clinical manifestations are less severe than those of classical galactosemia. Mental retardation and liver disease do not appear to be significant. Cataract formation is a serious consequence with early onset. Thalhammer's [109] and Kerr's [113] infants had transient hepatosplenomegaly, although Cook's [112] and Kerr's [113] infants were detected because of hyperbilirubinemia. Linneweh's [110] infant had a family history of cataracts, as did the original patients of Gitzelmann [18]. All of the infants developed early changes of cataract formation while receiving milk feedings. These resolved promptly after the infants were given low-galactose feedings.

Monteleone's [114] large kindred included 2 heterozygotes with cataracts and 6 of 10 siblings with cataracts in the third or fourth decade of life. The latter were not characterized by enzyme studies.

Laboratory Tests

Thalhammer [109] noted a delay in the accumulation of blood galactose and galactosuria. He found low values for galactose on fasting blood samples early in the morning and suggested that the optimal time to screen for excessive blood galactose was 1 hour after the second morning feed. Cook [112] noted a low blood glucose value of 32 mg/100 ml (1.8 mM) when his patient was 8 weeks of age, receiving a cow's milk formula. Blood galactose was 44 mg/100 ml simultaneously. The mechanism of the hypoglycemia is unclear.

Therapy

Therapy should be instituted promptly when either disorder is suspected. Proof of the specific enzymatic defect can then be obtained by analyzing the enzyme activities in red blood cells. A low galactose-lactose (milk) diet prevents the development of cataracts. Monteleone [114] suggested that dietary control of the heterozygote may also be important in preventing cataracts.

Genetics and Prevalence

The disorder appears to be an autosomal recessive trait. Mayes [120] estimated the frequency of galactokinase deficiency, based on the incidence of heterozygotes, as 1 in 40,000 to 1 in 50,000. Cook [112], however, suggested that Mayes overestimated the carrier frequency and indicated a more realistic incidence of 1 in 100,000.

Pathogenesis

The common pathogenetic mechanisms in classical galactosemia and galactokinase deficiency suggest that the metabolism of galactose to galactitol in the lens is responsible for cataract formation. The absence of liver disease and mental retardation, as well as of aminoaciduria, in galactokinase deficiency is consistent with the consideration that galactose-1-phosphate is the major toxic metabolite in classical galactosemia. Galactokinase activity has been studied in several tissues of the human fetus. While most tissues showed maximal activity at 28 weeks' gestation, the brain is constant and high [50,121].

The frequency of a deficiency of galactokinase as the etiologic factor in the cataracts of unknown origin is not well defined. In a survey of 210 persons who developed cataracts before the age of 40, Beutler and associates [122] assayed activities of galactokinase and of galactose-1-phosphate uridyl transferase in erythrocytes. Of 94 who developed cataracts before 1 year of age, 2 had a total deficiency of galactokinase and the remaining 92, a statistically significant reduction of enzyme activity. In contrast, those who developed cataracts in later life showed no abnormality in galactokinase activity. However, 2 had abnormalities of transferase activity, with no activity in one and a reduction to 15 percent of normal in the other. The significance of partial enzyme deficiencies as demonstrated in red blood cells may be due to variants and will require further surveys of large populations and detailed genetic analyses.

All neonates should be screened for these readily detected enzyme defects.

Case Report (Patient 8-1): A Fatal Case of Galactosemia Presenting as Sepsis and Meningitis[1]

This male infant was the 3,459-gm product of an uncomplicated term pregnancy, born to a 25-year-old gravida III para II, abortus I mother with blood type A, Rh negative, who had no venereal disease, and was rubella immune. After the birth of her first child 5 years previously, the mother had received Rh$_0$ (D) immune globulin (RhoGAM). The patient was delivered by cesarean section because of cephalopelvic disproportion. The Apgar scores were 8 at 1 minute and 9 at 5 minutes. After his first feeding at 12 hours, the baby vomited yellow material; thereafter, he fed poorly. At 36 hours of age, he became jittery; serum glucose concentration was 35 mg/dl (1.9 mM). After intravenous administration of 15 ml 10 percent dextrose in water, serum glucose concentration was normal and the baby was no longer tremulous. White blood cell count and serum electrolyte values were normal. During the next 18 hours, he twice vomited bile-stained material, but he did pass several meconium-containing stools. Roentgenograms of the abdomen showed only dilated loops of small bowel. Feeding was stopped, and the infant was transferred to Rhode Island Hospital at 52 hours of age.

On admission, he had jaundice and was moderately active, with stable vital signs. He weighed 3.46 kg, was 50 cm long, and head circumference was 36 cm. He had a grade II/VI systolic murmur at the left upper sternal border. The liver was palpable 1.5 cm below the right costal margin, there were no abdominal masses, and the spleen was not enlarged. The bowel sounds were faint, and the rectal examination yielded normal findings. There was third-degree hypospadias; the left testis was undescended, and the right partly descended. Findings on neurologic examination were normal except that a Moro response could not be elicited and his cry was high-pitched. The WBC count was 14,700/mm^3, with 82 percent polymorphonuclear leukocytes, 19 percent bands, and 8 percent monocytes. Blood type was A, Rh

---

[1]Modified from Dennehy PH, O'Shea PA, Abuelo DN. A newborn infant with bilious vomiting and jitteriness. *J Pediatr.* 1985,106:161–166.

positive. Urinalysis showed normal findings except that the sediment contained 15–20 WBC per high-powered field, rare red cells, and many bacteria. The blood glucose concentration was 90 mg/dl (5.0 mM), sodium 136 mEq/L, potassium 4.9 mEq/L, chloride 109 mEq/L, and carbon dioxide 17 mM/L. The glucose concentration fell to 43 mg/dl (2.4 mM). Total serum bilirubin concentration was 13.1 mg/dl, with direct-acting bilirubin 2.1 mg/dl. Chest roentgenograms, intravenous pyelogram, and voiding cystourethrogram all showed normal findings. Barium swallow, upper gastrointestinal series, and barium enema revealed no obstruction. Karyotype was 46,XY.

With a nasogastric tube in place, the baby was given 10 percent dextrose intravenously at 50–100 ml/kg/day (3.5–6.9 mg/kg/min) until 5 days of age, when feeding was reinstituted with Enfamil 20. No further vomiting occurred, but he again fed poorly. At 6 days of age, the baby again became tremulous; lumbar puncture yielded xanthochromic fluid with a glucose concentration of 1 mg/dl (0.06 mM), protein 160 mg/dl, RBC 330/mm³, and no white cells; Gram stain was negative. Counterimmunoelectrophoresis showed no bacterial antigens. On the next day, the patient began to have seizures and cyanosis, and blood began to ooze from all of his needle puncture sites. He went into shock and became comatose. Blood pressure was 38/18, pulse 170 bpm, temperature ~36°C. After tracheal intubation and mechanical ventilation, his blood gas values were pH 7.17, PO_2 20, and total CO_2 8 mM/L; FiO_2 was 45 percent.

Ampicillin (200 mg/kg/day) and gentamicin (7.5 mg/kg/day) were given. He received vitamin K, fresh-frozen plasma, packed red blood cells, and dopamine at a dose of 5 to 12 mg/kg/min. Despite all of these measures, he developed oliguria followed by anuria, and blood continued to ooze from needle puncture sites. A gram-positive coccus was cultured from the blood, and methicillin was added to the treatment. A computerized tomographic scan of the head showed no ventricular shift or dilation and no hemorrhage. He was given a double-volume exchange transfusion. Two days before death, SGOT activity was 299 IU/L, alkaline phosphatase 25 IU/L, bilirubin 6.2 mg/dl, ammonia 73 ug/dl, and SGPT 80 IU/L.

At the age of 10 days, the baby developed fixed and dilated pupils and died.

At autopsy, there were no dysmorphic features. The baby had acute meningitis and severe acute hypoxic and ischemic brain injury. Postmortem blood cultures failed to grow any organism, but the gram-positive coccus cultured premortem from blood was a group D streptococcus. Therefore, it is reasonably certain that this infant's death resulted from group D streptococcal meningitis and septicemia.

The liver was large and bright yellow, with patchy parenchymal collapse, fibrosis, and nodular regeneration, all much more striking in the left lobe. Microscopically, there was extensive panlobular fatty change. In the left lobe, there was extensive parenchymal collapse, with both fine and coarse areas of scarring in a pattern suggestive of postnecrotic cirrhosis. Regenerative nodules varied from 1 or 2 mm up to 1 cm and were abundant. The right lobe was also cirrhotic, but the pattern was micronodular and the fibrosis much less. Cholestasis and pseudoacinar change were prominent. The extrahepatic and intrahepatic biliary ducts were normal; there was a variable degree of ductular proliferation in proportion to the scarring.

There are two metabolic conditions that characteristically cause the hepatic changes seen in this infant: galactosemia and hereditary fructose intolerance. Babies with fructose intolerance do not develop cirrhosis unless they have been fed fructose, and this infant never received fructose. In view of the high incidence of neonatal meningitis and septicemia in galactosemia, the evidence pointing to that disorder became even more compelling.

Subsequently, enzyme assays of erythrocytes from the parents showed approximately 50 percent activity of galactose-1-phosphate uridyl transferase. The next pregnancy resulted in an affected infant who was diagnosed in utero at amniocentesis. The mother was fed a galactose-limited diet, as was the newborn.

Comment

Sepsis in the first week of life should raise the index of suspicion for the rare association with galactosemia. Lactose (galactose) feeds should be avoided until a definitive screening study has been performed.

A urinalysis measuring both total reducing sugars (Clinitest tablets) and glucose (glucose oxidase strip) may have suggested the possible diagnosis once milk feedings were given. This should always be done in the neonate with jaundice, vomiting, and failure to thrive.

• Summary

Galactosemia is an autosomal recessive defect in the specific enzyme, galactose-1-phosphate uridyl transferase. Manifestations in early infancy may relate to liver disease, failure to thrive, cataracts and mental retardation. Mellituria and aminoaciduria are present. Avoidance of galactose (lactose) prevents progression of the symptoms and permits normal growth. Early recognition of this problem in the newborn period and meticulous dietary control are essential to minimize the toxic effects of the accumulation of galactose-1-phosphate. Psychosocial mental and neurologic abnormalities may occur even with early rigid dietary management.

Several variants of the transferase deficiency are recognized: The Duarte variant with 50 percent of normal activity has no clinical manifestations, while the Negro variant may have classical galactosemia but an ability to metabolize galactose by alternate pathways.

A rare occurrence is the absence or uridine diphosphate galactose-4-epimerase which is associated with classical symptoms of galactosemia. Treatment is a galactose-restricted diet, but includes a small quantity of galactose intake to provide for synthesis of sphingolipids.

Galactokinase deficiency (galactose diabetes) is an autosomal recessive defect. The only clinical manifestation is cataracts. Galactokinase deficiency may be unrecognized for many years unless a urinalysis for reducing substances after lactose ingestion or routine enzyme screening in red blood cells is performed.

REFERENCES

1. VON REUSS A. Zuckerausscheidung im Saughlingsalter. *Wein Med Wochenschr.* 1908;58:799.
2. GÖPPERT F. Galacktosurie nach Milchzuckergabe bei angeborenem, familiärem, chronischem Leberleiden. *Berl Klin Wochenschr.* 1917;54:473.
3. MASON HH, TURNER ME. Chronic galactemia: report of case with studies on carbohydrates. *Am J Dis Child.* 1935;50:359.
4. GOLDBLOOM A, BRICKMAN HF. Galactemia. *J Pediatr.* 1946;28:674.
5. DONNELL GN, LANN SH. Galactosemia. *Pediatrics.* 1951;7:503.
6. KOMROWER GM, SCHWARZ V, HOLZEL A, GOLDBERG L. A clinical and biochemical study of galactosemia. *Arch Dis Child.* 1956;31:254.
7. HSIA DY-Y, WALKER FA. Variability in the clinical manifestations of galactosemia. *J Pediatr.* 1961;59:872.
8. HSIA DY-Y. Clinical variants of galactosemia. *Metabolism.* 1967;16:419.
9. NADLER HL, INOUYE T, HSIA DY-Y. Classical galactosemia: A study of fifty-five cases. In: Hsia DY-Y, ed. Galactosemia. Springfield, Ill.: Charles C Thomas, Pubs., 1969;127.
10. GREENBERG CR, DILLING LA, THOMPSON R, et al. Newborn screening for galactosemia: a new method used in Manitoba. *Pediatrics.* 1989;84:331.
11. SEGAL S. Disorders of galactose metabolism. In: Scriver CR, Beaudet AL, Sly WS, Valle D, eds. *The Metabolic Basis of Inherited Disease.* 6th ed. New York: McGraw-Hill, Inc., 1989;453.
12. TOWNSEND EH JR, MASON HH, STRONG PS. Galactosemia and its relation to Laennec's cirrhosis; review of literature and presentation of 6 additional cases. *Pediatrics.* 1951;7:760.
13. FANCONI G. Hochgradige Galaktose Intoleranz (Galaktose Diabetes) bei einem kunde mit neurofibromatosis Recklinghausen. *Jahrbuch fur kinderheilkunde.* 1933;138:1.
14. BEUTLER E, BALUDA MC, STURGEON P, DAY RW. The genetics of galactose-1-phosphate uridyl transferase deficiency. *J Lab Clin Med.* 1966;68:646.
15. MELLMAN WJ, TEDESCO TA, BAKER L. A new genetic abnormality. *Lancet.* 1965;1:1395.
16. GITZELMANN R. Deficiency of erythrocyte galactokinase in a patient with galactose diabetes. *Lancet.* 1965;2:670.
17. CUATRECASAS P, SEGAL S. Galactose conversion to D-xylulose: An alternate route of galactose metabolism. *Science.* 1966;153:549.
18. GITZELMANN R. Hereditary galactokinase deficiency; a newly recognized cause of juvenile cataracts. *Pediatr Res.* 1967;1:14.
19. LELOIR LF. The metabolism of hexosephosphates. In: McElroy WD, Glass B, eds. *Symposium on Phosphorus Metabolism. Vol. 1.* Baltimore: Johns Hopkins University Press, 1951;67.
20. LELOIR LF. Enzymatic transformation of uridine diphosphate glucose into a galactose derivative. *Arch Biochem.* 1951;33:186.
21. EISENBERG F JR, ISSELBACHER KJ, KALCKAR HM. Studies on metabolism of carbon-14-labelled galactose in a galactosemic individual. *Science.* 1957;125:116.
22. SEGAL S, BLAIR A, TOPPER YJ. Oxidation of carbon[14] labelled galactose by subjects with congenital galactosemia. *Science.* 1962;136:150.

23. NG WG, BERGREN WR, DONNELL GN. Galactose-1-phosphate uridyl transferase activity in galactosemia. *Nature.* 1964;203:845.

24. ISSELBACHER KJ. Evidence for an accessory pathway of galactose metabolism in mammalian liver. *Science.* 1957;126:652.

25. GITZELMANN R, CURTIUS HC, MULLER M. Galactitol excretion in the urine of a galactokinase-deficient man. *Biochem Biophys Res Commun.* 1966;22:437.

26. ELLIS C, WILCOX AR, GOLDBERG DM. Experience of routine live-birth screening for galactosemia in a British hospital, with emphasis on heterozygote detection. *Arch Dis Child.* 1972;47:34.

27. LEVY HL, SEPE SJ, SHIH VE, VAWTER GF, KLEIN JO. Sepsis due to Escherichia coli in neonates with galactosemia. *N Engl J Med.* 1977; 297:823.

28. PESCE MA, BODOURIAN SH. Clinical significance of plasma galactose and erythrocyte galactose-1-phosphate measurements in transferase-deficient galactosemia and in individuals with below-normal transferase activity. *Clin Chem.* 1982;28(2):301.

29. NG WB, LEE JES, LIN J, et al. Laboratory confirmation of galactosemia. In: Nyhan WL, ed. *Advances in Neonatal Screening.* Norwalk: Appleton-Century, 1984;401.

30. GITZELMANN R. Newborn screening for inherited disorders of galactose metabolism. In: Bickel H, Guthrie R, Hammersen G, eds. *Neonatal Screening for Inborn Errors of Metabolism.* Berlin: Springer-Verlag, 1980;67.

31. PAIGEN K, PACHOLEC F, LEVY HL. A new method of screening for inherited disorders of galactose metabolism. *J Lab Clin Med.* 1982; 99:895.

32. BOWLING FG, BROWN ARD. Development of a protocol for newborn screening for disorders of the galactose metabolic pathway. *J Inher Metab Dis.* 1986;9:99.

33. NG WB, KAWAMURA M, DONNELL GN. Galactosemia screening: methodology and outcome from worldwide data collection. In: Therrell BL, Jr, ed. *Advances in Neonatal Screening.* New York: Elsevier Science Publ., 1987;243.

34. RITTER JA, CANNON EJ. Galactosemia with cataracts; report of a case, with notes on physiopathology. *N Engl J Med.* 1955;252:747.

35. ROE TF, HALLATT JG, DONNELL GN, NG WG. Childbearing by a galactosemic woman. *J Pediatr.* 1971;78:1026.

36. HOLZEL A. Some aspects of galactosemia. *Mod Probl Paediatr.* 1959; 4:388. (Biblio-Paediatrica, fasc. 70.)

37. DONNELL GN, COLLADO M, KOCH R. Growth and development of children with galactosemia. *J Pediatr.* 1961;58:836.

38. HUGH-JONES K, NEWCOMB AL, HSIA DY-Y. The genetic mechanism of galactosemia. *Arch Dis Child.* 1960;35:521.

39. MORTENSEN O, SØNDERGAARD G. Galactosemia (Progress in Pediatrics). *Acta Paediatr.* 1954;43:467.

40. ISSELBACHER KJ. Galactosemia. In: Stanbury JB, Wyngaarden JB, and Fredrickson DS, eds. *The Metabolic Basis of Inherited Diseases.* New York: McGraw-Hill Book Co., Inc., 1960;208.

41. BORDEN M. Screening for metabolic disease in abnormalities. In: Nyhan WL, ed. *Amino Acid Metabolism in Clinical Medicine.* Norwalk: Appleton-Century, 1984;401.

42. DAHLQVIST A, SVENNINGSEN NW. Galactose in the urine of newborn infants. *J Pediatr.* 1969;75:454.

43. KIRKMAN HN. Galactosemia. Symposium on hereditary metabolic diseases. *Metabolism.* 1960;9:316.

44. HSIA DY-Y. Clinical variants of galactosemia. *Metabolism.* 1967;16:419.

45. NADLER HL, INOUYE T, HSIA DYY. Clinical galactosemia: a study of fifty-five cases. In: Hsia DYY, ed. *Galactosemia.* Springfield: Charles C. Thomas, 1969;127.

46. SHIN YS, RIETH WE, SCHAUB J. Prenatal diagnosis of galactosemia and properties of galactose-1-phosphate uridyl transferase in erythrocytes of galactosemic variants as well as in human fetal and adult organs. *Clin Chim Acta.* 1983;128:271.

47. ROLLAND MO, MANDOU G, FARRIAUX JP, DORCHE C. Galactose-1-phosphate uridyl transferase activity in chorionic villus: A first trimester prenatal diagnosis of galactosemia. *J Inher Metab Dis.* 1986;9:284.

48. ALLEN JT, GILLETT M, HOLTON JB, KING GS, PETTIT B. Evidence of galactosemia in utero. *Lancet.* 1980;1:603.

49. JAKOBS C, WARNER TG, SWEETMAN L, NYHAN WL. Stable isotope dilution analysis of galactitol in amniotic fluid: an accurate approach to the prenatal diagnosis of galactosemia. *Pediatr Res.* 1984;18(4):714.

50. SHIN-BUEHRING YS, BEIER T, TAN A, OSANG M, SCHAUB J. The activity of galactose-1-phosphate uridyl transferase and galactokinase in human fetal organs. *Pediatr Res.* 1977;11:1045.

51. DAHLQVIST A. Test paper for galactose in urine. *Scand J Clin Lab Invest.* 1966;18:Suppl 92:101, *Scand J Clin Lab Invest.* 1968;22:87.

52. KELLY S. Septicemia in galactosemia: *JAMA* 1971;216:330.

53. SHIH VE, LEVY HL, KAROLKEWICZ BA, HOUGHTON S, EFRON ML, ISSELBACHER KJ, BEUTLER E, MacCREATY RA. Galactosemia screening of newborns in Massachusetts. *N Engl J Med.* 1971;284:753.

54. HAWORTH JC, MacDONALD MS. Reducing sugars in the urine and blood of premature babies. *Arch Dis Child.* 1957;32:417.

55. IRONS M, LEVY HL, PUESCHEL S, CASTREE K. Accumulation of galactose-1-phosphate in the galactosemic fetus despite maternal milk avoidance. *J Pediatr.* 1985;107(2):261.

56. GITZELMANN R, HANSEN RG. Galactose biogenesis and disposal in galactosemics. *Biochim Biophys Acta.* 1974;372:374.

57. GITZELMANN R, AURICCHIO S. The handling of soya α-galactosides by a normal and a galactosemic child. *Pediatrics.* 1965;36:231.

58. HOLZEL A, KOMROWER GM, SCHWARZ V. Low-lactose milk for congenital galactosaemia. *Lancet.* 1955;269:92. (Letter to the Editor.)

59. KOCH R, ACOSTA P, RAGSDALE N, DONNELL GN. Nutrition in the treatment of galactosemia. *J Am Diet Assoc.* 1963;43:216.

60. DONNELL GN, BERGREN WR, BRETTHAUER RK, HANSEN RG. The enzymatic expression of heterozygosity in families of children with galactosemia. *Pediatrics.* 1960;25:572.

61. MEERA KHAN P, ROBSON EB. Report of the committee on the genetic constitution of chromosome 9, Cytogen. *Cell Genet.* 1978;22:106.

62. LEVY HL, HAMMERSEN G. Newborn screening for galactosemia and other galactose metabolism defects. *J Pediatr.* 1978;92:871.

63. REICHARDT JKV, BERG P. Cloning and characterization of a cDNA encoding human galactose-1-phosphate uridyl transferase. *Mol Biol Med.* 1988;5:107.

64. REICHARDT JKV. Galactosemia is caused by missense mutations: molecular studies and implications for therapy. Presented at the symposium "Galactosemia: New Frontiers in Research". Sponsored by NICHHD and the Children's Hospital Los Angeles, April 1989. (Personal communication.)

65. MEDLINE A, MEDLINE NM. Galactosemia: Early structural changes in the liver. *Can Med Assoc J.* 1972;107:877.

66. BELL LS, BLAIR WC, LINDSAY S, WATSON SJ. Lesions of galactose diabetes; pathological observations. *Arch Pathol.* 1950;49:393.

67. CROME L. A case of galactosaemia with the pathological and neuropathological findings. *Arch Dis Child.* 1962;37:415.

68. LEVY HL, DRISCOLL SG, PORENSKY RS, WENDER DF. Ovarian failure in galactosemia. *N Engl J Med.* 1984;310:50.

69. SCHWARZ V, GOLDBERG L, KOMROWER GM, HOLZEL A. Some disturbances of erythrocyte metabolism in galactosemia. *Biochem J.* 1956;62:34.

70. KALCKAR HM, ANDERSON EP, ISSELBACHER KJ. Galactosemia, a congenital defect in a nucleotide transferase: A preliminary report. *Proc Natl Acad Sci.* 1956;42:49.

71. ISSELBACHER KJ, ANDERSON EP, KURAHASHI K, KALCKAR HM. Congenital galactosemia, a single enzymatic block in galactose metabolism. *Science.* 1956;123:635.

72. KAUFMAN FR, NG WG, XU YK, et al. Treatment of patients (PTS) with classical galactosemia (G) with oral uridine. *Pediatr Res.* 1989;25 (4):142A.

73. MITCHELL HS. Cataracts in rats fed on galactose. *Proc Soc Exp Biol Med.* 1935;32:971.

74. CRAIG JM, MADDOCK CE. Observations on nature of galactose toxicity in rats. *Arch Pathol.* 1953;55:118.

75. LERMAN S. The lens in human and experimental galactosemia. *NY J Med.* 1962;62:785.

76. LERMAN S. The lens in congenital galactosemia. *Arch Ophthalmol.* 1959;61:88.

77. KINOSHITA JH. Selected topics in ophthalmic biochemistry. *Arch Ophthalmol.* 1963;70:558.

78. SIDBURY JB JR. The enzymatic lesions in galactosemia. *J Clin Invest.* 1957;36:929. (Abstract.)

79. CUSWORTH DC, DENT CE, FLYNN FV. Amino-aciduria in galactosemia. *Arch Dis Child.* 1955;30:150.

80. HSIA DY-Y, HSIA HH, GREEN S, KAY M, GELLIS SS. Amino-aciduria in galactosemia. *Am J Dis Child.* 1954;88:458.

81. URBANOWSKI JC, COHENFORD MA, LEVY HL, CRAWFORD JD, DAIN JA. Nonenzymatically galactosylated serum albumin in a galactosemic infant. *N Engl J Med.* 1982;306:84.

82. CORADELLO H, POLLAK A, SCHEIBENVEITER S, LEGENSTEIN E, LEVIN S, LUBEC G. Nichtenzymatische glykosylierung von hämoglobin und serumprotein bei kindern mit galaktosämie. *Wiener Klinische Wochenschrift.* 1983;95(22):804.

83. KOMROWER GM, LEE DH. Long-term follow-up of galactosemia. *Arch Dis Child.* 1970;45:367.

84. FISHLER K, DONNELL GN, BERGREN WR, KOCH R. Intellectual and personality development in children with galactosemia. *Pediatrics.* 1972;50:412.

85. FISHLER K, KOCH R, DONNELL GN, WENZ E. Developmental aspects of galactosemia from infancy to childhood. *Clin Pediatr.* 1980; 19:38.

86. GITZELMANN R, STEINMANN B. Galactosemia: how does long-term treatment change the outcome? *Enzyme.* 1984;32:37.

87. JAN JE, WILSON RA. Unusual late neurological sequelae in galactosemia. *Dev Med Child Neurol.* 1973;15:72.

88. PACKMAN S, LO W, SCHMIDT K, et al. Neurologic sequelae in galactosemia. In: Therrell BL, Jr., ed. *Advances in Neonatal Screening.* New York: Elsevier Science Publishers, 1987;261.

89. FRIEDMAN JH, LEVY HL, BOUSTANY R-M. Late onset of distinct neurologic syndromes in galactosemic siblings. *Neurology.* 1989;39: 741.

90. WAISBREN SE, NORMAN TR, SCHNELL RR, LEVY HL. Speech and language deficits in early-treated children with galactosemia. *J Pediatr.* 1983;102:75.

91. TEDESCO TA, MORROW G III, MELLMAN WJ. Normal pregnancy and childbirth in a galactosemic woman. *J Pediatr.* 1972;81:1159.

92. KAUFMAN FR, KOGUT MD, DONNELL GN, GOEBELSMANN U, MARCH C, KOCH R. Hypergonadotropic hypogonadism in female patients with galactosemia. *N Engl J Med.* 1981;304:994.

93. CHEN YT, MATTISON DR, SCHULMAN JD. Hypogonadism and galactosemia. *N Engl J Med.* 1981;305:464.

94. ROBINSON ACR, DOCKERAY CJ, CULLEN MJ, SWEENEY EC. Hypergonadotrophic hypogonadism in classical galactosaemia: evidence for defective oogenesis. Case report. *Br J Obstet Gynaecol.* 1984;91:199.

95. KAUFMAN FR, DONNELL GN, ROE TF, KOGUT MD. Gonadal function in patients with galactosaemia. *J Inher Metab Dis.* 1986;9:140.

96. FRASER JS, SHEARMAN RP, WILCKEN B, BROWN A, DAVIS K. Failure to identify heterozygotes for galactosaemia in women with premature ovarian failure. *Lancet.* 1987;ii:566.

97. BEUTLER E, BALUDA MC. An improved method for measuring galactose-1-phosphate uridyl transferase activity of erythrocytes. *Clin Chim Acta.* 1966;13:369.

98. MATHAI CK, BEUTLER E. Electrophoretic variation of galactose-1-phosphate uridyl transferase. *Science.* 1966;154:1179.

99. GITZELMANN R, POLEY JR, PRADER A. Partial galactose-1-phosphate uridyl transferase deficiency due to a variant enzyme. *Helv Paediatr Acta.* 1967;22:252.

100. LEVY HL, SEPE SJ, WALTON DS, et al. Galactose-1-phosphate uridyl transferase deficiency due to Duarte/galactosemia variation: Clinical and biochemical studies. *J Pediatr.* 1978;93:390.

101. KELLY S. Significance of the Duarte/classical galactosemic genetic compound. *J Pediatr.* 1979;92:937.

102. SEGAL S, BLAIR A, ROTH H. The metabolism of galactose by patients with congenital galactosemia. *Am J Med.* 1965;38:62.

103. GITZELMANN R, HANSEN RG. Galactose metabolism, hereditary defects and their clinical significance. In: Burman D, Holton JB, Pennock CA, eds. *Inherited Disorders of Carbohydrate Metabolism.* Lancaster: MTP Press Ltd, 1980;61.

104. GITZELMANN R. Deficiency of uridine diphosphate galactose 4-epimerase in blood cells of an apparently healthy infant. *Helv Paediatr Acta.* 1972;27:125.

105. HOLTON JB, GILLETT MG, MacFAUL R, YOUNG R. Galactosaemia: a new severe variant due to uridine diphosphate galactose-4-epimerase deficiency. *Arch Dis Child.* 1981;56:885.

106. BRANDT NJ, FORLAND A, MIKKELSEN M, NIELSEN A, TALSTRUP N. Galactosemia locus and the Down's syndrome chromosome. *Lancet.* 1963;2:700.

107. DAHLQVIST A, HALL B, KALLEN B. Blood galactose-1-phosphate uridyl transferase activity in dysplastic patients with and without chromosomal aberrations. *Hum Hered.* 1969;19:628.

108. GITZELMANN R, WELLS HJ, SEGAL S. Galactose metabolism in a patient with hereditary galactokinase deficiency. *Eur J Clin Invest.* 1974; 4:79.

109. THALHAMMER O, GITZELMANN R, PANTLITSCHKO MD. Hypergalactosemia and galactosuria due to galactokinase deficiency in a newborn. *Pediatrics.* 1968;42:441.

110. LINNEWEH F, SCHAUMLOFFEL E, VETRELLA M. Galaktokinase-defekt bei einem Neugeborenen. *Klin Wochenschr.* 1970;48:31.

111. DAHLQVIST A, GAMSTORP I, MADSEN H. A patient with hereditary galactokinase deficiency. *Acta Paediatr Scand.* 1970;59:669.

112. COOK JGH, DON NA, MANN TP. Hereditary galactokinase deficiency. *Arch Dis Child.* 1971;46:465.

113. KERR MM, LOGAN RW, CANT JS, HUTCHISON JH. Galactokinase deficiency in a newborn infant. *Arch Dis Child.* 1971;46:864.

114. MONTELEONE JA, BEUTLER E, MONTELEONE PL, UTZ CL, CASEY EC. Cataracts, galactosuria, and hypergalactosemia due to galactokinase deficiency in a child. *Am J Med.* 1971;50:403.

115. MCVIE R, DEUTSCHE MA, OLAMBIWONNU NO, FRASIER SD, DONNELL GN. Galactokinase deficiency: Clinical and biochemical studies in identical twins. *Clin Res.* 1971;19:216.

116. NG WG, DONNELL GN, BERGREN WR. Galactokinase activity in human erythrocytes of individuals at different ages. *J Lab Clin Med.* 1965;66:115.

117. VIGNERON C, MARCHAL C, DEIFTS C, VIDAILHET M, PIERSON M, NEIMAN N. Deficit partiel et transitoire en galactokinase erythrocytaire chez un nouveau-ne. *Arch Fr Pediatr.* 1970;27:523.

118. GITZELMANN R, ILLIG R. Inability of galactose to mobilize insulin in galactokinase-deficient individuals. *Diabetologia.* 1969;5:143.

119. GITZELMANN R. Hereditary galactokinase deficiency. *Citation Classics in Current Contents.* 1987;30:14.

120. MAYES JS. Screening for heterozygotes of the galactose enzyme deficiencies. In: Hsia DY-Y, ed. Galactosemia. Springfield, Ill.: Charles C Thomas, Pubs., 1969;291.

121. SHIN-BUEHRING YS, STUEMPFIG L, POUGET E, RAHM P, SCHAUB J. Characterization of galactose-1-phosphate uridyl-transferase and galactokinase in human organs from the fetus and adult. *Clin Chim Acta.* 1981;112:257.

122. BEUTLER E, MATSUMOTO F, KUHL W, KRILL A, LEVY N, SPARKES R, DEGNAN M. Galactokinase deficiency as a cause of cataracts. *N Engl J Med.* 1973;288:1203.

C H A P T E R   9

HEREDITARY FRUCTOSE INTOLERANCE

Three distinct entities that result from abnormalities in the metabolism of fructose have been recognized: (1) essential or benign fructosuria [1], (2) hereditary fructose intolerance [2,3], and (3) fructose-1,6-diphosphatase deficiency [4]. Only hereditary fructose intolerance (HFI) and those aspects of the other two defects necessary for a differential diagnosis are discussed here. Detailed reviews have been presented by Perheentupa, Raivio, and Nikkila [5], Nikkila and Huttunen [6], Froesch [7], and, most recently, Gitzelmann, Steinmann, and Van Den Berge [8].

In 1956, Chambers and Pratt described an adult with an "idiosyncrasy to fructose" [2]. The following year, Froesch, Prader, and associates [3] were the first to describe fully the typical syndrome of HFI, to find that the administration of fructose lowered the blood glucose in affected patients, and to postulate that the primary defect was the absence of fructose-1-phosphate aldolase in the liver. Subsequently, over 150 patients with HFI have been reported from around the world [5–21], indicating a wide distribution of this genetic defect, except for Israel [22]. The frequency of HFI is estimated to be 1:20,000 people in Switzerland by Gitzelmann and Baerlocher [23].

Clinical manifestations occur only after the ingestion of fructose or fructose-containing food, e.g., sucrose (table sugar: a glucose/fructose disaccharide), fruits, honey, and similar foods. Another source of fructose may be sorbitol, a sugar alcohol quantitatively converted to fructose in the liver [7,24]. Sorbitol may be an ingredient of "diabetic" chocolate or a sugar substitute in intravenous infusion solutions. The severity and type of clinical presentation depend upon the quantity of fructose in the diet and the age of the patient. Thus, the young infant is more vulnerable and may present with a serious chronic disease that begins with vomiting, failure to thrive, and hypoglycemia with the introduction of fructose in the diet and progresses rapidly to liver damage [3,9–12,23] with hepatomegaly, jaundice, elevated serum levels of hepatic enzymes, hypoalbuminemia, ascites, and even death [18,25–27]. At least six deaths in infancy due to unrecognized HFI were reported between 1968 and 1972 [18,19,25–27].

Some infants have been able "to convey their distaste for sweet-tasting foods" at a relatively young age to a sensitive, alert mother and remain healthy [5]. A strong aversion for any sweet foods develops in all children and adults with HFI.

After infancy, abdominal pain, nausea, vomiting, malaise, excessive sweating, tremor, confusion, coma, and convulsions may follow the ingestion of foods containing fructose. In adults, the continuous intake of fructose may result in renal tubular dysfunction and hypokalemia [28–30], leading to renal calculi [31], polyuria, and periodic or progressive weakness or paralysis [32].

It should be emphasized that fructosuria is not a constant finding and occurs only after the ingestion of fructose.

Although multiple forms of aldolase have been found in diverse tissues [33,34], the primary enzyme defect has been shown to be an absence of activity of aldolase, type B in liver [34–39], in intestinal mucosa [7,40], and in the renal cortex [41]. Cross and associates [42] identified the first mutation in the structural gene for B aldolase. The antibody to normal B aldolase cross-reacts with extracts of liver from some patients with HFI [39,43,44] and may even activate the mutant enzyme [45,46] (see the section on molecular genetics below).

In HFI, the secondary hypoglucosemia that follows the ingestion or administration of parenteral fructose is due to an inhibition of hepatic glucose release and is accompanied by a fall in serum inorganic phosphorus [5,7,25,35] and by a rise in serum magnesium [24,25] and uric acid [24,47]. There is no hyperglycemic response to glucagon [12,13,35]. Infusing galactose either with [48] or after [13] fructose results in elevating the blood glucose, but glycerol and dihydroxyacetone do not induce a rise in glucose [26,48]. In the majority of families studied, an autosomal recessive mode of inheritance has been suggested.

• Clinical Manifestations

A variety of clinical signs and symptoms have been described in patients with HFI [49,50]. The manifestations depend upon age, se-

verity of the disease, the quantity and duration of the fructose ingestion or administration, and other still undetermined factors. If fructose-
containing foods are avoided, the patients remain completely well and
free of symptoms.

Young Infants [5,9,10,14,18–27,33,38,40,45,46,51–60]

The most severe manifestations of this syndrome may occur in the
young infant who is given either sucrose (as the carbohydrate supplement to his artificial formula), fruits, or fruit juices. Breast-fed infants
remain symptom-free. Generally, the firstborn infant with the disease
may die or may suffer more than subsequently affected siblings who
profit from the experience of the parents and the physician with the
first child.

In the first few weeks to months of life, the infant may have
anorexia, prolonged vomiting, failure to thrive, and hypochromic
anemia. The vomitus may be projectile, blood-stained, or just "spit-
ting up." Periodic attacks of hypoglucosemia with apneic spells, occasional unconsciousness, and convulsions have been reported
[5,8,9,10,14,25,52]. On examination, the infants are usually cachec-
tic and stunted in growth. Jaundice, hepatomegaly and, less often,
splenomegaly may occur. If fructose-containing foods are continued, the disease progresses to more serious signs of liver failure [3,9–
12,23], including hypoalbuminemia, abdominal distention with ascites, generalized edema, and deficiencies of hepatic coagulation factors. Hemorrhagic manifestations have been prominent in some infants
who have had prolonged prothrombin times, plus reductions in factors V, VII, X, and fibrinogen, as well as elevations in factor VIII
[27,56]. Some of these abnormalities in coagulation factors have been
induced acutely following a diagnostic fructose tolerance test [58].
These infants may have elevated serum levels of bilirubin, serum enzyme activities (SGOT, SGPT, etc.), and amino acids (tyrosine and
methionine) [53–55]. On occasion, a severe metabolic acidosis may
occur that is in part due to renal tubular dysfunction [25,28–30] and
in part to the hyperlactic acidemia [12,13]. Albuminuria and aminoaciduria are usual. It must be reemphasized that a positive urine
test for reducing sugars or fructosuria is not invariably present and
may only appear after a significant exposure to fructose.

The liver, at biopsy prior to dietary therapy or at autopsy, shows
extensive abnormal changes by both light and electron microscopy.
These changes include focal areas of necrosis with or without storage
material, widening and proliferation of biliary ducts, tubular formations extending through hepatic lobules, atypical pigments within the
lumen of the pseudoacini, fatty degeneration of the peripheral lobules,
and portal fibrosis [18,61], as well as biliary cirrhosis [25].

Some infants may have milder signs and symptoms if only minimal amounts of fructose are offered or if their disease is less marked.
Thus, the clinical syndrome of HFI in the infant may be highly variable.

Early diagnosis of this condition is mandatory. If unrecognized
or allowed to go untreated, death can ensue [18,25–27]. All the clinical and all the abnormal laboratory findings appear to be reversible
once fructose has been removed from the diet. Striking improvement
can occur dramatically within 24–48 hours ("L'amelioration clinique
est spectaculaire" [54]). Thus, as in the infant suspected of having
galactosemia, "any infant with an enlarged liver and proteinuria—or
aminoaciduria . . ." plus vomiting, failure to thrive, and jaundice
". . . is so suspect of having HFI that fructose should be excluded
from the diet until the diagnosis has been ruled out." Similarly, parenteral fructose should be given only to patients "positively known
to tolerate sugar" [5].

The more seriously ill infants have been reported from Europe
[9,10,12,18,25,27]. One explanation might be that, in Europe, sucrose is used more commonly as the carbohydrate added to artificial
feeding than in the United States, where corn syrups containing dex-
trins or maltose are used.

In instances in which the affected infants can reject or select foods,
they develop a profound aversion to and distaste for anything sweet,
thus protecting themselves from the toxic effects of fructose. This is
particularly true in the adult, in whom a chronic syndrome has never
been reported, because he has learned what food to avoid. Some parents have recognized their infants' aversion to sweets as early as the
first months of life, and one mother solved the problem for her daugh-
ter with HFI by breast-feeding her for 2½ years (Patient 7 in [25]).

The Older Child and Adult

After the first year, vomiting may occur periodically and be attributed
to ketosis [62], which may simulate ketogenic hypoglycemia. In the
older child and adult with HFI, fructose taken orally produces a varying response. Some patients may have severe epigastric pain, nausea,
bloating, vomiting, and even diarrhea, with or without the symptoms
specifically associated with hypoglycemia. Others, especially adults,
may have little gastrointestinal discomfort and manifest only a delayed hypoglucosemic response. Phillips et al. [63] reported proteinuria and striking changes by electron microscopy in a liver biopsy
obtained 2 hours after the ingestion of 50 gm of fructose by an adult
man with HFI. They found that "concentric and irregularly disposed
membranous arrays occurred in the glycogen areas of most hepatocytes and were associated with marked rarefaction of hyaloplasm.

Many of the membranous formations resemble cytolysomes. It is concluded that the lesions are a manifestation of focal cytoplasmic degeneration and a consequence of fructose toxicity in these patients. It is suggested that the formation of the lesions is related to the intracellular accumulation of substrates." Renal calculi [31] may be found with polyuria. Periodic or progressive weakness and paralysis [32] have also been seen in some adults.

Of interest, no severe gastrointestinal reactions, except for mild epigastric discomfort, have been observed following intravenous administration of fructose in patients with HFI. Yet the onset of hypoglucosemia is essentially at the same time as that following oral fructose [35]. Of note, epigastric pain of short duration has also occurred in 12 of 19 normal adults after 50 gm of fructose were rapidly infused intravenously within a period of 20 minutes [64].

Failure to thrive, associated with recurrent vomiting, hepatomegaly, and frequently pronounced dysfunction of the liver and the renal tubule, is characteristic of the chronic form of HFI in infancy. In contrast, older children have been reported to have subtle biochemical and clinical abnormalities. Thus, hypoglycemia is not present, while hyperuricemia and hypermagnesemia are associated with increased urinary excretion rates for uric acid and magnesium. The most evident finding is severe growth retardation which may respond dramatically with catch-up growth to rigid restriction of dietary fructose (approximately 40 mg per kilogram per day) [65].

The patients with HFI usually have excellent teeth, with a minimal number of caries [7,13,25,35]. This is especially evident when patients are compared to nonaffected siblings.

• Diagnosis

The diagnosis of HFI is dependent upon a high index of suspicion and a careful nutritional history [66]. In contrast to the infant with galactosemia (see Chapter 8), the neonate with HFI remains perfectly well on breast feedings. In the infant, the onset of anorexia, vomiting, failure to thrive, drowsiness, and coma date from the introduction of fructose into the diet. With continued fructose feeding, hepatomegaly, jaundice, hemorrhagic manifestations, ascites, edema, and regression of neuromotor function can occur. Proteinuria and aminoaciduria are common. Reducing sugars are present in the urine only following the ingestion of fructose and must be distinguished from glucosuria. Infants with HFI have been considered to have pyloric stenosis, galactosemia, hereditary tyrosinemia or "acute tyrosinosis," hemorrhagic disease of the newborn, hepatitis, congenital cirrhosis, cytomegalic inclusion disease, or toxoplasmosis.

In the symptomatic young infant, a fructose-free diet must be instituted at once as a diagnostic-therapeutic test. A low blood glucose concentration, an elevated blood fructose concentration, and fructosuria following the administration of fructose establish the diagnosis. A complete reversal of symptoms occurs when fructose is eliminated from the diet.

In the older child and adult, there is a history of symptoms only following the ingestion of fructose-containing foods, as well as a marked avoidance of sweets.

Laboratory Diagnosis of HFI

Intravenous Fructose Tolerance Test

In the asymptomatic individual, an intravenous fructose tolerance test (0.25 g/kg/5 min) will produce a fall in plasma inorganic phosphorus [5,7,25,35] and prolonged hypoglucosemia; the latter may be overlooked unless a method specific for measuring glucose alone rather than all reducing sugars is used (see p. 64) (Fig. 9-1). A rise in plasma magnesium [24,25] and uric acid [24,47] occurs as well. Because of the severe and often prolonged intestinal symptoms associated with the oral test, the intravenous test should be used in establishing the diagnosis, if at all possible. Fructosuria may be present after the tolerance test, but the amount detectable in the urine does not exceed 3–5 percent of the administered load [12].

Biopsy and Enzyme Activity Analysis

Characteristically, in liver [34,35,37–39,45], kidney [41], and intestine [40], the activity of aldolase B with fructose-1-P as substrate is markedly reduced to 0–12 percent of normal. In liver, the enzyme activity with fructose-1,6-diphosphate as substrate varies from 25–87 percent of normal. Thus, Schapira et al. [1,38,39] emphasized that the mean ratio of the activities, utilizing F-1-P and F-D-P as substrates, which in normal adult liver is 1.0 to 1.1, was 5.5 and always greater than 3 in patients with HFI, as originally reported by Hers and Joassin [34]. Since the responses to a fructose-free diet and to intravenous fructose are specific, biopsies are not necessary for clinical diagnosis but may be essential for basic biochemical investigations (see below).

Molecular Genetic Analysis

Definitive diagnosis may be made utilizing leukocytes and identifying the gene abnormality on chromosome 9 [67].

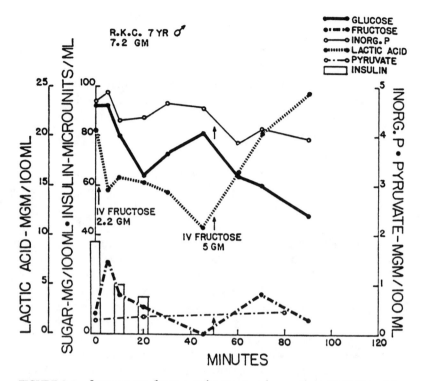

FIGURE 9-1. Intravenous fructose tolerance test in a patient (R.K.C.) with HFI, resulting in a fall in the levels of glucose, inorganic phosphorus, and insulin. Significant elevations of fructose and lactic acid levels occurred simultaneously. (Reprinted by permission of the *New England Journal of Medicine* 269;1271, 1963.)

· Therapy

Therapy is simple and consists of the total elimination of fructose and all potential sources of fructose from the diet. (See Appendixes II and III for fructose-free diet.) Strict instruction with attention to detail and to the minor manifestations of HFI must be provided for the patient and his family. For example, potatoes may be a significant source of fructose, depending upon the manner in which they are harvested, cooked, and stored [68]. If allowed to stand at room temperature for more than ten days, the fructose content diminishes significantly [68]. Certain vegetables, including broccoli, cucumber, gourds, and some brands of peas and rhubarb, contain a relatively small concentration of sucrose or fructose [69]. Obviously, each must be tested before being given to small infants. Among fruits that may contain low concentrations of fructose are avocados and some lemons.

It should be emphasized that the patient with HFI must only be given glucose when parenteral fluids are indicated. Invert sugar, sorbitol, or levulose must never be given in parenteral fluids to such a patient since each can produce profound illness and even death [19].

Intravenous glucose is given to treat the acute symptoms due to hypoglucosemia if the patient is given or inadvertently eats food containing fructose. There is no specific therapy for the intestinal manifestations. Some patients, as they become older, can tolerate small, but increasing amounts of fructose.

• Molecular Genetics

Hereditary fructose intolerance conforms to an autosomal recessive mode of inheritance [3] in almost all families reported. The exact genetic analysis of affected families is now possible with molecular genetic techniques applied to white cell DNA. Population studies with these new molecular probes are being carried out by Cross and associates [70].

Fructose-1,6-bisphosphate aldolase consists of four identical 40,000 dalton subunits in a tetrameric form. The three forms (A, B, and C) are distinguished by electrophoretic and catalytic properties. The isozymes are expressed in specific tissue patterns; thus, aldolase A is found in developing embryo and increases greatly in adult muscle. In contrast, aldolase B is dominant, while aldolase A is repressed in adult liver, kidney, and intestine. Finally, aldolase C is found equally with A in brain and nervous tissue.

In a remarkable series of observations, Cross et al. [42] identified a molecular lesion in the aldolase B gene from an affected person. They found a G → C transversion in exon 5 that creates a new recognition site for the restriction enzyme Ahall and results in an amino acid substitution (Ala → Pro) at position 149 of the protein within a region critical for substrate binding. These techniques were then used to specifically identify the genetic defects in HFI. They [70] subsequently studied 50 subjects and found the Ala → Pro in 67 percent of alleles, while another mutation (Ala 174 Asp) was found in 16 percent. A third mutation (L288 delta C) carried a single base pair deletion, causing a frame shift. Other mutations are likely.

• Pathogenesis

Before discussing the enzymatic deficiency and its secondary consequences in HFI, a simplified description of the normal metabolism of fructose is presented. As illustrated in Figure 9-2, fructose may be phosphorylated in the liver, kidney, and intestine by a specific fructokinase at the 1-position or by a nonspecific hexokinase at the 6-

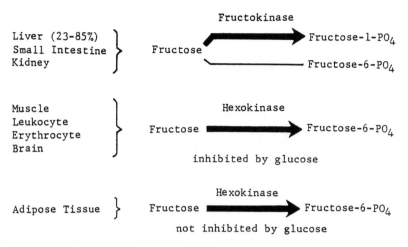

FIGURE 9-2. Normal fructose metabolism.

position. In other tissues of the body, phosphorylation of fructose occurs only at the 6-position. Glucose inhibits the phosphorylation of fructose in muscle, erythrocytes, leukocytes, and brain but not in adipose tissue [71,72]. The rapid uptake of fructose by adipose tissue is via a specific transport system that appears to operate independently of glucose or insulin [71]. Although fructose can be utilized in vitro by brain in the absence of glucose, fructose is unable to alleviate hypoglycemic manifestations in vivo because of its inability to cross the blood–brain barrier, according to Park et al. [73].

In the liver, kidney cortex, and mucosa of the small intestine, fructose-1-phosphate (F-1-P), in the presence of aldolase B, is split into the two trioses, glyceraldehyde and dihydroxyacetone phosphate, which may then enter the glycolytic cycle (Fig. 9-3). Evidence has been obtained that liver aldolase in rabbit exists in a complex formation with fructose-1,6-bisphosphatase and acts in a coordinated manner in gluconeogenesis [74].

Aldolase type B in liver both cleaves the phosphorylated hexoses F-1-P and F-1,6-diphosphate (FDP) equally and condenses the triosephosphates, glyceraldehyde phosphate and dihydroxyacetone phosphate, to FDP [75,76]. Normally, the cleaving activity ratio F-1-P/FDP is 1:2. Similar reactions occur in the mucosa of the small intestine and in the cortex of the kidney [30]. In contrast, aldolase type A or muscle type has a low affinity for F-1-P, while aldolase type C has an intermediate one.

Fructose-6-phosphate can be converted to glucose-6-phosphate by glucose phosphate isomerase or by being phosphorylated again by phosphofructokinase and ATP to FDP in the pathway common to the catabolism of glucose, galactose, and glycogen (Fig. 9-3). The FDP is also split to dihydroxyacetone phosphate and glyceraldehyde phosphate by aldolase B. FDP aldolase activity is diminished to a significantly lesser degree than that of F-1-P aldolase so that the activity ratio against the specific substrates exceeds 5.0.

The aldolases have been isolated from diverse tissues and characterized biochemically and immunologically. Enzyme activity has been studied, as has genetic material. In studies in the rat, mRNA specific for aldolase B has been shown to vary with starvation and intake of carbohydrate. In vivo regulation of the aldolase B gene expression differs strongly in the liver, kidney, and small intestine [77]. In the liver, the synthesis of the mRNA requires the presence of dietary carbohydrates, the cessation of glucagon release, and the presence of permissive hormones, including insulin for glucose- and maltose-fed

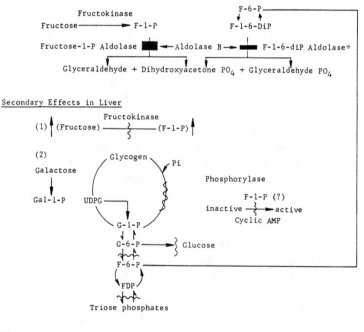

FIGURE 9-3. Hereditary fructose intolerance showing primary and secondary abnormalities.

rats, but excluding it for fructose-fed animals. In the small intestine, the presence of both dietary carbohydrates and insulin (for maltose-fed rats) is required, but glucagon and cAMP are devoid of any effect. In the kidney, the synthesis of the mRNA is constitutive, poorly modulated by the diet, and unaffected by hormonal status.

The complete amino acid sequence for human aldolase B was derived from cDNA and genomic clones [78]. The amino acid and nucleotide sequences of aldolase were found to be strongly conserved even between different isozymes.

All the evidence supports the concept that the primary enzymatic deficiency in HFI is a marked reduction in the activity of aldolase B in hepatic parenchymal cells [1,34,35,37] and also in the cells of the intestinal villi [7,40] and renal cortex [30] (Fig. 9-3). As a result of the enzyme deficiency, fructose-1-phosphate is not cleaved and accumulates in the liver, kidney, and intestine. The FDP is split by the aldolase A and aldolase C that have been shown to be present in livers from patients with HFI [38,45]. The abnormality involves the structural gene for aldolase B.

The genetically distinct cytosolic isoenzyme, aldolase B, expressed exclusively in liver, kidney, and intestine was investigated in three affected individuals from a nonconsanguineous kindred by Cox and associates [79]. The molecular basis of the enzymic defect was evaluated by diverse techniques, including: affinity chromatography, immunodiffusion gels, immunoaffinity chromatography, radioimmunoassay, and electrofocussing. They concluded that there is synthesis of an immunoreactive, but functionally and structurally modified enzyme variant that results from a restricted genetic mutation.

They further noted that the catalytic properties of the enzyme were profoundly modified in terms of both substrate affinity and absolute specific activity. Apparent specific activity for F-1-P cleavage was estimated to be reduced by almost an order of magnitude by radioimmunoassay and 100-fold by direct chemical assay. The enzyme determinations presented suggested that aldolase B in HFI has a very high FDP/F-1-P activity ratio and that the residual F-1-P aldolase activity in tissues is almost entirely accounted for by the presence of interfering amounts of isoenzymes A and C. In contrast, approximately one-half of the liver FDP aldolase in HFI is due to the presence of modified aldolase B.

As a consequence of the basic enzymatic deficiency, a series of metabolic events occurs following the administration of fructose to a patient with HFI. Some are due to the accumulation of F-1-P with the sequestering of inorganic phosphate (P_i) leading to intracellular deficiencies of both P_i and ATP. Others are the result of secondary inhibitions of critical steps in glycolysis, glycogenolysis, gluconeogenesis, and other homeostatic mechanisms within the cell that result in hypoglucosemia and acidosis.

Oberhaensli et al. [80] have observed an increase in sugar phosphates and decrease in inorganic phosphate in the liver of patients with hereditary fructose intolerance given small amounts of fructose before study by ^{31}P magnetic resonance spectroscopy.

As F-1-P accumulates in the cell, there is an inhibition of fructokinase [3,35], accounting for the high blood levels of fructose. Ultimately, 80–90 percent of the fructose is utilized, probably in the adipose tissue [35]. The mechanisms of the gastrointestinal symptoms remain obscure, although the accumulation of fructose-1-phosphate in the brush border of the small intestine may be responsible.

With the rise in blood fructose concentration (Fig. 9-1), there is a fall in P_i and an elevation of Mg^{++} that suggest a significant depletion, even if temporary, of intracellular ATP and P_i. As a consequence, there is an increased degradation of AMP to inosine 5'-phosphate and uric acid [81]; the latter increases in both plasma and urine [5,24]. Blood lactate concentration is also increased as a result of multiple interactions that include (1) competition for excretion with uric acid, (2) a secondary reaction to the renal tubular acidosis [28–32,42,82], and (3) secretion of epinephrine [5]. The elevations noted in free fatty acids (FFA) appear to be secondary to the hypoglucosemia, insulinopenia, and hepatocellular dysfunction. It is noteworthy that, although the elevation in lactate levels was not blocked, that of FFA was blocked by the simultaneous administration of glucose and fructose [5].

The exact metabolic defects responsible for the low levels of blood glucose are being elucidated. The data indicate that the hypoglucosemia results from a block in hepatic glucose output due to the secondary inhibition of both glycogenolysis and gluconeogenesis and not from an increase in the peripheral utilization of glucose. Two studies support the concept of a block in hepatic glucose output. First, Dubois et al. [14] demonstrated a decreased rate of disappearance of intravenous glucose administered after fructose. In addition, the slope of the decline in specific activity of radioactive glucose given intravenously diminished significantly after fructose administration, indicating that dilution of the glucose pool by nonlabeled hepatic glucose was markedly reduced. Second, whereas the patient with HFI responds to glucagon with a significant hyperglycemia when he is either fasting or at the end of a glucose tolerance test, he does not show a hyperglycemic response to glucagon after the ingestion of fructose [12,13,35] (Fig. 9-4). Additional evidence against an increased utilization of glucose is a lack of change or actual fall in the level of

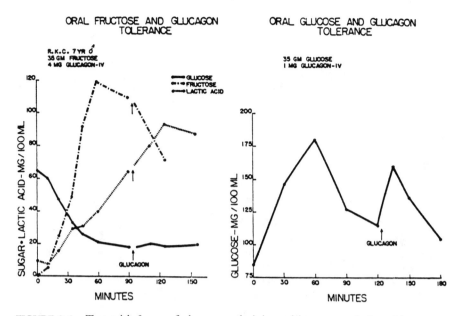

FIGURE 9-4. Test with 1 mg of glucagon administered intravenously in subject R.K.C., resulting in no elevation in the blood level of glucose 90 minutes after fructose given by mouth. However, 2 hours after the ingestion of glucose, 1 mg of glucagon produced significant hyperglycemia. (Reprinted by permission of the *New England Journal of Medicine* 269;1271, 1963.)

plasma insulin as measured by immunoassay after fructose [13,35,83] (see Fig. 9-1).

The site of the secondary enzymatic blocks in the liver responsible for the hypoglucosemia has also been investigated. In studies in vitro, F-1-P inhibited phosphoglucomutase [84]. However, the increase in the level of blood glucose after intravenous galactose indicates that the secondary block in glucose output is not due to the inhibition of phosphoglucomutase or glucose-6-phosphatase [13,48] (Fig. 9-5) or to the depletion of ATP. In addition, Hers [85] and others [25,55] have reported an increase in glucose-6-phosphatase activity in HFI livers. Therefore, it would appear that the increased fructose-1-phosphate and the deficiency in P_i inhibit glycogenolysis at the activation or action of phosphorylase. Fructose-1-phosphate, in the presence of low concentrations of P_i, competitively inhibits phosphorylase a activity [86–88], thus explaining the block in glycogenolysis. Of interest, an infusion of sodium phosphates sufficient to maintain normal plasma levels of P_i given with fructose does not prevent hypoglucosemia in patients with HFI [5,52].

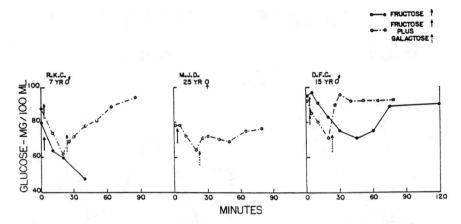

FIGURE 9-5. Intravenous administration of galactose in three patients with hereditary fructose intolerance, producing a prompt rise in the level of blood glucose previously depressed by intravenously infused fructose. The duration of the hypoglycemia was shortened after galactose administration, as compared with that after fructose alone. (Reprinted by permission of the *New England Journal of Medicine* 269;1271, 1963.)

An inhibition of hepatic gluconeogenesis contributes to the hypoglucosemia as well. Neither dihydroxyacetone phosphate nor glycerol can correct the hypoglucosemia following fructose [48]. Thus, the block in gluconeogenesis could be present between the triose condensing activity of aldolase B and the formation of glucose-6-phosphate. Apparently, there is a secondary inhibition of both glucose phosphate isomerase [89] and the triosephosphate condensing activity of aldolase B [90] by F-1-P. In addition, the condensing activity is further affected by adenosine 5-phosphate [90]. Although the inhibition of the aldolase may be more complete, that of the glucose phosphate isomerase is not without clinical significance. Using trace quantities of fructose-6-^{14}C and lactate-1-^{14}C, Landau et al. [91] found that 12–20 percent of a fructose load is phosphorylated to fructose-6-phosphate in patients with HFI, whereas none was metabolized via this pathway in normal controls. Thus, glucose phosphate isomerase would be critical in converting this intermediate to glucose. In conclusion, both the inhibition in glycogenolysis and gluconeogenesis effectively shut down hepatic glucose output after fructose administration in patients with HFI. The rate of onset of hypoglucosemia, which appears to be more rapid in younger patients, is the result of the degree of block in hepatic glucose output plus the rate of peripheral utilization.

Morris and associates [28,29,41] found extensive renal abnormalities following the administration of oral or intravenous fructose in subjects with HFI. These abnormalities included a variety of tubular defects, e.g., impaired reabsorption of phosphate, amino acid, glucose, and uric acid, indicating a complex dysfunction of the proximal renal tubule. In addition, they noted an acidification defect in which a decrease in proximal tubular reabsorption of bicarbonate exceeded 15 percent at normal plasma bicarbonate concentrations. During mild hyperchloremic acidosis associated with the administration of ammonium chloride and at plasma bicarbonate concentrations of 18–20 mEq/liter, urinary pH exceeded 6.0, and urinary excretion of net acid (titratable acid and ammonium ion minus bicarbonate) was inappropriately low for the degree of acidosis.

Glomerular filtration rate was not affected. Titratable acid excretion was increased by infused phosphate, but urinary pH remained elevated. When plasma bicarbonate was decreased to less than 14 mEq/liter, urinary pH was reduced to less than 5, and excretion rates of titratable acid and ammonium were not reduced. These observations indicate that a hydrogen ion gradient can be normally developed in the distal tubule and that net acid excretion can be maintained, provided that there is not an excess of bicarbonate in early distal tubular fluid. The primary acidification defect appears to be a limitation of proximal bicarbonate reabsorption so that excessive bicarbonate remains in the tubular fluid reaching the distal acidification site. The secretion of distal H^+ is insufficient to titrate this bicarbonate, so that there is a high urinary pH, bicarbonate wasting, and limited net hydrogen excretion unless severe acidosis occurs.

In later studies, Morris noted that parathyroid function was a modulating factor [82]. In a patient with HFI and hypoparathyroidism, fructose administration did not induce bicarbonate wasting until parathormone was administered. The biochemical mechanism(s) involved are unclear, but they may involve renal adenylyl cyclase in some indirect manner.

Enzyme studies of tissues that metabolize fructose have indicated differences between kidney cortex and medulla [30]. Fructokinase and triokinase are present in cortex but absent from medulla. Aldolase B was present in high concentration in medulla. In contrast, aldolase A was present in both areas of the kidney. The ratio of aldolase A-to-B activity was high in medulla (approximately 20:1). These observations support the hypothesis that the tubular defect in HFI is proximal and related to an accumulation of fructose-1-phosphate in tubular cells. They also are consistent with the suggestion that gluconeogenesis in the kidney occurs primarily in the cortex.

Thus, the patient with HFI manifests a wide variety of metabolic aberrations when given fructose. Additional investigations of these various parameters in patients with this congenital enzymatic defect may elucidate fundamental mechanisms in carbohydrate metabolism.

• Benign or Essential Fructosuria

Essential fructosuria, a relatively rare disorder of metabolism, has been estimated to occur in 1:130,000 of the general population. This condition is considered to be inherited as an autosomal recessive trait [92]. Since the patient is asymptomatic and the condition is harmless, the actual incidence may be higher. The primary enzymatic disorder is a deficiency of the enzyme fructokinase (1) (Fig. 9-2, reaction 1) that results in abnormally elevated levels of fructose in the blood, leading to fructosuria. In contrast to those with HFI, the patients with essential fructosuria are well and have no clinical disease.

• Fructose-1,6-Diphosphatase Deficiency

Fructose-1,6-diphosphatase deficiency [4], an enzymatic cause of fasting hypoglucosemia and metabolic acidosis with an increased anion gap, is associated with hepatomegaly, but no aversion for sweet-tasting foods. Hypoglycemia with a fall in serum inorganic phosphate follows an oral fructose tolerance test in these patients. Liver failure and the acute gastrointestinal clinical manifestations of the patient with HFI do not occur (see Chapters 7 and 10).

Case Report (Patient 9-1): An Infant with HFI Diagnosed Following the Intake of Unsweetened Apple Juice at 8 Weeks of Age

A female infant was born on January 20, 1980 after an unremarkable, full-term pregnancy. Delivery was vaginal breech with nuchal cord. Apgar scores were 3 at 1 min, 8 at 5 min and 10 at 10 min. Her weight was 7 lb, 7 oz (3.37 kg) and length 20 in (50.8 cm). Her examination was normal, and she required no special care. At 6 weeks of age, at a routine pediatric well baby visit, she was vaccinated for diptheria-pertussis-tetanus (DPT) and polio vaccine live oral (OPV) uneventfully. She had been taking Enfamil, 4 oz every 3–4 hours, and had a small supplement of cereals.

On the evening of admission (March 30, 1980) at 8 weeks of age, she was given 4 oz (120 ml) of apple juice for the first time. Within 1 hour she "fell asleep," became pale, and diaphoretic. When she was unarousable, she was taken by ambulance to the local hospital. Initial laboratory studies indicated a blood glucose of 24 mg/dl (1.33 mM), blood urea nitrogen (BUN) 11 mg/dl, sodium 138, chloride 104, potassium 3.6 mEq/L, and CO_2 14 mM/L. She was given 10 percent dextrose intravenously and became responsive. A lumbar puncture revealed no cells, a protein value of 26 mg/dl, and a glucose concentration of 25 mg/dl (1.39 mM). The gram stain was negative. White blood cell count was 6,900/mm³ with 22 segmented forms, 4 bands, 73 lymphocytes, and 1 eosinophil. Blood cultures, obtained on two occasions, showed no growth. The patient was transferred to the Rhode Island Hospital, with intravenous 20 percent dextrose being administered at the rate of 20 ml/hr (12.8 mg/kg/min). It is noteworthy that the apple juice did not have added sugar or sweeteners.

Family history indicated that the mother (5 ft, 0 in) and father (5 ft, 7 in) were both 33 years of age. There were no known metabolic disturbances on either side of the family. Subsequently, their second child, a son, was normal after a controlled challenge with fructose.

On physical examination, her temperature was 96.8°F, pulse 124/min, respirations 60/min with crying, and a systolic blood pressure 114 mmHg. Weight was 11 lb, 8 oz (5.2 kg) (75th percentile), length was 61 cm (95th percentile), and head circumference was 38.5 cm (50th percentile). Physical examination was unremarkable except for the liver which was definitely enlarged at 4 cm below the costal margin, smooth, and nontender.

The baby was given maintenance intravenous dextrose, 10 percent in 0.2 normal saline at 85 cc/kg/day (6 mg/kg/min). The blood glucose levels stabilized between 90–100 mg/dl (5–5.6 mM). The urines were negative for glucose, reducing sugars, and ketones throughout. The chemistries on admission were plasma glucose concentration of 405 mg/dl (22.5 mM) (post-therapy), BUN 14 mg/dl, creatinine 0.7 mg/dl, sodium 137, chloride 106, potassium 5.3 mEq/L, CO_2 13 mM/L, and serum calcium was 10.7 mg/dl. The initial impression was sepsis.

The next day, serum sodium concentration was 139, chloride 110, potassium 4.3 mEq/L, and CO_2 20 mM/L. The uric acid was noted to be 4.4 mg/dl. The history of the unsweetened apple juice was obtained from the mother. The initial differential diagnoses for hepatomegaly with an anion gap acidosis and hypoglycemia included: type I glycogen storage disease, fructose 1, 6 diphosphatase deficiency, hereditary fructose intolerance, galactosemia, possible insulinoma, possible hypothyroidism, and possible hypoadrenalism. The initial SGOT was 70 IU. The baby had an intravenous glucagon tolerance test (0.15 mg glucagon) which showed a prompt rise in glucose levels from a normal fasting of 85 mg/dl (4.7 mM) to 108 mg/dl (6.0 mM) at 15 minutes. Hereditary fructose intolerance was postulated. The baby was given fructose, 1.75 gm/kg orally as a 15 percent fructose solution, a dose estimated to be comparable to 4 oz of apple juice (Fig. 9-6). Within 50 minutes, the baby became diaphoretic, tachypneic to 70–80 breaths/min, and less responsive. The CO_2 fell from 20 to 15 mM/L and the glucose concentration from 84 to 25 mg/dl (4.7 to 1.4 mM). The baby also vomited part of the initial fructose feed, had borborygmi and flatulence. The study was aborted promptly, with intravenous dextrose via an indwelling peripheral venous catheter already in place. Urinary amino acids were unremarkable.

She was discharged with dietary advice, i.e., a fructose- and sucrose-free diet. At follow-up, her weights gradually declined across growth grids, but remained at the 25th percentile; in contrast, length (height) fell to below the 5th percentile by age 3½ years. Growth at age 9 years is 6.7 cm/yr (Fig. 9-7). She is a bright girl and participates in dancing and soccer. She handles minor illnesses well. She remains both clinically and biochemically normal.

At age 6 years, she was with her family at a fast-food restaurant. Her food was delayed, and she was extremely hungry. The tray contained her diet

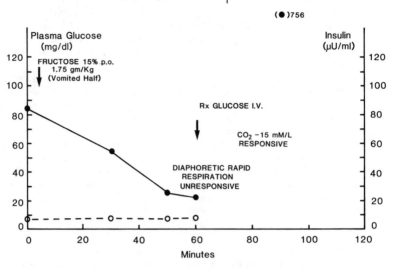

FIGURE 9-6. Hypoglycemic response (Patient 9-1) to oral fructose equivalent to the amount in the unsweetened apple juice that produced the initial symptomatic hypoglycemia at age 2 months. Note the rapidity of the response.

coke alongside her brother's regular coke. She inadvertently consumed the entire *regular* coke. She shortly vomited, became groggy, lethargic, and fell asleep. She was brought to the emergency room at the Rhode Island Hospital where the parents advised strongly that she receive intravenous dextrose. She is noted to have a strong aversion for sugar and most sweet foods.

Leukocytes harvested in August 1989 were studied by Dean Tolan. Using the polymerase chain reaction, he identified the nucleotide defect (noted above) which results in a specific amino acid substitution (Ala → Pro) in the aldolase B protein.

Comment

This infant represents a case of acute onset of hereditary fructose intolerance. She had two significant hypoglycemic episodes in the first 6 years of life. Her short stature may be in part genetic. Her intellectual development has been unaffected by either the hypoglycemic episodes or the dietary restrictions.

Case Report (Patient 9-2): A Male with HFI, Illustrating the Difficulty of Making a Diagnosis

A male AGA infant was born at 36 weeks' gestation, weighing 4 lb, 13 oz (2.36 kg) to unrelated parents. He initially lost approximately 8 percent of

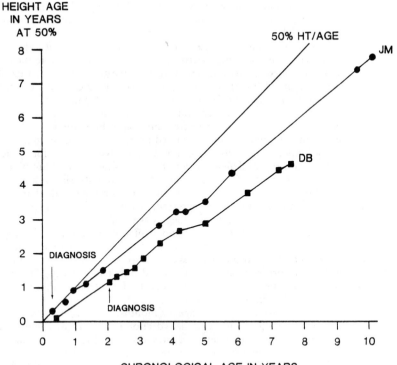

FIGURE 9-7.   Delayed growth in height in both Patients 9-1 and 9-2 even with fructose restriction.

his birth weight, to 4 lb, 7 oz, and was discharged at age 2 weeks at a weight of 4 lb, 11 oz.

Enfamil formula feedings were tolerated well until approximately three months of age. At 3 months old, he was admitted to the Rhode Island Hospital because of projectile vomiting shortly after most of his daily feedings. Stool frequency had decreased. He did not have fever at home. The patient's mother later recalled that she had tried to introduce fruit juices into the patient's diet at about this age. He would vomit shortly after virtually every fruit juice feeding.

On admission at 3 months, his weight was 9 lb, 2 oz (4.14 Kg), length 21½ in (54.6 cm), and head circumference 38 cm. All measurements were just below the 5th percentile for age. He had signs of mild dehydration. No abdominal masses were palpable. Barium swallow and upper GI radiologic procedures did not reveal any abnormalities. Admission studies revealed the following serum concentrations: glucose 72 mg/dl (4 mM), Na 140 mEq/L, K 5.1 mEq/L, Cl 104 mEq/L, CO_2 20 mM/L. A urinalysis obtained at the time of admission had a pH of 8, with no protein, glucose, or ketones detected. Total reducing substances were also negative. He was discharged with the impression that he had a minor gastroesophageal reflux.

At 4½ months of age, he was admitted to a Florida hospital for vomiting and diarrhea. Chest and upper GI series radiographs revealed no abnormalities. No definitive diagnosis was given.

He was hospitalized again at age 4¾ months at the Rhode Island Hospital. Persistent vomiting, diarrhea, and failure to thrive were the reasons for admission. Growth parameters were now weight of 9 lbs, 14 oz (4.48 kg), length 22 in (55.9 cm), and head circumference 39 cm. All were proportionate, but well below the 5th percentile for age. Hepatomegaly was noted for the first time. Serum concentrations of glucose, electrolytes, total protein, albumin, blood urea nitrogen, creatinine, and thyroxine were all within normal limits. A urine sample contained no traces of protein, glucose, ketones, occult blood, or total reducing substances. Screening tests for cystic fibrosis, alpha-1 antitrypsin deficiency, and hepatitis showed no abnormalities. However, SGOT and SGPT were elevated to 194 and 90 IU/L, respectively. Total and direct bilirubin levels were normal. By the time of discharge, his hepatomegaly appeared to have regressed. A tentative diagnosis of viral-induced vomiting, diarrhea, and hepatomegaly was made.

Over the ensuing months, the patient vomited consistently after feedings of fruit juice, applesauce, or other fruit products. Eventually, he refused to eat fruits and fruit products, as well as sweets. The mother tried to tell several health care professionals that her child didn't like sweets. She was usually told that she must be operating under a misconception, that no child didn't like or would refuse to eat sweets.

In February of 1984, at age 19 months, he was hospitalized in Boston, Massachusetts, for mild acute dehydration secondary to vomiting and diarrhea. Slow growth parameters, a microcytic and hypochromic anemia, and a liver edge palpable 2 cm below the right costal margin were noted. The patient's failure to thrive was attributed to poor caloric intake. Feeding difficulties secondary to poor maternal–child relationship were postulated. An extensive psychosocial workup was undertaken based on this premise.

The patient's next admission was at the Rhode Island Hospital in August of 1984. He was 25 months old. The purpose of the admission was to evaluate his persistent failure to thrive and hepatosplenomegaly. His growth parameters were now even further below the 5th percentile than on previous measurements: weight 18 lb, 13 oz (8.53 kg), length 30.3 inches (77 cm). His liver edge was palpable 3–4 cm below the right costal margin, and a spleen tip was also palpable. His CBC revealed a microcytic, hypochromic anemia with the following values: hematocrit 29.8 percent, hemoglobin 10.2 gm/dl, MCV 68 fl, MCH 23.4 pg. A urine sample contained elevated concentrations of several different acidic and neutral amino acids. Greater than two-fold elevations of concentrations for hydroxyproline, proline, valine, and leucine were found.

A careful nutritional history taken by the metabolism fellow and nutritionist independently revealed the previously ignored aversion to sweets.

An oral fructose tolerance test (1.2 gm/kg) produced classical changes in concentrations of plasma glucose, whole blood lactate, serum uric acid, and serum inorganic phosphorous that occur in hereditary fructose intolerance (Fig. 9-8). Within 45 minutes, concentrations of plasma glucose fell from 62 mg/dl to 25 mg/dl (3.6 to 1.4 mM), blood lactate rose from 9.8 mg/dl to 41.2 mg/dl, plasma phosphate fell from 4.6 mg/dl to 3.9 mg/dl, plasma uric acid rose from 6.3 mg/dl to 12.6 mg/dl, and plasma magnesium rose from 1.9 mg/

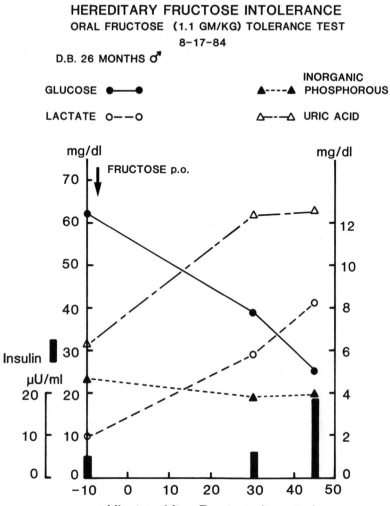

HEREDITARY FRUCTOSE INTOLERANCE
ORAL FRUCTOSE (1.1 GM/KG) TOLERANCE TEST
8-17-84

D.B. 26 MONTHS ♂

GLUCOSE ●——●

LACTATE ○——○

INORGANIC
▲----▲ PHOSPHOROUS

△—·—△ URIC ACID

FIGURE 9-8. Hypoglycemic response to oral fructose in a previously undiagnosed boy (Patient 9-2) with unrecognized prior hypoglycemic episodes.

dl to 2.4 mg/dl. By 30 minutes, he was pale, cool, diaphoretic, and sleepy. By 45 minutes, he was pale, "cold and clammy," lethargic, and difficult to arouse. The parents then recognized these signs and symptoms as similar to those he had had on several previous occasions. The test was terminated by intravenous dextrose via an indwelling catheter inserted previously. He responded promptly.

The family was instructed in the use of a fructose-restricted diet. No further symptoms occurred. He has continued to grow slowly. At 7⁷/₁₂ years, his height is below the 3rd percentile (equivalent to a 4½-year-old at the 50th percentile); weight is also below the 5th percentile (equivalent to a 3³/₁₂-year-old at the 50th percentile). His height growth is 4.6 cm/yr (Fig. 9-7). Both parents are under 5 ft tall.

Leukocytes were obtained for molecular genetic studies in August 1989. To date, the defect has not been detected by Dean Tolan (Boston University).

Comment

A careful nutritional history is the cornerstone for diagnosis in several inherited metabolic diseases, of which hereditary fructose intolerance is preeminent. His diagnosis was presumably delayed because of unfamiliarity with a rare disease. In contrast to Patient 9-1, the absence of the signs and symptoms of hypoglycemia further complicated diagnosis. This child represents chronic HFI with growth delay. His later course has been complicated in that he failed to show catch-up growth after dietary therapy and no explanation has been found. His recent electrolytes and urinary amino acids were normal.

This case history clearly emphasizes the importance of listening carefully to parents.

• Summary

Hereditary fructose intolerance, a relatively new metabolic disorder, has been estimated to occur in 1:20,000 persons, with a worldwide distribution. The defect in HFI appears to be a marked reduction in the activity of aldolase B in liver, kidney, and intestine, resulting in epigastric pain, bloating, nausea, and vomiting after the ingestion of fructose, and severe hypoglucosemia with its concomitant drowsiness, coma, and convulsions as a result of a secondary block in hepatic glucose output. A careful history makes the presence of this condition self-evident, and appropriate carbohydrate tolerance tests confirm the diagnosis.

If unrecognized in early infancy, hereditary fructose intolerance can be responsible for severe failure to thrive, protracted vomiting, hepatomegaly, stunted growth and development, liver failure, and, ultimately, death. Therefore, since all of these complications are reversible with removal of fructose from the diet, it is critical that the diagnosis be made and therapy instituted promptly in young infants. Thus, in reporting the death of a 3-year-old girl following intravenous fructose given postoperatively, Danks, Connellan, and Solomon [19] emphasized that "this case serves as a tragic reminder that the rarity of a disease is little consolation to those who suffer from it."

REFERENCES

1. SCHAPIRA F, SCHAPIRA G, DREYFUS JC. La lesion enzymatique de la fructosurie benigne. *Enzymol Biol Clin.* 1962;1:170.
2. CHAMBERS RA, PRATT YTC. Idiosyncrasy to fructose. *Lancet.* 1956;2:340.
3. FROESCH ER, PRADER A, LABHART R, STUBER HW, WOLF HP. Die hereditare Fructoseintoleranz, eine bisher nicht bekannte kongenitale Stoffwechselstorung. *Schweiz Med Wochenschr.* 1957;87:1168.
4. BAKER L, WINEGRAD AL. Fasting hypoglycemia and metabolic acidosis associated with deficiency of hepatic fructose-1,6-diphosphatase activity. *Lancet.* 1970;2:13.
5. PERHEENTUPA J, RAIVIO KO, NIKKILA EA. Hereditary fructose intolerance. *Acta Med Scand (Suppl.).* 1972;542:65.
6. NIKKILA EA, HUTTUNEN JK. Clinical and metabolic aspects of fructose. *Acta Med Scand (Suppl.).* 1972;542:1.
7. FROESCH ER. Essential fructosuria and hereditary fructose intolerance. In: Stanbury JB, Wyngaarden JB, Fredricks DS, eds. *The Metabolic Basis of Inherited Disease, 2nd ed.* New York: McGraw-Hill Book Co, 1972;131.
8. GITZELMANN R, STEINMANN B, VAN DEN BERGHE G. Disorders of fructose metabolism. In: Scriver CR, Beaudet AL, Sly WS, Valle D, eds. *Metabolic Basis for Inherited Disease, 6th ed.* New York: McGraw-Hill Book Co, 1989;399.
9. JEUNE M, PLANSON E, COTTE J, BONNEFOY S, NIVELON JL, SKOSOWSKY J. L'intolerance hereditaire au fructose. *Pediatrie.* 1961;16:605.
10. LELONG M, ALAGILLE D, GENTIL J, COLIN J, TUPIN J, BOUQUIER J. Cirrhose hepatique et tubulopathie par absence congenitale de l'aldolase hepatique. *Bull Mem Soc Med Hop Paris.* 1962;113:58.
11. LELONG M, ALAGILLE D, GENTIL J, et al. L'intolerance hereditaire au fructose. *Arch Fr Pediatr.* 1962;19:841.
12. PERHEENTUPA J, PITKANEN E, NIKKILA EA, SOMERSALO O, HAKOSALO J. Hereditary fructose intolerance. A clinical study of four cases. *Ann Paediatr Fenn.* 1962;8:221.
13. CORNBLATH M, ROSENTHAL IM, REISNER SH, WYBREGT SH, CRANE RK. Hereditary fructose intolerance. *N Engl J Med.* 1963;269:1271.
14. DUBOIS R, LOEB H, OOMS HA, GILLET P, BARTMAN M, CHAMPENOIS A. Etude, d'un cas d'hypoglycemie fonctionelle par intolerance au fructose. *Helvet Paediatr Acta.* 1961;16:90.
15. WOLFE H, ZSCHOCKE E, WEDEMEYER FW, HUBNER W. Angeborene hereditaire Fructose-intoleranze. *Klin Wochenschr.* 1959;37:693.
16. CORSINI F. L'intolleranza congenita al fruttosio. *Clin Pediatr (Bologna).* 1960;42:716.
17. DOHERTY RA, WILLIAMS HE, FIELD RA. Hereditary fructose intolerance. *J Pediatr.* 1963;63:721. (Abstract.)
18. LINDEMANN R, GJESSING LR, MERTON B, HALVORSEN S. Amino acid metabolism in hereditary fructosemia. *Acta Paediatr Scand.* 1970;59:141.
19. DANKS DM, CONNELLAN JM, SOLOMON JR. Hereditary fructose intolerance: Report of a case and comments on the hazards of fructose infusion. *Aust Paediatr J.* 1972;8:282.
20. KOHLIN P, MELIN D. Hereditary fructose intolerance in four Swedish families. *Acta Paediatr Scand.* 1968;57:24.

21. BAERLOCHER K, GITZELMANN R, STEINMANN B. Clinical and genetic studies of disorders in fructose metabolism. In: Burman D, Holton JB, Pennock CA, eds. *Inherited Disorders of Carbohydrate Metabolism.* Lancaster: MTP Press Ltd, 1980;163.

22. STEINITZ H, MIZRAHY O. Essential fructosuria and hereditary fructose intolerance. *N Engl J Med.* 1969;280:222. (Letter to the Editor.)

23. GITZELMANN R, BAERLOCHER K. Vorteile und nachteile der fructose in der nahrung. *Padiat Forbildiung Praxis.* 1973;37:40.

24. STEINMAN B, BAERLOCHER K, GITZELMANN R. Hereditare stoerungen des fruktosestoffwechsels: Belastungproben mit Fruktose, Sorbitol und Dihydroxyaceton. *Nutr Metab.* 1975;18 (Suppl 1):115.

25. LEVIN B, SNODGRASS GJAI, OBERHOLZER VG, BURGESS EA, DOBBS RH. Fructosaemia. *Am J Med.* 1968;45:826.

26. RENNERT OM, GREER M. Hereditary fructosemia. *Neurology.* 1970;20:421.

27. CAIN AAR, RYMAN BE. High liver glycogen in hereditary fructose intolerance. *Gut.* 1971;12:929.

28. MORRIS RC JR. An experimental renal acidification defect in patients with hereditary fructose intolerance. II. Its distinction from classic renal tubular acidosis, its resemblance to the renal acidification defect associated with the Fanconi syndrome of children with cystinosis. *J Clin Invest.* 1968;47:1648.

29. MORRIS RC JR. Renal tubular acidosis. *N Engl J Med.* 1969;281:1405.

30. KRANHOLD JF, LOH D, MORRIS RCJ. Renal fructose metabolizing enzymes: significance in hereditary fructose intolerance. *Science.* 1969;165:402.

31. HIGGINS RB, VARNEY JK. Dissolution of renal calculi in a case of hereditary fructose intolerance and renal tubular acidosis. *J Urol.* 1966;95:291.

32. MASS RE, SMITH WR, WALSH JR. The association of hereditary fructose intolerance and renal tubular acidosis. *Am J Med Sci.* 1966;251:516.

33. PENHOET E, RAJKUMAR R, RUTTER WJ. Multiple forms of fructose diphosphate aldolase in mammalian tissue. *Proc Natl Acad Sci USA.* 1966;56:1275.

34. HERS HG, JOASSIN G. Anomalie de l'aldolase hepatique dans l'intolerance au fructose. *Enzymol Biol Clin.* 1961;1:4.

35. FROESCH ER, WOLFE HP, BAITSCH H, PRADER A, LABHART A. Hereditary fructose intolerance. An inborn defect of hepatic fructose-1-phosphate splitting aldolase. *Am J Med.* 1963;34:151.

36. METAIS P, JUIF J, SACREZ R. Etude biochemique d'un cas d'intolerance hereditaire au fructose. *Ann Biol Clin.* 1962;20:801.

37. NIKKILA EA, SOMERSALO O, PITKANEN E, PERHEENTUPA J. Hereditary fructose intolerance, an inborn deficiency of liver aldolase complex. *Metabolism.* 1962;11:727.

38. SCHAPIRA F, DREYFUS JC. L'aldolase hepatique dans l'intolerance au fructose. *Rev Fr Etud Clin Biol.* 1967;12:486.

39. SCHAPIRA F, NORDMANN Y, GREGORI C. Hereditary alterations of fructose metabolizing enzymes. *Acta Med Scand (Suppl).* 1972;542:77.

40. NISELL J, LINDEN L. Fructose-1-phosphate aldolase and fructose-1,6-diphosphate aldolase in the mucosa of the intestine in hereditary fructose intolerance. *Scand J Gastroenterol.* 1968;3:80.

41. MORRIS RC JR, EUKI I, LOH D, EANES RZ, MCLIN P. Absence of renal fructose-1-phosphate aldolase activity in hereditary fructose intolerance. *Nature (London).* 1967;214:920.

42. CROSS NCP, TOLAN DR, COX TM. Catalytic deficiency of human aldolase B in hereditary fructose intolerance caused by a common missense mutation. *Cell.* 1988;53:881.

43. SCHAPIRA F, NORDMANN Y, DREYFUS JC. La lesion biochimique de l'intolerance au fructose. Detection immunologieque d'une aldolase modifiee. *Rev Fr Etud Clin Biol.* 1968;13:267.

44. SCHAPIRA R, HATZFELD A, GREGORI C. Studies on liver aldolases in hereditary fructose intolerance. *Enzyme.* 1974;18:73.

45. GITZELMANN R, STEINMANN B, BALLY C, LEBHERZ HC. Antibody activation of mutant human fructose diphosphate aldolase B in liver extracts of patients with hereditary fructose intolerance. *Biochem Biophys Res Comm.* 1974;59:1270.

46. SCHAPIRA F. Kinetic and immunological abnormalities of aldolase B in hereditary fructose intolerance. *Proc Biochem Soc.* March 1975; *Abstracts of Communications.* 1975;3:232.

47. PERHEENTUPA J, RAIVIO K. Fructose-induced hyperuricaemia. *Lancet.* 1967;2:528.

48. GENTIL C, COLIN J, VALETTE AM, ALAGILLE D, LELONG M. Etude du metabolisme glucidique au cours de l'intolerance hereditaire au fructose. Essai d'interpretation de l'hypoglucosemie. *Rev Fr Etud Clin Biol.* 1964;9:596.

49. ENDRES W, SIERCK T, SHIN YS. Clinical course of hereditary fructose intolerance in 56 patients. *Acta Paediatr Jpn.* 1988;30:452.

50. ODIEVRE M, GENTIL C, GAUTIER M, ALAGILLE D. Hereditary fructose intolerance in childhood. *Am J Dis Child.* 1978;132:605.

51. LEVIN B, OBERHOLZER VG, SNODGRASS GJAI, STIMMLER L, WILMERS MJ. Fructosaemia, an inborn error of fructose metabolism. *Arch Dis Child.* 1963;38:220.

52. DESBUQUOIS B, LARDINOIS R, GENTIL C, ODIEVRE M. Effets d'une surcharge en phosphate de sodium sur l'hypoglucosemie. *Arch Fr Pediatr.* 1969;26:21.

53. GRANT DB, ALLEXANDER FW, SEAKINS JWT. Abnormal tyrosine metabolism in hereditary fructose intolerance. *Acta Paediatr Scand.* 1970;59:432.

54. WILLEMS C, HEUSDEN A, RENSON P, LEGAT C, MONARD Y, STAINER L. Hypertyrosinemie avec hypermethioninemie neonatale dans un cas d'intolerance au fructose. *Helv Paediatr Acta.* 1971;26:467.

55. RAJU L, CHESSELLS JM, KEMBALL M. Manifestation of hereditary fructose intolerance. *Br Med J.* 1971;2:446.

56. DOMINICK H-CHR, HOSEMANN R, DIEKMANN L. Fructose-intoleranz bei 2 geschwistern. Biochemische und histologische untersuchungen. *Monatsschr Kinderheilkd.* 1972;120:32.

57. STAMPFLER G, HEUMANN G, SCHNEEGANS E. Intolerance hereditaire au fructose et anomalies de la crase sanguine. *Pediatrie.* 1972;27:169.

58. BAGNELL P, HUG G, WALLING L, SCHUBERT WK. Biochemical and morphological observations in severe infantile fructose intolerance. *Pediatr Res.* 1974;8:430. (Abstract.)

59. BAERLOCHER K, GITZELMANN R, STEINMANN B, GITZELMANN-CUMARA-SAMY N. Hereditary fructose intolerance in early childhood: a major diagnostic challenge. *Helv Paediat Acta.* 1978;33:465.

60. MERCIER JC, BOURRILLON A, BEAUFILS F, ODIEVRE M. Intolerance hereditaire au fructose a revelation precoce. *Arch Franz Ped.* 1976;33:945.

61. ROSSNER JA, FEIST D. Hereditare fructose intoleranz. *Verh Dtsch Ges Pathol.* 1971;55:376.

62. CHAPTAL J, JEAN R, BONNET H, CASTEL J, MOREL G. Vomissement acetonemiques symptomatiques d'une intolerance congenitale au fructose chez deux soeurs. *Arch Fr Pediatr.* 1968;25:745.

63. PHILLIPS JJ, LITTLE JA, PTAK TW. Subcellular pathology of hereditary fructose intolerance. *Am J Med.* 1968;44:910.

64. SAXON L, PAPPER S. Abdominal pain occurring during the rapid administration of fructose solutions. *N Engl J Med.* 1957;256:132.

65. MOCK DM, PERMAN JA, THALER MM, MORRIS RC JR. Chronic fructose intoxication after infancy in children with hereditary fructose intolerance. *N Engl J Med.* 1983;309:764.

66. STEINMANN B, GITZELMANN R. The diagnosis of hereditary fructose intolerance. *Helv Paediat Acta.* 1981;36:297.

67. TOLAN DR, PENHOET EE. Characterization of the human aldolase B gene. *Mol Biol Med.* 1986;3:245.

68. KLIMMT G, HUBSCHMANN K, GMYREK D. Untersuchungen zur verminderung des fructosegehalts der Kartoffel. Ein beitrag zur diatetischen behandlung der hereditaren fructoseintoleranz. *Monatsschr Kinderheilkd.* 1968;116:21.

69. PERHEENTUPA J. Fructose intolerance. In: Gardner LI, ed. *Endocrine and Genetic Diseases of Childhood and Adolescence, 2nd ed.* Philadelphia: W.B. Saunders Co, 1975;986.

70. CROSS NC, DEFRANCHIS R, SEBASTIO G, et al. Molecular analysis of aldolase B genes in hereditary fructose intolerance. *Lancet.* 1990;335:306.

71. FROESCH ER, GINSBERG JL. Fructose metabolism of adipose tissue. I. Comparison of fructose and glucose metabolism in epididymal adipose tissue of normal rats. *J Biol Chem.* 1962;237:3317.

72. FROESCH ER. Fructose metabolism in adipose tissue. *Acta Med Scand (Suppl)* 1972;542:37.

73. PARK CR, JOHNSON LH, WRIGHT JH JR, BATSEL H. Effect of insulin on transport of several hexoses and pentoses into cells of muscle and brain. *Am J Physiol.* 1957;191:13.

74. MacGREGOR S, SINGH VN, DAVOUST S, MELLONI E, PONTREMOLI S, HORECKER BL. Evidence for formation of a rabbit liver aldolase-rabbit liver fructose-1,6-bisphosphatase complex. *Proc Natl Acad Sci USA.* 1980;77:3889.

75. KALETTA-GMUNDER U, WOLF HP, LEUTHARDT F. Euber aldolasen. II. Chromatographische Trenning von 1-phosphofructaldolase und diphosphfructaldolase der Leber. *Helv Chem Acta.* 1957;40:1027.

76. PEANASKY RJ, LARDY HA. Bovine liver aldolase. I. Isolation, crystallization and some general properties. *J Biol Chem.* 1958;233:365.

77. MUNNICH A, BESMOND C, DARQUY S, et al. Dietary and hormonal regulation of aldolase B gene expression. *J Clin Invest.* 1985;75:1045.

78. ROTTMAN WH, TOLAN DR, PENHOET EE. Complete amino acid sequence for human aldolase B derived from cDNA and genomic clones. *Proc Natl Acad Sci.* 1984;81:2738.

79. COX TM, O'DONNELL MW, CAMILLERI M, BURGHES AH. Isolation and characterization of a mutant liver aldolase in adult hereditary fructose intolerance. *J Clin Invest.* 1983;72:201.

80. OBERHAENSLI RD, TAYLOR DJ, RAJAGOPALAN B, et al. Study of hereditary

fructose intolerance by use of ^{31}P magnetic resonance spectroscopy. *Lancet.* 1987;ii:931.

81. WOODS HF, EGGLESTON LV, KREBS HA. The cause of hepatic accumulation of fructose-1-phosphate on fructose loading. *Biochem J.* 1970; 119:501.

82. MORRIS RC JR, MCSHERRY E, SEBASTIAN A. Modulation of experimental renal dysfunction of hereditary fructose intolerance by circulating parathyroid hormone. *Proc Natl Acad Sci USA.* 1971;68:132.

83. SAMOLS E, DORMANDY TL. Insulin response to fructose and galactose. *Lancet.* 1963;1:478.

84. SIDBURY JB JR. Zur Biochemie der hereditaren fructoseintoleranz. *Helvet Paediatr Acta.* 1959;14:317. (Letter to the Editor.)

85. HERS H. Augmentation de l'activite de la glucose-6-phosphatase dans l'intolerance au fructose. *Rev Int Hepatol.* 1962;12:777.

86. THURSTON JH, JONAS EM, HAUHART RE. Decrease and inhibition of liver glycogen phosphorylase after fructose. *Diabetes.* 1974;23:597.

87. KAUFMANN U, FROESCH ER. Inhibition of phosphorylase-a by fructose-1-phosphate, d-glycerophosphate and fructose-1,6-diphosphate: Explanation for fructose-induced hypoglycemia in hereditary fructose intolerance and fructose-1,6-diphosphatase deficiency. *Eur J Clin Invest.* 1973;3:407.

88. VAN DEN BERGHE G, HUE L, HERS HG. Effect of the administration of fructose on the glycogenolytic action of glucagon. *Biochem J.* 1973;134:637.

89. ZALITIS J, OLIVER IT. Inhibition of glucose-phosphate isomerase by metabolic intermediates of fructose. *Biochem J.* 1967;102:753.

90. BALLY C, LEUTHARDT F. Aldolase and hypoglycemia in hereditary fructose intolerance. *Eur J Clin Invest.* (personal communication.)

91. LANDAU BR, MARSHALL JS, CRAIG JW, HOSTETLER KY, GENUTH SM. Quantitation of the pathways of fructose metabolism in normal and fructose-intolerant subjects. *J Lab Clin Med.* 1971;78:608.

92. LASKER M. Essential fructosuria. *Hum Biol.* 1941;13:51.

C H A P T E R   10

DEFECTS

IN

GLUCONEOGENESIS

• Primary Defects

Defects in all four key enzymes in the pathway of gluconeogenesis have now been described. Deficiency of glucose-6-phosphatase activity is the most frequent (see glycogen storage disease, Chapter 7), followed by fructose-1,6-diphosphatase. Deficiencies of the other two, phosphoenolpyruvate carboxykinase and pyruvate carboxylase activity, are much less frequent. Lactic acidosis is common to all, while hypoglycemia occurs consistently only in the first two conditions, along with hepatomegaly.

Pyruvate Carboxylase Deficiency

Pyruvate carboxylase is one of a family of carboxylases that contain biotin [1]. It controls the first step in gluconeogenesis, i.e., pyruvate to oxaloacetate, and is allosterically activated by acetyl CoA. As a result of this defect, hypoglycemia would be expected to occur after a fast sufficient to deplete hepatic glycogen stores [2,3]. In fact, only half the cases reported have been hypoglycemic. One theoretical explanation is that the glycerol derived from lipolysis enters the gluconeogenic pathway beyond the enzymatic defect and provides substrate for glucose formation.

Two clinical entities have been described [3,4]. The original North American reports included infants with chronic or recurrent lactic acidosis, seizures, hypotonia, and delayed neurologic development. Hypoglycemia was not a constant finding. The acidosis was at times intractable to sodium bicarbonate therapy. In contrast, infants have been reported from France with a similar clinical presentation, plus evidence of liver disease with elevated blood ammonia and plasma citrulline levels. The onset was early and progression to death rapid. In the former group, lactate-to-pyruvate ratios (L/P) were normal, whereas in the latter the L/P was elevated. This altered redox state was also seen in elevated acetoacetate-to-3-hydroxybutyrate ratios. Plasma amino acids have not been remarkable; in particular, alanine concentrations have been high, normal, or low.

Molecular studies with cultured skin fibroblasts indicated that the patients with hyperammonemia did not synthesize a protein of the correct subunit molecular weight (M_r 125 K daltons) corresponding to pyruvate carboxylase [5]. In addition, they had no cross-reacting material (CRM) to antiserum against pyruvate carboxylase, whereas all the other patients did have CRM. They postulated two different mutations in the pyruvate carboxylase gene: one results in the synthesis of a relatively inactive pyruvate carboxylase protein CRM (+ve) and the other in the lack of expression of the gene in the form of a recognizable protein CRM (−ve).

Therapy is directed against the acidosis with sodium bicarbonate (massive amounts may be required) and the hypoglycemia with parenteral glucose. Biotin has been effective in other carboxylase deficiencies, but has not been in this disorder.

Hepatic Phosphoenolpyruvate Carboxykinase (PEPCK) Deficiency

Fiser et al. [6] have reported a 9-month-old Mexican-American female with episodic hypoglycemia first documented in the immediate neonatal period. Hormone concentrations were not remarkable; neither were the responses to fructose, galactose, or glycerol. Fasting alanine levels were high, but alanine administration failed to increase the low plasma glucose levels. A liver biopsy at 5½ months of age indicated normal glycogenolytic and gluconeogenic enzyme activities, except for reduced pyruvate carboxylase and markedly low or undetectable PEPCK. Hommes and associates [7] have studied two unrelated infants who had an onset of hypoglycemia at 3 months and 19 months, respectively. The first infant had a large tongue and a grossly enlarged liver. Serum transaminase levels were elevated in both. The usual causes of hypoglycemia were ruled out, and the course was one of rapid deterioration. Liver obtained at biopsy (first case) or immediately postmortem (in both) did not show abnormalities of the enzymes of glycogen metabolism; however, PEPCK activity was only detectable at low levels. The grossly fatty livers found at postmortem were considered to be due to increased fatty acid synthesis and related to decreased gluconeogenesis and modification of citrate-malate metabolism and the availability of acetyl CoA. Whether this enzyme defect is primary or secondary is unknown. Furthermore, the relationship to acquired liver disease per se is unclear. These patients indicate the importance of hormone, substrate, and liver enzyme assays in defining the etiology of hypoglycemia.

Vidnes and Søvik [8] have studied three infants with persistent hypoglycemia, but normoinsulinemia. In two, there was reduced incorporation of ^{14}C-alanine to glucose. A defect in gluconeogenesis was postulated (but not proven), possibly at phosphoenolpyruvate carboxykinase or pyruvate carboxylase. In one, they [9] found an abnormal subcellular distribution of PEPCK with virtually no activity being detected in the extramitochondrial fraction of a liver homogenate.

PEPCK is a critical rate limiting enzyme in the control of hepatic gluconeogenesis. It is coupled with pyruvate carboxylase to effect conversion of pyruvate to phosphoenolpyruvate via oxaloacetate. In its absence, glucose cannot be synthesized from precursor lactate or alanine. Because the enzyme is distributed both in the cytosol and mitochondria, biochemical analysis is difficult. As with other defects in gluconeogenesis, the metabolic lactic acidosis may be severe.

There are insufficient numbers of reported cases to provide a genetic analysis.

Sudden infant death syndrome (SIDS) has been attributed to hypoglycemia secondary to a defect in gluconeogenesis by Lardy [10]. PEPCK has been studied in livers from infants dying unexpectedly due to SIDS. No abnormal activities have been noted. Sturner and Susa [11] have studied 52 infants ages 3 weeks to 7 months. Although the activity of phosphoenolpyruvate carboxykinase in liver was significantly reduced in SIDS ($p < 0.001$) and in SIDS with other findings ($p < 0.01$) compared to non-SIDS deaths, no differences were found in vitreous glucose concentration (a reflection of plasma glucose concentration) or liver glycogen. It is unlikely that hypoglycemia due to a defect in gluconeogenesis is of etiologic significance in SIDS.

Hepatic Fructose-1,6-Diphosphatase Deficiency

In 1970, an unusual form of hypoglycemia associated with ketosis was first reported by Baker and Winegrad [12]. Unlike other forms of "ketotic" hypoglycemia, lactic acidosis was noted as well. The triad could be induced by fasting, by feeding a high-fat diet or by the administration of fructose, glycerol, or sorbitol.

Since the original report, other infants and children have been described with similar findings [13–23] and variable degrees of deficiencies in enzyme activity [16,21,24,25]. This disorder is unique to infancy. Sixty percent of affected subjects are female. At least half the cases reported had an onset in the newborn period with symptomatic hypoglycemia and/or acidosis. Since a nonfructose, high-carbohydrate intake may be protective, these infants do better on breast milk, which contains 6–8 percent lactose (glucose-galactose). Any event that limits intake and/or results in hypercatabolism, such as an intercurrent infection with fever, may produce hypoglycemia and metabolic acidosis. Hepatomegaly with a fatty liver may be present. Glucose administration is critical since these infants may rapidly succumb to hypoglycemia and severe lactic acidosis if the condition is not recognized. The firstborn affected infant is at greater risk for a fatal outcome because of failure to diagnose the initial serious event. In contrast, affected siblings are likely to have a benign course, including normal growth and development.

The aversion for sweets (sucrose) and the abdominal cramps so characteristic of hereditary fructose intolerance (see Chapter 9) do not occur in these patients. In addition, patients with HFI do not develop hypoglycemia with fasting. These observations are important in the differential diagnosis.

The pathogenesis of this disorder has been defined by studies in individual patients by Baker and Winegrad [12] and Pagliara et al. [13]. The major event is a total failure of gluconeogenesis as a result of the absence of the key enzyme, fructose-1,6-diphosphatase, in liver, although muscle is unaffected. As a result, functional studies by substrate loading with fructose, glycerol, alanine, sorbitol, or dihydroxyacetone fail to elevate blood glucose concentrations and indeed may result in hypoglycemia and lactic acidosis (Fig. 10-1). At this time, plasma insulin and magnesium levels are low, while plasma FFA, ketones, phosphate, and uric acid levels are elevated. The latter is presumably due to renal tubular transport competition. In contrast, galactose is converted to glucose without difficulty. The subjects are variably sensitive to short overnight fasts and may not respond to glucagon since hepatic glycogen is depleted. Glucogenic amino acid concentrations, especially alanine, are elevated at the time of hypoglycemia. Increased urinary glycerol excretion during fasting has been observed [26].

The diagnosis may be established by demonstrating the enzyme deficiency in liver [12,13] or jejunal mucosa [16].

The use of leukocytes for assay of fructose-1,6-diphosphatase has been the subject of minor technical controversy [18,27]. It is apparent that meticulous attention to details of pH and instrumentation are

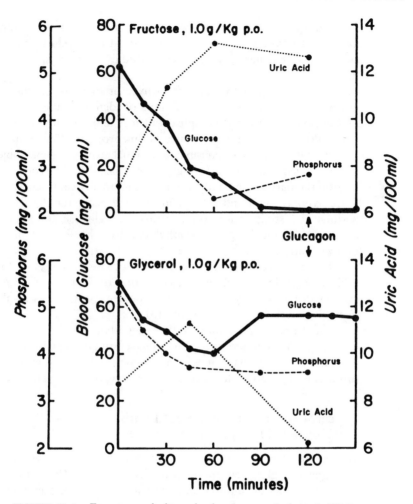

FIGURE 10-1. Fructose and glycerol tolerance tests in hepatic FDPase deficiency. (From Baker and Winegrad. *Lancet.* 1970;2:13, with permission.)

essential for the development of a sensitive analysis. At least two techniques have been reported with relative similarities in the results [28,29].

Variability of clinical responses to functional testing makes a definitive diagnosis dependent upon tissue enzyme analysis. However, a presumptive diagnosis is possible, utilizing fructose and glycerol tolerance tests [12] (see Fig. 10-1). The mechanisms responsible for the hypoglycemia that occurs in the postabsorptive state following the administration of fructose or glycerol are not well delineated.

There is speculation concerning the role of phosphorylated intermediates that possibly inhibit glycogenolysis at the level of phosphorylase activity. Further specific in vitro studies are necessary to clarify this observation.

The enzyme is either absent in liver or markedly reduced. The normal enzyme contains four subunits of identical molecular weight 36,000. Its regulation is complex, but it is allosterically inhibited by AMP. Proteolytic degradation affects this property; thus limited proteolysis may in part be responsible for residual activity in some subjects.

Management, once the diagnosis has been made, requires alertness on the part of the family and physician to any catabolic situation. Since hypoglycemia and lactic acidosis may occur rapidly with short periods of fasting or infection, intravenous glucose and sodium bicarbonate should be given prophylactically whenever an untoward event is anticipated.

Treatment consists of a diet free of sucrose, fructose, or sorbitol and not high in protein. A diet consisting of 56 percent calories as carbohydrate, 32 percent fat, and 12 percent protein has resulted in normal growth and development [13].

The number of families studied suggests a simple autosomal recessive mode of inheritance. Preliminary studies suggest that intermediate levels of enzyme activity are present in liver and in white cells of parents. No molecular defect has been reported as yet.

Glycerol Intolerance in a Child with Intermittent Hypoglycemia

Glycerol is a major three-carbon intermediate of glycolysis that can participate in gluconeogenesis in the liver as well. The following patient represents an unusual abnormality in glycerol metabolism inconsistently resulting in significant hypoglycemia.

A 3-year-old boy was investigated for numerous episodes of fatigue, irritability, pallor, and sweating, which began at 11 months of age, when he had an episode of symptomatic hypoglycemia with ketonuria [30]. He had euphoria, mental confusion, drowsiness, nausea, and vomiting 1–5 hours after oral administration of glycerol in doses of 0.5–1.0 g/kg. Orally administered MCT (1 g/kg) had similar effects. On one occasion, oral glycerol also provoked hypoglycemia, as did a 16½-hour fast. Intravenously administered glycerol (0.09 g/kg) induced an immediate loss of consciousness from which he recovered spontaneously after 30 minutes; there were no changes in blood glucose concentrations. Intravenously administered fructose (0.25 g/kg) was tolerated normally. Leukocytes showed normal activities for

FDPase, glycerol kinase, and glycerol phosphate dehydrogenase. The restriction of dietary intake of fat has been associated with a marked improvement in physical and mental activities. These observations indicated a unique, yet undefined intolerance to glycerol, which suggests caution in the diagnostic use of glycerol in the investigation of hypoglycemia as well as in the therapy of increased intracranial or intraocular pressure.

At follow-up at 5½ years of age, this patient appeared completely normal except for occasional episodes of lethargy and unresponsiveness with normal blood sugars. Concurrently, he had low levels of dopamine beta hydroxylase activities in plasma which fell further following glycerol. This occurrence suggested a defect in the dopamine-epinephrine pathway at the sympathetic nerve endings.

Gitzelmann has suggested that this is an undiagnosed example of FDPase deficiency. However, blood lactate levels were 7–14 mg/dl and did not increase following IV fructose, IV glycerol, or oral glycerol. Although hepatic enzymes were not measured, leukocytes were shown to have normal levels of FDPase.

Wapnir et al. [31] reported a patient whose glycerol intolerance was associated with moderately swollen mitochondria in hepatocytes. Enzyme studies indicated deficient cytosolic and mitochondrial α-glycerol phosphate dehydrogenases, reduced liver fructose-diphosphatase, and increase sensitivity of the latter to inhibition by α-glycerophosphate. This patient improved with a 6-week course of folic acid therapy and did not have recurrence of his hypoglycemia [32].

• Secondary Defects in Gluconeogenesis

Defects in Fatty Acid Metabolism: Hypoketonemia Associated with Normoinsulinemia and Hypoglycemia

The past 15 years have been noteworthy for the identification of several newly recognized syndromes in infancy associated with recurrent hypoglycemia, hypoketonemia, normoinsulinemia, and often a Reye's-like syndrome [33]. The presentation requires differentiation from primary hyperinsulinemia and its associated hypoglycemia and hypoketonemia (discussed in Chapter 5). Among the syndromes described are specific defects in long-chain acyl CoA dehydrogenase (LCAD), medium-chain acyl CoA dehydrogenase (MCAD), short-chain acyl CoA dehydrogenase (SCAD), multiple acyl CoA dehydrogenases (MAD), carnitine acyl transferase (CAT), and 3-hydroxy,3-methyl glutaryl CoA lyase.

TABLE 10-1. Features of medium-, long-, and short-chain acyl-CoA dehydrogenase deficiencies

MANIFESTATIONS	MCAD	LCAD	SCAD
Induced by fasting			
Vomiting	+	+	+
Coma	+	+	+
Nonketotic hypoglycemia	+	+	−
Fatty hepatomegaly	+	+	?
Dicarboxylic aciduria	+	+	+/−
Chronic abnormalities			
Carnitine deficiency	+	+	+
Cardiomyopathy	−	+	−
Muscle weakness	−	+	−
Retardation	−	−	+
Autosomal recessive inheritance	+	+	+

(From Stanley. *Adv Pediatr.* 1987;34:59–88, with permission.)

Stanley has summarized the pertinent findings among the three specific dehydrogenases in Tables 10-1 and 10-2 [33]. The pathway for mitochondrial fatty acid oxidation is presented in Figure 10-2.

TABLE 10-2. Clinical features of genetic enzyme defects in fatty acid oxidation

DEFICIENCY*	MAINLY MUSCLE		MAINLY LIVER		MAINLY CNS
	Weakness	Rhabdomyolysis	Coma	Acidosis	Retardation
CPT					
Adult	−	+	−	−	−
Infantile	−	−	+	−	−
ACD					
MCAD	−	−	+	−	−
LCAD	+	+/−	+	−	−
SCAD	+	−	+	+	+
MAD					
Mild	+/−	−	+	−	−
Severe	+	−	+	+	+
HMG-CoA lyase	−	−	+	+	−

(From Stanley. *Adv Pediatr.* 1987;34:59–88, with permission.)
*ACD = acyl-CoA dehydrogenase; MCAD = medium chain acyl-CoA dehydrogenase; LCAD = long-chain acyl-CoA dehydrogenase; SCAD = short-chain acyl-CoA dehydrogenase; MAD = multiple acyl-CoA dehydrogenase; HMG-CoA = beta-hydroxy-beta-methylglutaryl-CoA

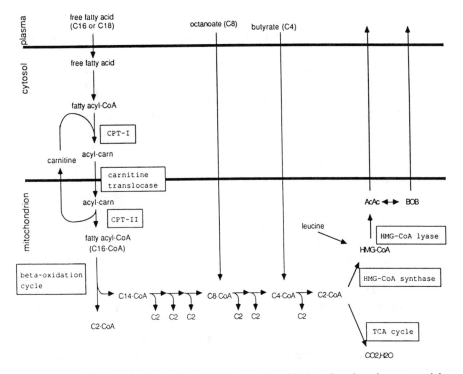

FIGURE 10-2. Pathway of mitochondrial fatty acid oxidation showing the sequential degradation of a typical, 16-carbon long-chain fatty acid (palmitate) to 2-carbon acetyl-CoA units, which are then used for ketone synthesis (in liver) or oxidized in the tricarboxylic acid cycle (in muscle). (From Stanley. *Adv Pediatr.* 1987;34:59–88, with permission.)

Carnitine Palmitoyl Transferase Deficiency

Carnitine palmitoyl transferase (CPT) is essential to the transport of long-chain fatty acids (C12–C16) from cytoplasm to mitochondrion where beta-oxidation occurs. There are two forms of the enzyme; CPT-I is located on the cytosolic face of the inner mitochondrial membrane where the long-chain acyl CoA reacts with carnitine to form acyl carnitine. This latter compound is transported across the mitochondrial membrane by a specific translocase. In the mitochondrion matrix, a related CPT-II restores the acyl CoA, while carnitine is free to shuttle back to the outer membrane. Since long-chain fatty acids are important sources of energy in diverse tissues (e.g., liver, muscle, heart, brain), a genetic defect in CPT-I or II would be expected to have a variety of manifestations. Other functions are described for carnitine, in particular, the mass action effect of carnitine in establishing the steady-state intramitochondrial ratio of acyl-CoA/CoASH [34].

CPT-I deficiency in the adult form has been characterized by episodes of muscle pain and myoglobinuria associated with exercise. Excessive myoglobinuria may result in acute renal failure. Clinically, this entity must be differentiated from muscle phosphorylase deficiency (type V glycogen storage disease) and from phosphofructokinase deficiency. Myoglobinuria may occur in childhood, but the diagnosis is rarely made before 16 years of age. Hypoglycemia and coma are not a feature of this disorder.

In contrast, marked hypoglycemia, which is associated with hepatic CPT-I deficiency, has been reported in two sisters at age 8 months, one of whom died [35]. A 20-hour fast resulted in the development of hypoglycemia (109–34 mg/dl [6.1 mM–1.9 mM]), a rise in plasma free fatty acids (0.01–3.5 mEq/L), but persistently low ketone bodies (beta-hydroxybutyrate 2.8 mg/dl, acetoacetate 2.7 mg/dl) (Fig. 10-3). Administration of medium-chain triglycerides produced a rise in both plasma glucose concentration and ketoacids. A liver biopsy indicated a nonspecific steatosis without visible mitochondrial abnormalities. Liver homogenate contained no CPT activity but did have 3-hydroxybutyrate dehydrogenase activity, a marker of

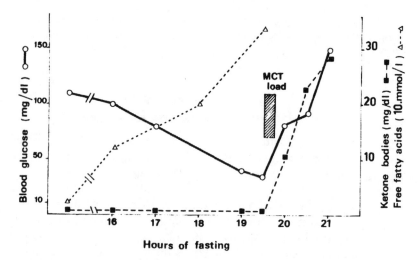

FIGURE 10-3. Plasma glucose, ketones, and free fatty acids concentrations during prolonged fast. Plasma glucose (○) declines, but total ketone bodies (■) do not increase despite elevated plasma nonesterified fatty acid (△) concentrations. MCT load restores normal plasma ketone body and glucose values. (From Bougneres et al. *J Pediatr.* 1981;98:742, with permission.)

the inner mitochondrial membrane. Bougneres et al. [35] have suggested that the hypoglycemia is secondary to a failure of gluconeogenesis due to decreased hepatic production of acetyl CoA and NADH.

Medium-Chain Acyl CoA Dehydrogenase Deficiency

The medium-chain acyl CoA dehydrogenase defect has been reported in over 100 infants. The onset is usually associated with a catabolic state (fasting or an intercurrent infection), episodic vomiting, lethargy, hepatomegaly, and coma (Tables 10-1 and 10-2). The onset is sufficiently nonspecific to include Reye's syndrome in the differential diagnosis [36,37]. Some fatalities have been classified as sudden infant death syndrome. The associated laboratory findings include hypoglycemia, hypoketonemia (absent urinary ketones, low plasma beta-hydroxybutyrate concentrations), and normal or low plasma insulin concentrations.

Specialized analyses of urine are required to identify the abnormal medium-chain dicarboxylic aciduria. Rinaldo et al. [38] have developed a stable-isotope dilution measurement of urinary n-hexanoylglycine and 3-phenylpropionylglycine which is highly specific for MCAD. Bhuijan et al. [39] have devised a simple, inexpensive method for the detection of octanoyl-carnitine in urine by reverse-phase, high-performance, thin-layer chromatography of the p-bromophenacyl derivative. Among the metabolites previously reported are dicarboxylic acids (adipate, suberate, sebacate, and unsaturated sebacate), hydroxyacids, suberylglycine, and octanoyl-carnitine. Octanoyl-carnitine has been identified in urine by fast atom bombardment-mass spectroscopy [40].

Treem et al. [41] have differentiated MCAD and LCAD from Reye's syndrome based on the younger age at presentation, history of unexplained death of a sibling, a previous episode of lethargy, and hypoglycemia or acidosis precipitated by fasting stress. In addition, serum transaminase levels are normal or minimally elevated, as are prothrombin times in MCAD. Light microscopic alterations in the liver include steatosis, which may be either macro-or microvesicular. The characteristic mitochrondrial changes noted by electron microscopy in Reye's syndrome are not usually evident in acyl CoA dehydrogenase deficiency.

A secondary carnitine deficiency may complicate the basic problem. Diagnosis of this abnormality may be obscured during illness and fasting; however, in the fed state, plasma total carnitine concentrations are low. Stanley [33] has summarized secondary carnitine deficiency syndromes. He has emphasized that total plasma carnitine concentration is approximately 30 percent of normal, while liver and muscle total carnitine contents are similarly reduced to 25 and 20 percent of normal. The urine contains the acyl carnitine: octanoyl carnitine.

Cultured skin fibroblasts and peripheral mononuclear leukocytes have been studied successfully in establishing the diagnosis of MCAD [42].

Strauss et al. [43] have recently reported on the molecular analysis of medium-chain acyl CoA dehydrogenase deficiency. Yokota et al. [44] have sequenced polymerase chain reaction (PCR)–amplified variant medium-chain acyl CoA dehydrogenase cDNAs in cultured fibroblasts from three MCAD-deficient patients. An A to G transition was identified at position 985 of the coding region that causes a lysine-304 to glutamate substitution of the mature protein. This provides another precise technique for diagnosis.

Therapy

There is no specific therapy for MCAD deficiency. Once the initial biochemical abnormalities are defined, hypoglycemia should be treated with a minibolus (0.25 gm/kg IV dextrose, followed by a continuous infusion at 6–8 mg/kg/min). Elevation of the plasma glucose concentration and the associated increase in endogenous insulin secretion should be important in suppressing lipolysis, thus diminishing free fatty acid mobilization and accumulation of the metabolites secondary to the MCAD deficiency. The abnormalities can be minimized by avoiding fasting. Intercurrent infections, especially with vomiting, should be carefully and frequently monitored for hypoglycemia so that parenteral dextrose may be given before symptoms occur.

Long-Chain Acyl CoA Dehydrogenase Deficiency

Although LCAD patients may present with all the findings noted above for MCAD subjects (including hepatomegaly), they tend to present at an earlier age, usually under 6 months [45]. A significant difference between LCAD and MCAD is the involvement of muscle, both skeletal and cardiac, in the former. As with MCAD, a secondary carnitine deficiency may complicate the presentation. Intermittent myopathic episodes have been reported in association with muscle pain and myoglobinuria. Urinary ketones are absent, but dicarboxylic acids are increased. These include C12–C16 dicarboxylic acids in addition to C6–C10. This autosomal recessive disorder is much less frequent than MCAD and can be diagnosed by enzyme studies of fibroblasts, white blood cells, or liver.

Short-Chain Acyl CoA Dehydrogenase Deficiency

This is the rarest of the acyl CoA dehydrogenase deficiencies described to date, which may be related to the severity of the onset which often is unrecognized in early infancy [33]. The findings are nonspecific but include several of the features found in MCAD and LCAD. These include vomiting, coma, and progressive muscle weakness. In contrast to the other disorders, marked developmental delay may be found. A secondary carnitine deficiency can be documented in plasma and muscle. Urinary organic acid analyses indicate increased concentrations of ethylmalonic, butyric, butyrylglycine, and methyl succinic acids, but not the medium-chain dicarboxylic acids observed in MCAD or LCAD. This very rare metabolic disorder can be diagnosed by enzyme analysis of fibroblasts.

Recently, the molecular basis of human short-chain acyl CoA dehydrogenase deficiency has been defined through molecular cloning and identification of the nucleotide sequence of cDNAs encoding human short-chain acyl CoA dehydrogenase [46].

Multiple Acyl CoA Dehydrogenase Deficiency

The multiple acyl CoA dehydrogenase (MAD) disorders, which are characterized biochemically by the inability to metabolize all the acyl CoAs normally oxidized via the acyl CoA dehydrogenases, occur in two forms: severe (MAD-S) and mild (MAD-M) [47]. The severe forms have an onset in the neonatal period and consist of two subtypes, one of which has congenital anomalies. Late-onset MAD is mild. The clinical symptoms include varied degrees of hypoketotic hypoglycemia, acidosis, fatty changes in the liver, kidney, and sometimes heart. Urinary excretion of dethiolated acyl CoAs and their derived oxidation products is increased. Glutaric aciduria type II (MAD-S) is associated with increased urinary excretion of glutarate, ethylmalonate, isovalerate, α-methylbutyrate, isobutyrate, aliphatic dicarboxylic acids, and their derivatives. The name is derived from the predominant excretion of glutaric acid. MAD-M or ethylmalonic-adipic aciduria mild GA-II is associated with increased urinary excretion of ethyl-malonic acid, adipic acid, and hexanoylglycine. MAD-S patients usually do not survive the neonatal period.

The biochemical defects have been characterized in fibroblasts, in both groups of subjects.

Rhead and associates have studied mitochondrial fatty acid metabolism in fibroblasts [47,48]. They have developed a technique of fusion and complementation to identify the specific biochemical abnormalities. In addition to defects in the dehydrogenases, they have found decreased electron transfer flavoprotein (ETF) activities (29–51 percent of control) in five MAD-M cell lines, whereas in four MAD-S lines ETF was markedly reduced to 4–21 percent. They also identified two cell lines from MAD-S with an abnormality in electron transfer flavoprotein-ubiquinone oxido-reductase activities. Loehr et al. [49] have commented on heterogeneity of clinical and biochemical phenotypes and reported deficiency of electron transfer flavoprotein or electron transfer flavoprotein-ubiquinone oxido reductase activity in fibroblasts from 23 patients.

Therapy involves avoidance of fasting or catabolic states associated with infections or fever, as in the single acyl CoA dehydrogenase defects. Dextrose should be administered early in the course of an illness. Some patients with mild MAD have been responsive to riboflavin therapy. This therapy requires biochemical monitoring of the specific disorders.

Pathogenesis of Hypoglycemia in Defects of Acyl CoA Metabolism

No primary defect in glucose metabolism has been described in the defects of acyl CoA metabolism. The association of hypoglycemia with fasting or increased catabolism (accelerated starvation) is consistent with a defect in gluconeogenesis. The mechanisms suggested by Francois [50] to be operative in 3-hydroxy,3-methyl glutaryl CoA lyase deficiency may explain the mechanism here (see section on 3-OH,3CH$_3$ glutaryl CoA lyase, p. 373). As glycogen is depleted, hepatic glucose output diminishes. Under normal conditions of fasting, the high energy requirements of the brain are met by alternate substrates, including beta-hydroxybutyrate and lactate. In the absence of the former, the obligatory cerebral glucose requirement exceeds hepatic glucose production, resulting in hypoglycemia. An alternate or additional hypothesis places control in the hepatocyte where the initial step in gluconeogenesis requires activation of the enzyme pyruvate carboxylase to convert pyruvate to oxaloacetate. The carboxylase is activated by acetyl CoA. In the absence of acetyl CoA formation secondary to the defect in acyl CoA dehydrogenases, gluconeogenesis cannot be initiated. It is likely that both factors are operative: (1) defective gluconeogenesis and (2) defective ketone body formation, reducing alternate substrates for brain.

Carnitine Deficiency

Secondary carnitine deficiency (low plasma total carnitine concentrations) has been reported in a variety of metabolic disorders, including deficiencies of the long-chain, medium-chain, and short-chain acyl CoA dehydrogenases, but not in deficiency of the multiple acyl CoA dehydrogenases [33,51]. In addition, low levels have been reported in isovaleric acidemia, propionic acidemia, and methylmalonic aciduria [52]. Hoppel has recently reviewed the methodology for carnitine analysis of plasma and urine. He described a refined radioenzymatic method [34] and emphasized that the ratio of acyl carnitine to carnitine may be abnormally elevated in urine while plasma values are normal. Renal loss also has been noted in Fanconi syndrome and cystinosis [53]. Variable metabolites have been found in urine depending on the specific etiology. The significance of low plasma total carnitine levels is unclear. Thus, carnitine supplementation in the above disorders has not been associated with clear metabolic or clinical improvement.

In contrast to the secondary deficiency, primary carnitine deficiency appears to be very rare. Slonim et al. [54] described dietary-dependent carnitine deficiency as a cause of significant nonketotic hypoglycemia in an infant whose plasma glucose concentrations were 8 and 15 mg/dl (0.44 and 0.83 mM) at ages 9 and 12 weeks. The infant was normal at birth but developed a low-grade diarrhea at 4 weeks, which was treated with a soy-based formula deficient in carnitine. Each illness was associated with prostration, vomiting, and hepatomegaly. At 3 months, the infant's weight was at the 5th percentile, while length was at the 20th, and head circumference at the 15th percentile for age. Serum creatine phosphokinase and lactic dehydrogenase activities were markedly elevated, but serum ammonia was normal. Studies of response to fasting demonstrated a significant fall in plasma glucose concentration (87–43 mg/dl [4.8–2.4 mM]) after a 12-hour fast at 3 months of age, and (95–31 mg/dl [5.3–1.7 mM]) after a 17-hour fast at 6 months. Each episode was associated with very low plasma ketones and very high FFA concentrations. No evidence of hepatocellular damage was found on biopsy. Plasma and urinary carnitine concentrations were low until the diet was supplemented with carnitine. Following this therapy, her weight, length, and head circumference were all at the 15th percentile for age, and she (at age 7 months) tolerated a fast for 20 hours without hypoglycemia. Plasma beta-hydroxybutyrate concentration increased appropriately. The infant remained asymptomatic. Tissue carnitine content was not analyzed, nor were the enzymes involved in fatty acid transport and oxidation in liver and muscle. The mechanism for the hypoglycemia presumably is the same as that in carnitine acyl transferase I (see p. 363).

Treem et al. [55] have suggested that the diagnosis of primary carnitine deficiency requires (1) reduction in tissue carnitine levels sufficient to limit fatty acid oxidation, (2) evidence of impaired fatty acid oxidation, (3) correction of the disorder when carnitine levels are restored toward normal, and (4) no other primary defect in fatty acid oxidation. They described a 3½-month-old, previously well female who was found limp, unresponsive, and apneic after a prolonged overnight fast. Her pH was 7.17, pCO_2 60 mmHg, and plasma glucose concentration 7 mg/dl (0.39 mM). Electrolytes were normal, but serum ammonia was elevated. Total plasma carnitine concentrations ranged from undetectable to very low levels (2.2 µmol/L) on three occasions. Although the infant was treated with supplemental carnitine at 4 months, she had significant developmental delay and myoclonic seizures. Cultured skin fibroblasts had normal acyl CoA dehydrogenase activities. Liver and muscle had markedly reduced carnitine levels. With a 12-hour fast (terminated when the plasma glucose concentration was 51 mg/dl [2.8 mM]), plasma FFA concentration rose to 2.22 mM, while beta-hydroxybutyrate remained low (0.27 mM). Oral L-carnitine corrected the patient's impairment of hepatic fatty acid oxidation. Renal studies also showed a defect in carnitine transport, resulting in increased urinary losses. The studies of fibroblasts indicated a defect in the carrier mediated transport of carnitine. No satisfactory explanation (other than presented above, see CAT-I) for the hypoglycemia was provided (see p. 365).

• Defects in Amino Acid Metabolism

3-Hydroxy,3-Methyl Glutaryl CoA Lyase Deficiency: A Defect in Leucine Catabolism

In 1976, a 7-month-old male was recognized as having a Reye's-like syndrome of vomiting, coma, hepatomegaly, metabolic acidosis, hypoglycemia, and hyperammonemia [56]. Examination of the urine by gas chromatography-mass spectrometry (GC-MS) revealed a characteristic organic acid pattern of four metabolites proximal to the defect, i.e., 3-hydroxyisovaleric acid; 3-methylglutaric, 3-methylglutaconic acids I,II; and 3-hydroxy,3-methyl glutaric acid. The pathway for leucine catabolism is shown in Figure 10-4. The defect precludes the formation of acetoacetic acid, so hypoketonemia is also a feature.

By 1988, 18 cases were reported and summarized by Gibson et al. [57]. Vomiting and hepatomegaly were characteristic. Age of onset was in infancy, at 2 days to 19 months. Coma and lethargy were reported in half the cases. A severe metabolic acidosis with a large anion gap ($[Na + K] - [Cl + HCO_3]$) was consistently present, while hypoglycemia occurred in 15 (83 percent) patients. The hyper-

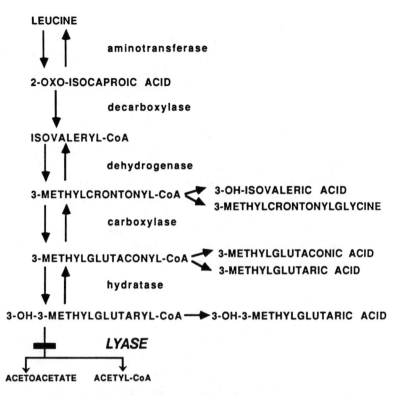

LEUCINE

aminotransferase

2-OXO-ISOCAPROIC ACID

decarboxylase

ISOVALERYL-CoA

dehydrogenase

3-METHYLCRONTONYL-CoA 3-OH-ISOVALERIC ACID
                        3-METHYLCRONTONYLGLYCINE

carboxylase

3-METHYLGLUTACONYL-CoA 3-METHYLGLUTACONIC ACID
                         3-METHYLGLUTARIC ACID

hydratase

3-OH-3-METHYLGLUTARYL-CoA ➤ 3-OH-3-METHYLGLUTARIC ACID

LYASE

ACETOACETATE   ACETYL-CoA

FIGURE 10-4. Pathway for leucine catabolism, indicating the site of the lyase block and the metabolites that appear in urine.

ammonemia present in half the patients, which was not as elevated as in Reye's syndrome, was variable, 29 to 1370 μmol/l. Although there is some disagreement regarding the interpretation of the urinary organic acid profile, most investigators consider it a reliable diagnostic indicator [58,59]. Organic acid(s) not of endogenous metabolic origin may also appear in urine. Techniques other than GC-MS have been reviewed by Gibson [57].

Therapy

Initial therapy is directed at providing glucose at high rates, 8–10 mg/kg/min, to provide substrate for brain and to minimize protein catabolism and leucine availability. Sodium bicarbonate therapy at 2–4 mEq/kg over the initial 4–6 hours in the intravenous fluids at 75 mEq/L is necessary to stabilize and correct the acidosis. Other sources of calories, including protein and fat, must be withheld initially. Maintenance electrolytes should be included once the acidosis is corrected.

Introduction of protein should be judicious at 0.25 gm/kg/day and increased gradually, not to exceed 1.0 gm/kg/day, before diagnosis is established. Once the characteristic urinary pattern has been found, then diet should consist of leucine-free formula (now available) or MSUD formula (maple syrup urine disease) which is devoid of the three branch chain amino acids (leucine, valine, isoleucine). If the latter is used, then valine and isoleucine should be supplemented at the levels found in infant formulas. Because leucine is an essential amino acid, a minimal amount must be provided for growth and synthesis of hemoglobin which contains 15 percent leucine (wt/wt). The recommendation for infants under 2 years is 100 mg/kg/day as a proprietary, defined nutrient formula. After age 2, the requirement is reduced on a weight basis to 80 mg/kg/day.

There is evidence that both total and free plasma carnitine are low in this disorder. At least one patient has been treated successfully with supplemental carnitine [60].

Genetics

This disorder affects males and females equally and is inherited as an autosomal recessive. The enzyme activity has been identified in liver, leukocytes, lymphocytes, skin fibroblasts, and placenta. While enzyme activity is very low in the homozygotes, activity is highly variable in the parents and siblings. Gibson et al. [61] have developed an improved assay for enzyme activity of leukocytes. The prospects for prenatal diagnosis are good but have not yet been achieved. The gene locus and molecular defect have not yet been identified.

Prognosis

Prognosis is generally good but has been variable. Of the 18 cases summarized, four died, and two had mental retardation as well as significant neurological residua. The majority are normal at follow-up. Intercurrent infection with hypoglycemia and metabolic acidosis is the greatest risk. Hospitalization with parenteral glucose is critical to minimize complications. Adverse reactions to immunizations have been described and warrant caution in management.

Pathogenesis of Hypoglycemia

The mechanism(s) responsible for the severe hypoglycemia have not been established [50]. It is likely that there is diminished hepatic glucose output secondary to a failure of gluconeogenesis. One suggestion is that the absence of lyase activity results in an altered accumulation of CoA derivatives of the abnormal organic acids which could lead to depletion of free Co ASH. A concomitant fall in the level of acetyl CoA, a key allosteric activator of gluconeogenesis, could be the controlling factor. Since this is a controlling cofactor for pyruvate carboxylase, it is likely that conversion to phosphoenolpyruvate is limited.

The rapidity of onset and severity of symptoms of hypoglycemia may be related to diminished cerebral alternate fuels, i.e., beta-hydroxybutyrate, so that glucose is the obligate source for brain energy. Francois [50] has infused one child with beta-hydroxybutyrate and prevented the fall in blood glucose concentration during fasting. When the child was normoglycemic, alanine produced a normal rise in glucose. This study was not repeated when the child was hypoglycemic. The exact mechanism involved remains obscure.

Case Report (Patient 10-1): Early Onset Presenting with Severe Acidosis, Prompt Diagnosis, and Subsequent Dietary and Crisis Management

M.C. was born June 2, 1986 of unrelated parents after an uneventful pregnancy and delivery. She was sent home at 2 days of age on formula feeds which she took poorly. By day 5, she was obtunded and poorly responsive. She had obvious hepatomegaly. Her pediatrician evaluated and treated her for sepsis. She was hemoconcentrated (Hb/Hct 20/62) and severely acidotic, pH 7.05, total CO_2 4.9 mM/L, anion gap 35 mEq/L. Initial plasma glucose concentration was 43 mg/dl (2.4 mM) and blood ammonia 175 ug/dl. She responded well to parenteral glucose and supplemental sodium bicarbonate. The initial urine was diagnostic for a defect in 3-hydroxy,3-methyl glutaryl CoA lyase deficiency (Fig. 10-5). The infant was fed limited amounts of Enfamil to provide leucine at 50 mg/kg/day. The remaining nutrient and calories were provided by an MSUD formula supplemented with isoleucine and valine. Sodium bicarbonate at 2 mEq/kg/day was provided as a prophylactic supplement against metabolic acidosis. This intake did not provide enough leucine either for normal growth or correction of the iatrogenic anemia (Hb 6.6 gm/dl), although acidosis and hypoglycemia were prevented. Leucine intake was increased stepwise to 100 mg/kg/day whereupon both growth and correction of the anemia occurred.

The infant thrived except for four intercurrent infections during the first 2 years. Two were minor and required no specific therapeutic intervention. The other two were similar major events which included: (1) febrile episodes (103° F) associated with minor respiratory symptoms and rapidly progressing to vomiting, (2) unresponsiveness and seizures within 12 hours, requiring hospitalization, (3) mild acidosis (total CO_2 > 18 mM/L), but (4) profound symptomatic hypoglycemia with plasma glucose concentration <10 mg/dl (0.56 mM). Therapy with parenteral glucose (0.5 gm/kg as a 25 percent solution), followed by a continuous infusion at 8 mg/kg/min, resulted in gradual clearing of the neurological symptoms over several hours. Blood ammonia concentrations were only mildly elevated. Serum amino acids showed a generalized increase, including leucine, similar to that noted at the time of diagnosis. Urinary organic acids showed a similar pattern but less marked than

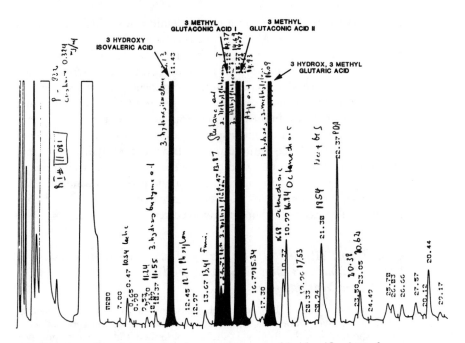

FIGURE 10-5. Gas chromatograph-mass spectrographic identification of urinary metabolites from a newborn with a defect in 3-hydroxy, 3-methyl glutaryl CoA lyase. (Dr. Kay Tanaka provided the GC-MS urine analysis.)

originally. These levels were grossly abnormal compared to the patterns obtained between illnesses. An EEG early in this admission showed marked left-sided slow delta wave activity consistent with a metabolic encephalopathy.

The family is highly alert to the risks of intercurrent infection, especially hypoglycemia. They have been taught home blood glucose monitoring. Baking soda (NaHCO$_3$) continues to be added to her MSUD formula. In order to diversify her intake, an exchange system has been devised in which leucine content of protein-containing foods are related to ml of Enfamil (leucine = 1.54 mg/ml). They have a copy of Pennington and Church (14th edition) which lists amino acid content of foods. Once a month, a 3-day prospective dietary record is analyzed for kilocalories and contents of protein, isoleucine, valine, and leucine.

Anthropometric measurements are normal at age 4 years, as are detailed behavioral and intellectual assessments. The earlier hepatomegaly has subsided. The EEG is normal. She has tolerated all of her immunizations without any untoward event.

Comment

This unusual patient was diagnosed and treated promptly in the newborn period. Problems were both iatrogenic (anemia, growth failure) and induced by the basic biochemical abnormality. Meticulous management of her ongoing growth as well as of intermittent crises (hypoglycemia) has resulted in a normal child by age 4 years.

Leucine-Induced Hypoglycemia

Leucine is unique among the essential amino acids because of the role of the branched chain amino acids (BCAA) in the glucose-alanine cycle. The BCAA are transaminated in muscle to provide pyruvate to alanine conversion. The latter is transported to the liver, where gluconeogenesis is increased. The BCAA carbon skeleton is further metabolized in muscle. In addition to a role in muscle protein turnover, leucine is also insulinogenic.

Congenital leucine-induced familial hypoglycemia, a very rare disorder, was first reported in 1956 by Cochrane, Payne, Simpkiss, and Woolf [62]. Leucine produced a marked fall in the blood sugar level in certain hypoglycemic infants in whom the number of convulsions had increased on a high-protein, low-carbohydrate diet. Subsequently, infants with spontaneous hypoglycemia have been found to be sensitive to leucine [63–65].

Leucine sensitivity with symptomatic hypoglycemia has been found to be associated with hyperinsulinemia, including "nesidioblastosis" or adenomata.

Clinical Manifestations

Classically, symptoms and signs occurred shortly after a high-protein meal and varied in severity from pallor and weakness to major convulsions. Prolonged fasting may also be associated with hypoglycemia. Ocular abnormalities, especially alternating esotropia and squint, were often observed.

Laboratory Findings

The only positive laboratory finding at the time of symptoms is a low level of glucose in blood or in cerebrospinal fluid. Neither acetone nor reducing substances have been reported in the urine.

These infants and children have plasma insulin determinations that are absolutely or relatively (insulin to glucose ratio) elevated.

Therapy

As in all significant acute hypoglycemic episodes, the immediate treatment is to supply glucose by administering parenteral glucose.

The long-term therapy is to provide a diet that contains minimal amounts of leucine, yet is adequate for growth (see Appendixes II, III). This is essentially a low-protein diet and has been described by Roth and Segal [66]. In addition, high carbohydrate feedings are provided from 20 to 30 minutes after meals, upon arising, and at bedtime as originally suggested by Cochrane et al. [62]. Recently, oral raw tapioca starch has been effective in preventing postabsorptive hypoglycemia [67].

Maple Syrup Urine Disease

Classic maple syrup urine disease (MSUD) was first described in 1954 by Menkes, Hurst, and Craig [68]. Additional reports followed shortly, as did the elucidation of the metabolic defect with identification of the ketoacids [69]. The onset is immediately after birth (within the first week), with poor feeding, vomiting, hypertonicity, and a shrill cry. In addition to various abnormalities of tone, seizures often occur. If treatment is not instituted, coma associated with increased intracranial pressure and a bulging fontanel results. If the infant survives, severe mental retardation occurs. These findings are associated with a recurrent ketoacidosis and urine with a characteristic odor. As in other disorders resulting in organic acid excretion, a simple way to improve sensitivity is to freeze the sample, thereby partially concentrating the organic acid in the supernatant for easier olfactory detection.

A number of variants have been described [70]. In one form of the disease, intermittent branch chain aminoaciduria, neurologic manifestations predominate and are precipitated by episodes of catabolism such as with infection, fever, starvation, or anesthesia. Clinically, ataxia and episodes of lethargy occur, which may progress to coma.

There appear to be two clinical forms of this subgroup, one without acidosis. A milder second form manifests itself in recurrent ataxia and psychomotor delay and has been found to be responsive to thiamine. Additional subgroups have been identified in association with the enzymes associated with the branch chain ketoacid dehydrogenase (BCKD) complex. Further subgroups have been identified by the use of polyclonal antibodies specific for BCKD.

Hypoglycemia

Donnell et al. [71] first reported hypoglycemia in MSUD in 1967. Their patient had fasting hypoglycemia and a flat oral glucose tolerance test which improved with control of the plasma amino acid profile. Haymond and associates [72] have studied extensively a female infant with classic thiamine-unresponsive MSUD during her 2 months of life. When the branched chain amino acids were increased, fasts as brief as 9 hours were associated with hypoglycemia and low blood lactate and alanine levels, but appropriate insulin, growth hormone, cortisol, and ketone concentrations. Intravenous glucagon or oral fructose resulted in normal glycemic responses. Alanine infusions did not elevate blood glucose levels but did result in a transient rise in glutamate and a marked sustained rise in glutamine values. They speculated that a defect in gluconeogenesis was related to a preferential shunting of 3-carbon substrates from gluconeogenic amino acids into glutamine, which resulted in decreased net oxaloacetate production and impaired gluconeogenesis.

In order for the three branch chain amino acids, leucine, isoleucine, valine, to be utilized or metabolized, they must first be transferred from the plasma or interstitium to the cytosol by a specific L transporter system [70]. An amino acid transferase then produces the three specific ketoacid analogs, which are then transported into the mitochondrial matrix. Here, the multienzyme complex branch chain alpha-ketoacid dehydrogenase is required for further metabolism. This is the site(s) of the defect in MSUD.

Frequency

Since the onset of symptoms is so rapid after birth (hours to days), neonatal screening for elevated plasma leucine concentration is essential for prompt diagnosis and early intervention with a diet extremely low in the branched chain amino acids. Screening utilizes *Bacillus subtilis*, which is incubated with a measured spot of dried blood and whose growth is dependent on leucine.

The frequency is highly variable, depending in part upon inbreeding; thus, a rate as high as 1/760 has been reported in Mennonites, while one as low as 1/290,000 was found in the New England Collaborative Study of a mixed population [73]. Bedside screening may be done as described by Menkes[1] [68].

Confirmation can be done by thin-layer chromatography or, more specifically, by gas chromatography and mass spectroscopy of urinary ketoacids. Prenatal diagnosis can be made by studies of either fibroblasts or chorionic villi for labelled ^{14}C-BCKA conversion to $^{14}CO_2$ [70].

MSUD appears to be transmitted as a simple autosomal recessive.

---

[1]A freshly prepared solution of 2 N HCl saturated with 2,4-dinitrophenylhydrazine is mixed with an equal volume of urine. At room temperature, after 2 minutes, the cloudy solution will contain bright yellow crystals in a positive test.

As yet, no chromosome location has been identified. Although several of the enzymes (proteins) have been isolated and characterized, specific molecular genetic abnormalities have not been found to date [74].

Therapy

Therapy requires meticulous attention to details of diet restriction with monitoring of blood and urine amino acids and ketoacids. Since the branched chain amino acids are essential for normal anabolic processes, including growth, a specific prescribed amount of each BCAA must be provided [70]. These requirements vary with age. Periods of catabolism as a result of infections, fever, or anorexia must be anticipated, monitored, and treated early with dextrose.

Branched Chain Organic Acidosis

Specific defects in the enzymes involved in the metabolism of the branched chain amino acids, leucine, valine, and isoleucine have now been recognized. Since most of these do not involve carbohydrate metabolism, they are not considered here.

Isovaleric Acidemia

Isovaleryl CoA dehydrogenase (IVD) deficiency can present acutely within a few days after birth with listlessness, lethargy, vomiting, dehydration, and seizures [75]. An abnormal odor ("sweaty feet") may be noticed due to isovaleric acid accumulation. A severe metabolic acidosis and ketonuria are present. A less severe form of this metabolic disorder occurs later in infancy and is only manifest during periods of catabolism, i.e., infections. In one such patient, hyperglycemia and metabolic acidosis required differentiation from diabetes mellitus with ketoacidosis.

Diagnosis is made from a characteristic pattern of urinary organic acids determined by gas chromatography and mass spectroscopy. The metabolites include isovaleryl-glycine and 3-hydroxyisovaleric acid.

The IVD gene has been assigned to chromosome 15 [76]. The nucleotide sequence of messenger RNA encoding human isovaleryl-coenzyme A dehydrogenase has been determined in fibroblasts [77]. Several mutations were identified and were consistent with a point mutation or small deletion.

Therapy involves restricting protein, minimizing endogenous catabolism with glucose, and treating the metabolic acidosis with sodium bicarbonate.

Deficiency of 3-Methyl Crotonyl CoA Carboxylase

This rare enzyme defect must be carefully identified biochemically to avoid confusion with the biotin-responsive multiple carboxylase(s) deficiencies [78]. The urinary organic acid patterns determined by GC-MS are distinctive for 3-hydroxy-isovaleric acid and 3-methylcrotonylglycine. The clinical presentation is no different from that of the other organic acidurias associated with hypoglycemia and with onset in early infancy. Intolerance to protein ingestion may be an important factor. Initially, the blood glucose concentration may be normal or low. Blood lactate concentration has been elevated.

Acutely, parenteral dextrose and sodium bicarbonate administration are indicated. Once stable, management involves dietary protein restriction (<2.0 gm/kg/day). In the absence of specific enzyme (liver, fibroblasts, leukocytes) analyses, treatment should include large doses of biotin.

3-Methylglutaconic Aciduria: 3-Methylglutaconyl CoA Hydratase Deficiency

This very rare defect has been identified in brothers with speech retardation, ages 5 and 7 years [79]. In one, fasting 18 hours produced hypoglycemia and a compensated metabolic acidosis. Urinary metabolites determined by GC-MS included: 3-methyl-glutaconic acid and 3-methylglutaric acid. No specific therapy beyond moderate restriction of protein intake is necessary.

Organic Aciduria with Variable Hypoglycemia

Two of the organic acidurias deserve comment because they may be secondarily associated with disturbances in carbohydrate metabolism. Propionyl-CoA carboxylase deficiency was originally described in great detail by Childs et al. as idiopathic hyperglycinemia and hyperglycinuria [80]. Observations over a 4½-year period in the original patient indicated that blood glucose levels were within normal limits under all conditions. However, further observations in other patients indicate that symptomatic hypoglycemia may occur. Robert et al. [81] reported a term newborn who developed a severe anion gap acidosis and protracted hypoglycemia by the third day of life which responded to parenteral glucose at 6 mg/kg/min. Propionyl CoA carboxylase was deficient in both leukocytes and fibroblasts. Severe metabolic acidosis due to ketonemia and a large anion gap is characteristic.

A defect in the glycine-cleavage system of brain has been reported [82]. Strychnine therapy has been inconsistent in its effect [83,84].

Another related disorder is methylmalonic acidemia, which also presents in the immediate neonatal period with ketosis and a severe metabolic acidosis. Hypoglycemia with seizures has been reported [85]; however, in an extensive review of 45 patients, Matsui did not list carbohydrate problems as significant [86]. The prenatal (6–12 weeks) diagnosis of methylmalonic acidemia and propionic acidemia has been made by measurement of methylmalonic and methylcitric acids, respectively, in amniotic fluid [87].

Hereditary Tyrosinemia

Hereditary tyrosinemia (formerly tyrosinosis) occurs in the neonatal period in either an acute or chronic form [88]. The onset of liver disease is associated with a cabbagelike odor. The acute form has a rapidly progressive course to death within 6 months unless a liver transplant is performed. Hyperplasia of the pancreas and hypoglycemia may be associated findings. The chronic form may also include hypoglycemia, but the primary findings are those of a severe nodular cirrhosis, a nephropathy leading to a Fanconi syndrome, and failure to thrive. There is also an increased risk of hepatic carcinoma.

The impaired metabolism of tyrosine differs from that in transient neonatal tyrosinemia in that the abnormality does not respond to ascorbic acid therapy. The increased urinary excretion of tryosyl derivatives is probably secondary to decreased activity of 4-hydroxyphenyl pyruvic acid oxidase. The primary defect, however, is now considered to be a deficiency in fumaryl acetoacetate hydroxylase. The exact toxic substrates involved have not been identified. The defect(s) is associated with increased plasma tyrosine and methionine concentrations, as well as hyperphosphatemia and a generalized aminoaciduria.

A defect in the last step of tyrosine metabolism (fumarylacetoacetase) has been found. Prenatal diagnosis is possible on cultured amniotic fluid cells [89].

The etiology of the hypoglycemia is not clear. Severe liver disease may result in defective glycogenesis, glycogenolysis, and gluconeogenesis. More specifically, pancreatic hyperplasia may result in hyperinsulinemia. In either situation, nutritional support with frequent feedings and monitoring of blood glucose concentration is important.

• Summary

Hypoglycemia, metabolic acidosis, and hepatomegaly can occur within hours after birth. Specific metabolic defects may be present in several disease pathways important to gluconeogenesis, including enzymes primarily concerned with gluconeogenesis, fatty acid metabolism, or specific amino acids (i.e., branched chain amino acids).

Clinical signs and symptoms should result in a high index of suspicion. Specific diagnosis requires quantification of metabolites in urine (e.g., gas chromatographic-mass spectroscopy for urinary organic acids) and/or plasma (e.g., amino acids). Enzyme analysis of leukocytes or skin fibroblasts may be necessary to establish a definitive diagnosis.

Management should be initiated concomitantly with diagnostic evaluation. Parenteral fluids with glucose and sodium bicarbonate therapy may be life-saving. Ultimate management depends upon understanding the pathogenetic mechanisms involved in specific metabolic defects.

REFERENCES

1. NYHAN WL. Inborn errors of biotin metabolism. *Arch Derm.* 1987;123:1696.
2. SAUDUBRAY J-M, MARSAC C, CHARPENTIER C, et al. Neonatal congenital lactic acidosis with pyruvate carboxylase deficiency in two siblings. *Acta Paediatr Scand.* 1976;65:719.
3. HOMMES FA, SCHRIJVER J, DIAS TL. Pyruvate carboxylase deficiency, studies on patients and on an animal model system. In: Burman D, Hallan JB, Pennook CA, eds. *Inherited Disorders of Carbohydrate Metabolism.* Baltimore: University Park Press, 1979;269.
4. HAWORTH JC, ROBINSON BH, PERRY TL. Lactic acidosis due to pyruvate carboxylase deficiency. *J Inher Metab Dis.* 1981;4:57.
5. ROBINSON BH, OCI J, SHERWOOD WG, et al. The molecular basis for the two different clinical presentations of classical pyruvate carboxylase deficiency. *Am J Hum Genet.* 1984;36:283.
6. FISER RH, MELSHER HL, FISCHER DA. Hepatic phosphoenolpyruvate carboxykinase deficiency: A new cause of hypoglycemia in childhood. *Pediatr Res.* 1974;8:432.
7. HOMMES KA, BENDIEN K, ELEMA JD, BREMER HJ, LOMBECK I. Two cases of phosphoenolpyruvate carboxykinase deficiency. *Acta Paediatr Scand.* 1976;65:233.
8. VIDNES J, SØVIK O. Gluconeogenesis in infancy and childhood. II. Studies on the glucose production from alanine in three cases of persistent neonatal hypoglycaemia. *Acta Paediatr Scand.* 1976;65:297.
9. VIDNES J, SØVIK O. Gluconeogenesis in infancy and childhood. III. Deficiency of the extramitochondrial form of hepatic phosphoenolpyruvate carboxykinase in a case of persistent neonatal hypoglycaemia. *Acta Paediatr Scand.* 1976;65:307.
10. LARDY HA, BENTLE LA, WAGNER MJ, et al. Defective phosphoenolpyruvate carboxykinase in victims of sudden infant death syndrome. National Institute of Child Health, Symposium on SIDS, July 1975.
11. STURNER WQ, SUSA JB. Sudden infant death and liver phosphoenolpyruvate carboxykinase analysis. *Foren Sci Internat.* 1980;16:19.
12. BAKER L, WINEGRAD AI. Fasting hypoglycemia and metabolic acidosis

associated with deficiency of hepatic fructose-1,6-diphosphatase activity. *Lancet.* 1970;2:13.

13. PAGLIARA AS, KARL IE, KEATING JP, BROWN BI, KIPNIS DM. Hepatic fructose-1,6-diphosphatase deficiency. A cause of lactic acidosis and hypoglycemia in infancy. *J Clin Invest.* 1972;51:2115.

14. BAERLOCHER K, GITZELMANN R, NÜSSLI R, DUMERMUTH G. Infantile lactic acidosis due to hereditary fructose-1,6-diphosphatase deficiency. *Helv Paediatr Acta* 1971;26:489.

15. HÜLSMANN WC, FERNANDES J. A child with lactic-acidemia and fructose diphosphatase deficiency in the liver. *Pediatr Res.* 1971;5:633.

16. GREENE HL, STIFEL FB, HERMAN RH. Ketotic hypoglycemia due to hepatic fructose-1,6-diphosphatase deficiency. Treatment with folic acid. *Am J Dis Child.* 1972;124:415.

17. MELANCON SB, KHACHADURIAN AK, NADLER HL, BROWN BI. Metabolic and biochemical studies in fructose-1,6-diphosphatase deficiency. *J Pediatr.* 1973;82:650.

18. MELANCON SB, NADLER HL. Detection of fructose-1,6-diphosphatase deficiency with use of white blood cells. *N Engl J Med.* 1972;286:731.

19. SAUDUBRAY JM, DREYFUS JC, CEPANEC C, LELOCH H, PHAM-HU-TRUNG, MOZZICONACCI P. Acidose lactique, hypoglycémie et hépatomégalie par deficit héréditaire en fructose-1,6-diphosphatase hépatique. *Arch Fr Pediatr.* 1973;30:609.

20. RETBI JM. Acidose lactique et hypoglycémie par déficit congénital en fructose-1,6-diphosphatase hépatique. *Thèse médicine.* Paris: René Descartes, 1972.

21. DEROSAS FJ, WAPNIR A, LIFSHITZ F, SILVERBERG M, OLSON M. Folic acid enhanced gluconeogenesis in glycerol-induced hypoglycemia and fructose-1,6-diphosphatase deficiency. The 56th Annual Meeting of The Endocrine Society, Atlanta, Georgia, June, 1974 (Abstract).

22. ODIEVRE M, MOATTI BN, DREYFUS JC, BEAUFILS F, LEJEUNE C, FEFFER J. Deficit en fructose-1,6-diphosphatase chez deux soeurs. *Arch Fr Pédiatr.* 1975;32:113.

23. HOPWOOD NJ, HOLZMAN I, DRASH AL. Fructose-1, 6-diphosphatase deficiency. *Am J Dis Child.* 1977;131:418.

24. HOMMES FA, CAMPBELL R, STEINHART C, ROESEL RA, BOWYER F. Biochemical observations on a case of hepatic fructose-1,6-diphosphatase deficiency. *J Inher Metab Dis.* 1985;8:169.

25. SHIN YS, ENDRES W, GERG J, et al. Three cases of fructose-1,6-disphosphatase deficiency: the biochemical and clinical variability. Personal communication, 1990.

26. DREMSEK PA, SACHER M, STOGMANN W, GITZELMANN R, BACHMANN C. Fructose-1,6-diphosphatase deficiency: glycerol excretion during fasting test. *Eur J Pediatr.* 1985;144:203.

27. CAHILL J, KIRTLEY ME. FDPase activity in human leukocytes. *N Engl J Med.* 1975;292:212.

28. MELANCON SB, NADLER HL. Letter to the Editor. *N Engl J Med.* 1975;292:212.

29. SCHRIJVER J, HOMMES FA. Activity of fructose-1,6-diphosphatase in human leukocytes. *N Engl J Med.* 1975;292:1298.

30. COWLES C, OZAND PT, SHUTTEE R, CORNBLATH M. Glycerol intolerance in a child with intermittent hypoglycemia. *J Pediatr.* 1975;86:43.

31. WAPNIR RA, LIFSHITZ F, SEKARAN C, TEICHBERG S, MOAK SA. Glycerol-induced hypoglycemia: a syndrome associated with multiple liver enzyme deficiencies. Clinical and in vitro studies. *Metabolism.* 1982;31:105.

32. FORT P, WAPNIR RA, DE ROSAS F, LIFSHITZ F. Long-term evolution of glycerol intolerance syndrome. *J Pediatr.* 1985;106:453.

33. STANLEY CA. New genetic defects in mitochondrial fatty acid oxidation and carnitine deficiency. *Adv Pediatr.* 1987;34:59.

34. HOPPEL CL. Determination of carnitine. In: Hommes FA, ed. Techniques in diagnostic human biochemical genetics: a laboratory manual. New York: Wiley-Liss, 1990, p. 309.

35. BOUGNERES PF, SAUDUBRAY JM, MARSAC C, BERNARD O, ODIEVRE M, GIRARD J. Fasting hypoglycemia resulting from hepatic carnitine palmitoyl transferase deficiency. *J Pediatr.* 1981;98:742.

36. STANLEY CA, COATES PM. Inherited defects of fatty acid oxidation which resemble Reye's syndrome. *J Natl Reye's Syndrome Fndn.* 1985;5:190.

37. BOUGNERES PF, ROCCHICCIOLI F, COLVRAA S, et al. Medium-chain acyl-CoA dehydrogenase deficiency in two siblings with a Reye-like syndrome. *J Pediatr.* 1985;106:918.

38. RINALDO P, O'SHEA JJ, COATES PM, HALE DE, STANLEY CA, TANAKA K. Medium-chain acyl-coA dehydrogenase deficiency. *N Engl J Med.* 1988;319:1308.

39. BHUIJAN AKMJ, WATMOUGH NJ, TURNBULL DM, AYSNLEY-GREEN A, LEONARD JV, BARTLETT K. A new simple screening method for the diagnosis of medium chain acyl-coA dehydrogenase deficiency. *Clin Chim Acta.* 1987;165:39.

40. MILLINGTON DS, ROE CR, MALTBY DA. Application of high resolution fast atom bombardment and constant B/E ratio linked scanning to the identification and analysis of acyl carnitines in metabolic disease. *Biomed Mass Spectrum.* 1984;11:236.

41. TREEM WR, WITZELBEN CA, PICCOLI DA, et al. Medium-chain and long-chain acyl coA dehydrogenase deficiency: clinical, pathological and ultrastructural differentiation from Reye's syndrome. *Hepatology.* 1986;6:1270.

42. COATES PM, HALE DE, STANLEY CA, CORKEY BE, CORTNER JA. Genetic deficiency of medium-chain acyl coenzyme A dehydrogenase: studies in cultured skin fibroblasts and peripheral mononuclear leukocytes. *Pediatr Res.* 1985;19:671.

43. STRAUSS AW, DURAN M, ZHANG ZF, ALPERS R, KELLY DP. Molecular analysis of medium chain acyl-CoA dehydrogenase deficiency. *Prog Clin Biol Res.* 1990;321:609.

44. YOKOTA I, YASHUHIRO I, COATES PM, TANAKA K. Molecular basis of medium chain acyl-Coenzyme A dehydrogenase deficiency. *J Clin Invest.* 1990;86:1000.

45. HALE DE, BATSHAW ML, COATES PM, et al. Long chain acyl coenzyme A dehydrogenase deficiency: an inherited cause of nonketotic hypoglycemia. *Pediatr Res.* 1985;19:666.

46. NAITO E, OZASA H, IKEDA Y, TANAKA K. Molecular cloning and nucleotide sequence of cDNA's encoding human short chain acyl-CoA dehydrogenase deficiency. *Prog Clin Biol Res.* 1990;321:625.

47. AMENDT BA, RHEAD WJ. The multiple acyl coenzyme A dehydrogenation disorders, glutaric aciduria type II and ethylmalonic-adipic aciduria. *J Clin Invest.* 1986;78:205.

48. MOON A, RHEAD WJ. Complementation analysis of fatty acid oxidation disorders. *J Clin Invest.* 1987;79:59.

49. LOEHR JP, GOODMAN SI, FRERMAN FE. Glutaric acidemia type II; heterogeneity of clinical and biochemical phenotypes. *Pediatr Res.* 1990;27:311.

50. FRANCOIS B, BACHMANN C, SCHUTGENS RBH. Glucose metabolism in a child with 3-hydroxy,3-methyl glutaryl coenzyme A lyase deficiency. *J Inher Metab Dis.* 1981;4:163.

51. NYHAN WL. Abnormalities of fatty acid oxidation. *N Engl J Med.* 1988;319:1344. (Editorial.)

52. WOLFF JA, THUY LP, HAAS R, CARROL JE, PRODANOS C, NYHAN WL. Carnitine reduces fasting ketogenesis in patients with disorders of proprionate metabolism. *Lancet.* 1986;1:289.

53. STEINMANN B, BACHMANN C, COLOMBO JP, GITZELMANN R. The renal handling of carnitine in patients with selective tubulopathy and with Fanconi syndrome. *Pediatr Res.* 1987;21:201.

54. SLONIM AE, BORUM PE, TANAKA K, et al. Dietary-dependent carnitine deficiency as a cause of nonketotic hypoglycemia in an infant. *J Pediatr.* 1981;99:551.

55. TREEM WR, STANLEY CA, FINEGOLD DN, HALE DE, COATES PM. Primary carnitine deficiency due to a failure of carnitine transport in kidney, muscle and fibroblasts. *N Engl J Med.* 1988;319:1331.

56. FAULL K, BOLTON P, HALPERN B, et al. Patient with defect in leucine metabolism. *N Engl J Med.* 1976;204:1012.

57. GIBSON KM, BREUER J, NYHAN WL. 3-hydroxy,3-methyl glutaryl coenzyme A lyase deficiency: review of 18 reported patients. *Eur J Pediatr.* 1988;148:180.

58. NORMAN EJ, DENTON MD, BERRY HK. Gas-chromatographic/mass spectrometric detection of 3-hydroxy,3-methyl glutaryl CoA lyase deficiency in double first cousins. *Clin Chem.* 1982;28:137.

59. ROE CR, MILLINGTON DS, MALTBY DA. Identification of 3-methyl-glutaryl carnitine. A new diagnostic metabolite of 3-hydroxy,3-methyl glutaryl-coenzyme A lyase deficiency. *J Clin Invest.* 1986;77:1391.

60. CHALMERS RA, STACEY TE, TRACEY BM, et al. L-carnitine in disorders of organic acid metabolism: response to L-carnitine by patients with methylmalonic aciduria and 3-hydroxy,3-methyl glutaric aciduria. *J Inher Metab Dis.* 1984;7(2):109.

61. GIBSON KM, LEE CF, KAMALI V, et al. 3-hydroxy,3-methyl glutaryl-CoA lyase deficiency as detected by radiochemical assay in cell extracts by thin-layer chromatography, and identification of three new cases. *Clin Chem.* 1990;36:297.

62. COCHRANE WA, PAYNE WW, SIMPKISS MJ, WOOLF LI. Familial hypoglycemia precipitated by amino acids. *J Clin Invest.* 1956;35:411.

63. GRUMBACH MM, KAPLAN SL. Amino acid and alpha-keto acid-induced hyperinsulinism in the leucine-sensitive type of infantile and childhood hypoglycemia. *J Pediatr.* 1960;57:346.

64. MABRY CC, DI GEORGE AM, AUERBACH VH. Leucine-induced hypoglycemia. I. Clinical observations and diagnostic considerations. *J Pediatr.* 1960;57:526.

65. GENTZ J, LEHMANN O, ZETTERSTRÖM R. Studies on leucine-induced hypoglycemia. *Acta Paediatr.* 1962;51:169.

66. ROTH H, SEGAL S. Dietary management of leucine-sensitive hypoglycemia. *Pediatrics.* 1964;34:831.

67. ROSE SR, CHROUSOS G, CORNBLATH M, SIDBURY J. Management of postoperative nesidioblastosis with zinc protamine glucagon and oral starch. *J Pediatr.* 1986;108:87.

68. MENKES JH, HURST PL, CRAIG JM. New syndrome: progressive familial infantile cerebral dysfunction associated with an unusual urinary substance. *Pediatrics.* 1954;14:42.

69. WESTALL RG, DANCIS J, MILLER S. Maple sugar urine disease. *Am J Dis Child.* 1957;94:571.

70. DANNER DJ, ELSAS LJ II. Disorders of branched chain amino acid and ketoacid metabolism. In: Scriver CR, Beaudet AL, Sly WS, Valle D, eds. *The Metabolic Basis of Inherited Disease.* 6th ed. New York: McGraw-Hill, Inc, 1989; 671.

71. DONNELL GN, LIEBERMAN E, SHAW KNF, KOCH R. Hypoglycemia in maple syrup urine disease. *Am J Dis Child.* 1967;113:60.

72. HAYMOND MW, KARL IE, FEIGIN RD, DeVIVO D, PAGLIARA AS. Hypoglycemia and maple syrup urine disease: Defective gluconeogenesis. *Pediatr Res.* 1973;7:500.

73. LEVY HC. Genetic screening. *Adv Hum Genet.* 1973;4:389.

74. HARRIS RA, ZHANG B, GOODWIN GW, et al. Regulation of the branched-chain alpha-ketoacid dehydrogenase and elucidation of a molecular basis for maple syrup urine disease. *Adv Enzyme Regul.* 1990;30:245.

75. TANAKA K, BUDD MA, EFRON ML, ISSELBACHER KJ. Isovaleric acidemia: a new genetic defect of leucine metabolism. *Proc Natl Acad Sci USA.* 1966;56:236.

76. MATSUBARA Y, INDO Y, NAITO E, et al. Molecular cloning and nucleotide sequence of cDNAs encoding the precursors of rat long chain acyl-coenzyme A, short chain acyl coenzyme A, and isovaleryl-coenzyme A dehydrogenases: sequence homology of four enzymes of the acyl-coA dehydrogenase family. *J Biol Chem.* 1989;264:16321.

77. MATSUBARA Y, ITO M, GLASSBERG R, SATYABHAMA S, IKEDA Y, TANAKA K. Nucleotide sequence of messenger RNA encoding human isovaleryl-coenzyme A dehydrogenase and its expression in isovaleric acidemia fibroblasts. *J Clin Invest.* 1990;85:1058.

78. NYHAN WL, SAKATI NA. *Diagnostic Recognition of Genetic Disease.* Philadelphia: Lea and Febiger, 1987;50.

79. SWEETMAN L. Branched chain organic acidurias. In: Scriver CR, Beaudet AL, Sly W, Valle D, eds. *The Metabolic Basis of Inherited Disease.* 6th ed. New York: McGraw-Hill Inc, 1989;791.

80. CHILDS B, NYHAN WL, BORDEN M, BARD L, COOKE RE. Idiopathic hyperglycinemia and hyperglycinuria: a new disorder of amino acid metabolism. *Pediatrics.* 1961;27:522.

81. ROBERT MF, SCHULTZ DJ, WOLF B, COCHRAN WD, SCHWARTZ AL. Treatment of a neonate with propionic acidaemia and severe hyperammonia by peritoneal dialysis. *Arch Dis Child.* 1979;54:962.

82. PERRY TL, URQUHART N, MCLEAN J, et al. Nonketotic hyperglycinemia. *N Engl J Med.* 1975;292:1269.

83. STEINMANN B, GITZELMANN R. Strychnine treatment attempted in new-

born twins with severe nonketotic hyperglycinemia. *Helv Paediat Acta.* 1979;34:589.

84. GITZELMANN R, STEINMANN B. Clinical and therapeutic aspects of non-ketotic hyperglycinemia. *J Inher Metab Dis.* 1982;5(2):113.

85. NYHAN WL, FAWCETT N, ANDO T, RENNERT OM, JULIUS RL. Response to dietary therapy in B12 unresponsive methylmalonic acidemia. *Pediatrics.* 1973;51:539.

86. MATSUI SM, MAHONEY MJ, ROSENBERG LE. The natural history of the inherited methylmalonic acidemias. *N Engl J Med.* 1983;308:857.

87. COUDE M, CHADEFAUX B, RABIER D, KAMOUN P. Early amniocentesis and amniotic fluid organic acid levels in the prenatal diagnosis of organic acidemias. *Clin Chim Acta.* 1990;187(3):329.

88. BABER MD. A case of congenital cirrhosis of the liver with renal tubular defects akin to those in the Fanconi syndrome. *Arch Dis Child.* 1956;31:335.

89. KUITTINGEN EA, STEINMANN E, GITZELMANN R, et al. Prenatal diagnosis of hereditary tyrosinemia by determination of fumarylacetoacetase in cultured amniotic fluid cells. *Pediatr Res.* 1985;19:334.

APPENDIX I

INTERFERENCE WITH GLUCOSE MEASUREMENT

More than 250 substances have been screened to ascertain whether they would interfere with glucose measurement when using the YSI Model 23A Glucose Analyzer. All the substances tested were found to be "noninterfering" at the highest naturally occurring plasma level that has come to our attention, and most were "noninterfering" at any reasonable concentration. We use the term "noninterfering" to mean that the substance by itself would give a reading smaller than 5 mg/dl glucose, and would affect the sensitivity of the Model 23A to glucose by less than 5 percent. However, several exogenous substances can interfere, and nothing should be added to specimens save those preservatives and anticoagulants recommended in the section entitled "Sample Handling and Collection."

Following is a list of substances of particular interest, or to which the Model 23A is especially sensitive, with the expected "interfering level" at which an error of 5 percent or 5 mg/dl glucose could occur. Except for heparin, all concentrations are in units of mg/dl. The Model 23A is "not suitable for use" with specimens containing substances at or above the "interfering level" tabulated. These numbers are only approximate because of instrument-to-instrument variability, and because linear response was assumed in making extrapolations from the level tested. In no circumstance should the user attempt to calculate a correction to the apparent glucose assay based upon these numbers.

Complete test results are available from Yellow Springs Instruments on request.

INTERFERENCE WITH GLUCOSE MEASUREMENT

TABLE 1. Interferences*

SUBSTANCE	FORMULA WEIGHT	LEVEL TESTED (mg/dl)	INTERFERING LEVEL (mg/dl)
Anticoagulants: The following are safe at the usual levels			
Sodium oxalate	134.01	1,000	11,000
Sodium fluoride	41.99	5,000	4,800
Heparin sodium		200 U/ml	1,800 U/ml
Dipotassium EDTA	404.46	2,000	5,200
Sodium citrate	294.1	5,000	31,000
Preservatives: The following do not interfere at usual levels; however, we have not evaluated their efficacy as preservatives or antiglycolytics			
2-Iodoacetamide	184.96	1,000	900
Iodoacetic acid	185.96	1,000	1,900
Sodium iodoacetate, free of iodine and iodide	207.93	2,000	8,000
Sodium tetraborate decahydrate	381.37	2,000	3,400
The following may interfere: Do not use			
Benzalkonium chloride	396.11	1,000	150
Methyl paraben	152.15	1,000	80
Phenol	94.11	50	1.6
Sodium azide	65.01	1,000	360
Thymol	150.22	100	75

All following substances are noninterfering at the highest naturally occurring plasma level that has come to our attention.

Substances of Particular Interest in Diabetes

Acetone	58.08	2,000	26,000
beta-Hydroxybutyric Acid	126.1	1,000	14,000
L-Leucine	131.2	1,000	21,000
Sorbitol	182.17	10,000	/ 14,000
Tolbutamide	270.34	1,000	2,200
D-Xylose	150.13	2,000	730

Endogenous Substances of General Interest

D(−)adrenaline	183.21	200	110
Ascorbic acid	176.12	200	280
Bilirubin (dissolved in DMSO)	584.7	40	140
L(+)cysteine hydrochloride	256.63	100	100
D(−)fructose	180.16	1,000	5,400
d-galactose	180.16	1,000	300
Gentisic acid	154.12	200	110
D(+)glucosamine hydrochloride	215.64	1,000	280
Glucose-6-phosphate	336.32	500	3,000
Glutathione, reduced	307.3	100	100

SUBSTANCE	FORMULA WEIGHT	LEVEL TESTED (mg/dl)	INTERFERING LEVEL (mg/dl)
d-Mannose	180.16	1,000	170
Tyrosine	181.2	200	160
Uric acid	168.11	100	400

Radiopaques: Safe even at high levels

Meglumine iodipamide	1,335.02	52,000	25,000
Meglumine iothalamate	809.13	60,000	29,000
Renografin (Squibb)	mixture	76,000 (solids)	22,000
Sodium methiodal	244.01	40,000	9,000

Lipids and Related Substances

Cholesterol (in isopropanol)	386.66	1,000	2,800
Cholesteryl octanoate (in isopropanol)	512.86	1,000	8,600
Cholic acid	408.58	2,000	16,000
Nonanoic acid (in isopropanol)	158.23	2,000	2,700
Octanol (in isopropanol)	130.23	2,000	500
Silicone oil (SF-90(50)) (in isopropanol)		2,000	18,000
Tripalmitin (in isopropanol)	807.3	1,000	2,100

Drugs, Poisons and Miscellaneous Exogenous Substances

Acetaminophen	151.16	325	7
Acetylsalicylic acid	180.16	1,000	4,000
p-Aminosalicylic acid	153.13	200	10
Catechol	110.11	5	0.3
Dextran	20,000	1,000	2,000
L-3,4-dihydroxyphenylalanine	197.2	100	1,400
2,3-dimercaptopropanol	124.2	100	5
Ethanol	46.07	5,000	28,000
Formaldehyde	30.03	370	42
Guaiacol	124.14	20	0.8
Hydrazine sulfate	130.12	10	1
Hydrogen peroxide	34.01	30	4.5
Hydroquinone	110.11	20	0.8
Hydroxylamine hydrochloride	69.49	1	0.15
Isoniazid	137.15	10	1.6
2-mercaptoethanol	78.13	100	1
Methylene blue	373.90	1,000	370
D-penicillamine	149.2	500	190
Potassium cyanide	65.12	200	50
Potassium iodide	166.02	20	14
Potassium thiocyanate	97.18	500	36
Pyridoxine hydrochloride	205.7	500	24
Salicylamide	137.14	50	2.2
Sodium nitrite	69.01	100	26

Continued on next page

INTERFERENCE WITH GLUCOSE MEASUREMENT

SUBSTANCE	FORMULA WEIGHT	LEVEL TESTED (mg/dl)	INTERFERING LEVEL (mg/dl)
Sodium salicylate	160.10	2,000	1,200
Sodium sulfide nonahydrate	240.18	2	0.8
2-thiouracil	128.15	10	0.6
Thiourea	76.12	10	0.5
o-tolidine dihydrochloride	285.22	50	20
o-toluidine	107.16	10	1

*This material is reproduced from the Yellow Springs Instrument 23A Glucose Analyzer Manual Regarding Interferences, with permission.

Note: Chlorpromazine, iodoacetamide, phloridzin and various mercurials have been reported to inhibit the transport of glucose through erythrocyte membranes in vitro, which could conceivably lead to erroneously low whole blood glucose readings by the YSI method. We have been unable to produce any error in our laboratory with reasonable levels of these materials, but it may nevertheless be prudent to determine glucose in plasma, rather than whole blood, for specimens in which these substances (or any other reported glucose transport inhibitors) are believed to be present.

A P P E N D I X   II

DIETS

FOR DISORDERS

OF CARBOHYDRATE

METABOLISM*

TABLE 1. Galactose-free diet

TYPE OF FOOD	FOOD TO INCLUDE	FOOD TO OMIT
Milk and milk products	None. Nutramigen to be used in place of milk.	All milk of any kind: skim, dried, evaporated, condensed. Cheeses. Ice cream, sherbets. Any food containing milk or milk products.
Meat, fish, fowl	Beef, chicken, turkey, fish, lamb, veal, pork, ham.	Creamed or breaded meat, fish, or fowl. Luncheon meats, hot dogs, liver sausage. Meats containing milk or milk products. Organ meats such as liver, pancreas, brain.
Eggs	All.	None.
Vegetables	Artichokes, asparagus, beets, green beans, wax beans, broccoli, cauliflower, celery, corn, chard, cucumber, eggplant, kale, lettuce, greens, okra, onions, parsley, parsnips, pumpkin, rutabagas, spinach, squash, tomatoes.	Sugar beets, peas, lima beans, soybeans, legumes. Creamed, breaded, or buttered vegetables. Any vegetables in which lactose has been added during processing.

Continued on next page

---

*Prepared by Miss Bernita A. Youngs, Chief Nutritionist, Maternity and Infant Care Project, Chicago Board of Health; Formerly, Clinic Dietitian, Research and Educational Hospitals, University of Illinois College of Medicine; 1966 and as modified 1976 by the authors.

TABLE 1. Continued

TYPE OF FOOD	FOOD TO INCLUDE	FOOD TO OMIT
Potatoes and substitutes	White potatoes, sweet potatoes, macaroni, noodles, spaghetti, rice.	Any creamed, breaded, or buttered; mashed. French fried potatoes and instant potatoes if lactose or milk has been added during processing.
Breads and cereals.	Any that do not contain milk or milk products.	Prepared mixes such as muffins, biscuits, waffles, pancakes; some dry cereals; instant cream of wheat. (Read labels *carefully*.) Dry cereals with added skim milk powder or lactose. Breads and rolls made with milk. Crackers.
Fats	Oils, shortenings, dressings that do not contain milk or milk products. Bacon.	Margarine, butter, cream, cream cheese. Dressings containing milk or milk products.
Soups	Clear soups, vegetable soups that do not contain peas or lima beans. Consommes.	Cream soups, chowders, commercially prepared soups that contain lactose.
Desserts	Water and fruit ices, jello, angel food cake, homemade cakes, pies, cookies from allowed ingredients.	Commercial cakes and cookies and mixes. Custard, puddings, ice cream made with milk. Anything containing chocolate.
Fruits	All fresh, canned, or frozen that are not processed with lactose.	Any canned or frozen that are processed with lactose.
Miscellaneous	Nuts, peanut butter, popcorn (unbuttered), pure sugar candy, jelly or marmalade, sugar, Karo, carob powder, chewing gum, olives.	Gravy, white sauce, chocolate, cocoa, toffee, peppermints, butterscotch, caramels, molasses candies, instant coffee, powdered soft drinks, monosodium glutamate, some spice blends.

Labels should be read carefully, and any products that contain milk, lactose, casein, whey, dry milk solids or curds should be omitted.

Lactate, lactic acid, lactalbumin, and calcium compounds *do not* contain lactose.

TABLE 2. Sucrose- and fructose-free diet

FOOD	AMOUNT	FOODS TO USE	FOODS TO AVOID
Milk	Any	Any.	None.
Meat, fish, poultry, cheese	Any	Beef, veal, lamb, pork, chicken, turkey, fish, cheese.	Ham, bacon, lunch meats, and any other meats in which sugar is used in processing.
Eggs	Any	Any.	None.
Vegetables	Any	Asparagus, cabbage, cauliflower, celery, green beans, green peppers, lettuce, spinach, wax beans.	All other vegetables.
Potato or substitute	Any	White potatoes,* macaroni, noodles, spaghetti, rice.	Sweet potatoes.
Fruits	None	None.	All fruits and fruit juices.
Bread	None	No bread. Soda crackers, saltines.	Any bread. Other crackers.
Cereal	Any	Cooked or ready-to-eat cereals (except sugar-coated cereals).	Sugar-coated cereals.
Fat	Any	Butter, margarine, oil, homemade mayonnaise or French dressing made without sugar.	Mayonnaise, salad dressings made with sugar.
Desserts	Any	Dietetic jello, dietetic ice cream, dietetic puddings.	All desserts containing sugar, such as cake, pie, cookies, candy, puddings, jello, ice cream, sherbet and others. Any desserts containing honey, fruit or fruit juice.
Miscellaneous	Any	Vegetable juices (no tomato). Coffee, tea. Salt, pepper, and other condiments. Broth, soups from allowed vegetables. Sugar substitute. Dietetic beverages.	Catsup, chili sauce, and other sauces containing sugar. Carbonated beverages. Sugar, honey, maple syrup, jam, jellies, preserves.

Labels of all canned, packaged or processed foods should be checked to be sure that sugar or fruit is not used.

*See Chapter 9, p. 327 for details.

DIETS FOR DISORDERS OF CARBOHYDRATE METABOLISM

TABLE 3. Leucine-restricted diet*

FOOD	AMOUNT	FOODS TO USE	FOODS TO AVOID
Milk	Only as indicated.	Special leucine-poor formula.	All milk: whole, skim, evaporated, condensed, dried, buttermilk. Milk products such as cheese. Foods prepared with milk, such as ice cream.
Eggs	None.	None.	Eggs or foods prepared with eggs.
Meat, fish, poultry or cheese	Only as indicated.	Beef, veal, lamb, pork, liver, chicken, turkey.	Any other meat or poultry, sausage, lunch meat, other meat products, except as allowed on individual meal plan. Cheese, fish.
Vegetables	As desired.	Fresh, frozen, canned, or juice. Asparagus, green beans, beets, cabbage, carrots, cucumbers, eggplant, onions, pumpkin, squash, tomatoes.	Peas, lima beans, kidney beans, soybeans, lentils, any other vegetables not listed to use. Vegetables prepared with cream sauce or breaded.
Potato or substitute	Only as indicated.	White potato, sweet potato.	Rice, noodles, spaghetti, macaroni.
Fruits	As desired.	Fresh, canned, frozen or juice. Any fruit.	Dried fruits.
Bread	Only as indicated.	White bread.	Any other bread such as whole wheat, rye, special breads, crackers, corn-bread, biscuits, etc.
Cereal	Only as indicated.	Cornflakes, cream of rice, pablum rice, shredded wheat.	Any other cereal.
Fats	As desired.	Butter, margarine.	
Desserts	As desired.	Cakes and cookies made without egg, milk or nuts. Sherbet made without milk. Gelatin.	Cakes, cookies, pies, puddings, ice cream. Any desserts made with milk, eggs or nuts.
Miscellaneous	As desired.	Carbonated beverages, jams, jelly, preserves. Sugar (glucose or sucrose).	Nuts.

The foods should be arranged into a meal plan in such a way that the prescribed amount of protein will be spaced to avoid an excess of leucine at one time, which would precipitate hypoglycemia. Three meals a day with a prescribed amount of sugar given upon rising, 20 to 30 minutes after breakfast, lunch, and supper and before sleep are necessary. Foods should be given in measured amounts to meet the calculated requirements for the individual child.

*Adapted from Roth and Segal. Dietary management of leucine-sensitive hypoglycemia. *Pediatrics.* 1964;34:831.

A P P E N D I X III

CARBOHYDRATE CONTENT OF FOODS*

*From Hardinge, Swarner, and Crooks. *J Am Diet Assoc.* 1965;46:198.

TABLE 1. More common carbohydrates in foods per 100 gm edible portion

FOOD	MONO-SACCHARIDES		REDUCING SUGARS* (gm)	DISACCHARIDES			POLYSACCHARIDES					
	Fructose (gm)	Glucose (gm)		Lactose (gm)	Maltose (gm)	Sucrose (gm)	Cellulose (gm)	Dextrins (gm)	Hemicellulose (gm)	Pectin (gm)	Pentosans (gm)	Starch (gm)
Fruits												
Agave juice	17.0		19.0	†								
Apple	5.0	1.7	8.3			3.1	0.4		0.7	0.6		0.6
Apple juice			8.0			4.2						
Apricots	0.4	1.9				5.5	0.8		1.2	1.0		
Banana												
Yellow green			5.0			5.1						8.8
Yellow			8.4			8.9						1.9
Flecked	3.5	4.5				11.9						1.2
Powder			32.6			33.2		9.6				7.8
Blackberries	2.9	3.2				0.2						
Blueberry juice, commercial			9.6			0.2						
Boysenberries			5.3			1.1				0.3		
Breadfruit												
Hawaiian			1.8			7.7						
Samoan			4.9			9.7						
Cherries												
Eating	7.2	4.7	12.5			0.1				0.3		
Cooking	6.1	5.5	11.6			0.1						
Cranberries	0.7	2.7				0.1						
Currants												
Black	3.7	2.4				0.6						
Red	1.9	2.3				0.2						
White	2.6	3.0										

Item							
Dates							
Invert sugar, seedling type	23.9			0.3			
Deglet Noor		24.9	16.2	45.4			3.0
Egyptian			35.8	48.5			
Figs, Kadota							
Fresh	8.2	9.6		0.9			0.1
Dried	30.9	42.0		0.1			0.3
Gooseberries	4.1	4.4		0.7			
Grapes							
Black	7.3	8.2		0.2			
Concord	4.3	4.8	9.5	0.2			
Malaga	8.0		22.2				
White	8.1						
Grapefruit	1.2	2.0		2.9		1.3	
Guava			4.4	1.9			
Lemon							
Edible portion			1.3	0.2	3.0		
Whole	1.4	1.4		0.4		0.7	
Juice	0.9	0.5		0.1	0.7		
Peel			3.4	0.1			
Loganberries	1.3	1.9		0.2			
Loquat							
Champagne		12.0		0.8			
Thales		9.0		0.9			
Mango			3.4	11.6			0.3
Melon							
Cantaloupe	0.9	1.2	2.3	4.4	0.3		
Cassaba,							
Vine ripened			2.8	6.2			
Picked green			3.2	3.9			
Honeydew							
Vine ripened			3.3	7.4			
Picked green			3.6	3.3			

Continued on next page

TABLE 1. Continued

	MONO-SACCHARIDES		REDUCING SUGARS*	DISACCHARIDES			POLYSACCHARIDES					
FOOD	Fructose (gm)	Glucose (gm)	(gm)	Lactose (gm)	Maltose (gm)	Sucrose (gm)	Cellulose (gm)	Dextrins (gm)	Hemicellulose (gm)	Pectin (gm)	Pentosans (gm)	Starch (gm)
Fruits												
Yellow	1.5	2.1				1.4						
Mulberries	3.6	4.4										
Orange												
Valencia (Calif.)	2.3	2.4	4.7			4.2	0.3					
Composite values	1.8	2.5	5.0			4.6			0.3	1.3	0.3	
Juice												
Fresh	2.4	2.4	5.1			4.7						
Frozen, reconstituted			4.6			3.2						
Palmyra palm, tender kernel	1.5	3.2				0.4						
Papaw (*Asimina triloba*) (North America)			5.9			2.7						
Papaya (*Carica papaya*) (tropics)			9.0			0.5						
Passion fruit juice	3.6	3.6				3.8						
Peaches	1.6	1.5	3.1			6.6		0.7		0.7		1.8
Pears												
Anjou	5.0	2.5	7.6			1.9				0.7		
Bartlett			8.0			1.5				0.6		
Bosc	6.5	2.6				1.7				0.6		
Persimmon			17.7									
Pineapple												
Ripened on plant	1.4	2.3	4.2			7.9						
Picked green			1.3			2.4						

Plums										
Damson	3.4	5.2	8.4		1.0					
Greengage	4.0	5.5			2.9					
Italian prunes	2.9	4.5	4.6		5.4		0.5		0.9	0.7
Sweet	1.3	3.5	7.4		4.4				1.0	2.0
Sour					1.5				1.0	0.1
Pomegranate			12.0		0.6					
Prunes, uncooked	15.0	30.0	47.0		2.0	2.8		10.7	0.9	
Raisins, Thompson seedless			70.0						1.0	
Raspberries	2.4	2.3	5.0		1.0				0.8	
Sapote	3.8	4.2		0.7						
Strawberries										
Ripe	2.3	2.6	3.8		1.4					
Medium ripe			4.8		0.3					
Tangerine	1.2	1.6	3.4		9.0	0.2		0.3		
Tomatoes										
Canned			3.0		0.3				0.3	
Seedless pulp			6.5		0.4	0.4			0.5	
Watermelon										
Flesh red and firm, ripe			3.8		4.0				0.1	
Red, mealy, overripe			3.0		4.9				0.1	
Vegetables										
Asparagus, raw	1.2				0.2			0.3		
Bamboo shoots			0.5			1.2				
Beans										
Lima										
Canned					1.4					
Fresh					1.4					
Snap, fresh			1.7		0.5	0.5	0.3	1.0	0.5	
Beets, sugar					12.9	0.9		0.8	1.2	2.0

Continued on next page

TABLE 1. Continued

FOOD	MONOSACCHARIDES		REDUCING SUGARS* (gm)	DISACCHARIDES			POLYSACCHARIDES					
	Fructose (gm)	Glucose (gm)		Lactose (gm)	Maltose (gm)	Sucrose (gm)	Cellulose (gm)	Dextrins (gm)	Hemicellulose (gm)	Pectin (gm)	Pentosans (gm)	Starch (gm)
Vegetables (continued)												
Broccoli							0.9		0.9		0.9	1.3
Brussels sprout							1.1		1.5			
Cabbage, raw			3.4			0.3	0.8		1.0			
Carrots, raw			5.8			1.7	1.0		1.7	0.9		
Cauliflower		2.8				0.3	0.7		0.6			
Celery												
Fresh			0.3			0.3						
Hearts			1.7			0.2						
Corn												
Fresh		0.5				0.3	0.6	0.1	0.9		1.3	14.5
Bran									77.1		4.0	
Cucumber			2.5			0.1						
Eggplant			2.1			0.6			0.5			
Lettuce			1.4			0.2	0.4		0.6			
Licorice root		1.4				3.2						22.0
Mushrooms, fresh			0.1				0.9		0.7			2.5
Onions, raw			5.4			2.9			0.3	0.6		
Parsnips, fresh						3.5						7.0
Peas, green						5.5	1.1		2.2			4.1
Potatoes, white	0.1	0.1	0.8			0.1	0.4		0.3			17.0
Pumpkin			2.2			0.6			0.5			0.1
Radishes			3.1			0.3			0.3	0.4		
Rutabagas		5.0				1.3					0.8	
Spinach			0.2				0.4		0.8			

Squash, Sweet potato, Beans, and Milk data (continued table — column headers appear on a preceding page).

Food										
Squash										
Butternut	0.2	0.1		0.4						2.6
Blue Hubbard	1.2	1.1		0.4						4.8
Golden crookneck			2.8	1.0	0.7					
Sweet potato										
Raw	0.3	0.4	0.8	4.1	0.6		1.4	2.2	1.6	16.5
Baked			14.5	7.2						4.0

Mature Dry Legumes

Food										
Beans										
Mung										
Black gram				1.6						
Green gram				1.8						
Navy				7.2	3.1	3.7	6.4		8.2	35.2
Soy			1.6	1.5	2.6	1.4	6.6		4.0	1.9
Cow pea				2.4	5.4		4.8			
Garbanzo (chick peas)										
Garden pea (*Pisum sativum*)‡				6.7	5.0		5.1			38.0
Horse gram (*Dolichos biflorus*)				2.7						
Lentils				2.1						28.5
Pigeon pea (red gram)				1.6						
Soybean										
Flour				6.8						
Meal				6.8						

Milk and Milk Products

Food		
Buttermilk		
Dry		39.9
Fluid, genuine and cultured		5.0

Continued on next page

TABLE 1. Continued

FOOD	MONO-SACCHARIDES Fructose (gm)	Glucose (gm)	REDUCING SUGARS* (gm)	DISACCHARIDES Lactose (gm)	Maltose (gm)	Sucrose (gm)	POLYSACCHARIDES Cellulose (gm)	Dextrins (gm)	Hemicellulose (gm)	Pectin (gm)	Pentosans (gm)	Starch (gm)
Milk and Milk Products *(continued)*												
Casein		0.1										
Ice cream (14.5% cream)				3.6		16.6						
Milk												
Ass				6.0								
Cow				4.9								
Dried												
Skim				52.0								
Whole				38.1								
Fluid												
Skim				5.0								
Whole				4.9								
Sweetened, condensed				14.1		43.5						
Ewe				4.9								
Goat				4.7								
Human												
Colostrum				5.3								
Mature				6.9								
Whey				4.9								
Yogurt				3.8								

Nuts and Nut Products

Almonds, blanched	0.2		2.3				2.1	
Chestnuts	2.2		3.6				1.2	18.0
Virginia	1.2		8.1				2.8	18.6
French	3.3		3.6		0.3		2.5	33.1
Coconut milk, ripe			2.6					
Copra meal, dried	1.2	1.2	14.3	15.6	0.6		2.2	0.9
Macadamia nut	0.3		5.5					
Peanuts	0.2		4.5	2.4	2.5	3.8		4.0
Peanut butter	0.9							5.9
Pecans			1.1				0.2	

Cereals and Cereal Products

Barley								
Grain, hulled				2.6		6.0	8.5	62.0
Flour	3.1						1.2	69.0
Corn, yellow				4.5		4.9	6.2	62.0
Flaxseed				1.8		5.2		
Millet grain							6.5	56.0
Oats, hulled						0.9	6.4	56.4
Rice								
Bran	1.4		10.6	11.4		7.0	7.4	
Brown, raw	0.1		0.8		2.1		2.1	69.7
Polished, raw	trace§		0.4	0.3	0.9		1.8	72.9
Polish	0.7						3.8	
Rye								
Grain				3.8		5.6	6.8	57.0
Flour	2.0						4.1	71.4
Sorghum grain							2.5	70.2
Soya-wheat (cereal)							3.3	46.4

Continued on next page

TABLE 1. Continued

FOOD	MONOSACCHARIDES		REDUCING SUGARS* (gm)	DISACCHARIDES			POLYSACCHARIDES					
	Fructose (gm)	Glucose (gm)		Lactose (gm)	Maltose (gm)	Sucrose (gm)	Cellulose (gm)	Dextrins (gm)	Hemicellulose (gm)	Pectin (gm)	Pentosans (gm)	Starch (gm)
Cereals and Cereal Products (*continued*)												
Wheat												
Germ, defatted			2.0			8.3					6.2	
Grain			2.0			1.5	2.0	2.5	5.8		6.6	59.0
Flour, patent					0.1	0.2		5.5			2.1	68.8
Spices and Condiments												
Allspice (pimenta)			18.0			3.0						
Cassia			23.3									
Cinnamon			19.3									
Cloves			9.0									2.7
Nutmeg			17.2									14.6
Pepper, black			38.6									34.2
Syrups and Other Sweets												
Corn syrup		21.2			26.4			34.7				
High conversion		33.0			23.0			19.0				
Medium conversion		26.0			21.0			23.0				
Corn sugar		87.5			3.5			0.5				
Chocolate, sweet dry						56.4						
Golden syrup			37.5			31.0						
Honey	40.5	34.2				1.9		1.5				
Invert sugar			74.0			6.0						

402 •

Jellies, pectin	11.3				40–65		
Royal jelly	9.8				0.9		
Jellies, starch					25–60		7–12
Maple syrup		1.5			62.9		
Milk chocolate			8.1		43.0		
Molasses	8.0	8.8			53.6		
Blackstrap	6.8	6.8	26.9		36.9		
Sorghum syrup		27.0			36.0		

Miscellaneous

Beer		1.5				2.8	0.3
Cacao beans, raw, Arriba	0.6	0.5	1.1		1.9		
Carob bean							
Pod		11.2			23.2		1.4
Pod and seeds		11.1			19.4		
Soy sauce	0.9						

*Mainly monosaccharides plus the disaccharides, maltose, and lactose.
†Blanks indicate lack of acceptable data.
‡Also known as Alaska pea, field pea, and common pea.
§Trace = less than 0.05 gm.

GLUCOSE RATES FOR INTRAVENOUS THERAPY WITH PRECAUTIONS RELATED TO HYPOPHOSPHATEMIA

• Hypophosphatemia

Prolonged therapy with glucose at high rates (over 10 mg/kg/min) may produce a decrease in both plasma potassium and phosphate that is due to cellular uptake of these ions.* Although maintenance-type fluids usually provide for the major cations and anions, they often do not provide inorganic phosphate. Recent studies have indicated that inorganic phosphate is critical to the formation of 2,3 diphosphoglycerate (DPG). The latter is an important ligand of hemoglobin, which affects oxygen affinity in the erythrocyte. Significant decreases in inorganic phosphate have been associated with decreased erythrocyte DPG and a shift of the oxygen dissociation curve to the left, thus resulting in a lower $P_{50}O_2$ and decreased availability of oxygen to tissues. Since this decrease cannot be judged clinically, we recommend the monitoring of plasma inorganic phosphate and the addition of

---

*Travis, Sugarman, Ruberg, et al. Alterations of red cell glycolytic intermediates and oxygen transport as a consequence of hypophosphatemia in patients receiving intravenous hyperalimentation. *N Engl J Med.* 1971;285:763; and Ricour, Millot, and Balsan. Phosphorus depletion in children on long-term total parenteral nutrition. *Acta Paediatr Scand.* 1975;64:385.

Glucose rates for intravenous therapy*

GLUCOSE RATE PER kg			ENERGY[†] PER kg (kcal/day)	VOLUME RATE AT PERCENT GLUCOSE CONCENTRATION				
(mg/min)	(g/hr)	(g/day)		5%	10%	15% (ml/kg/day)	20%	25%
4	0.24	5.76	23.0	115[‡]	58[§]	38	29	23
6	0.36	8.64	34.6	173	86	58	43	35
8	0.48	11.5	46.1	230	115	77	58	46
10	0.60	14.4	57.6	...	144	96	72	58
12	0.72	17.3	69.1	...	173	115	86	69
14	0.84	20.2	80.6	...	202	134	101	81
16	0.96	23.0	92.2	...	230	154	115	92
20	1.20	28.8	115.2	...	...	192	144	115
24	1.44	34.6	138.2	...	...	230	173	138

*Dextrose is glucose monohydrate with a molecular weight of 198 compared to 180 for anhydrous glucose. Since dextrose is the commercially available form, the approximations in this table are 18 ÷ 180 or 10% too low when dextrose is given.
[†]Calculated at the approximate energy value of 4.0 kcal/g for polysaccharide metabolized instead of the more exact value of 3.8 for glucose.
[‡]Double underlined values compare glucose rates and infusion concentrations at reasonable volumes for infants beyond the first day of life.
[§]Single underlined values similarly compare these for the initial day of life when fluid is restricted to approximately 60–65 ml/kg/day.

potassium phosphate to maintenance fluids, provided hyperkalemia is not present. Buffered potassium phosphate is available commercially or may be prepared from K_2HPO_4 2.0 g and KH_2PO_4 0.4 g, which together provide 26 mM potassium and 14.5 mM phosphate (in a molar ratio of 4:1 dibasic to monobasic). If these quantities are made up in 25-ml vials, then each ml would contain approximately 1 mM potassium and 0.6 mM buffered phosphate. These may be added to the parenteral glucose solution to provide 2–3 mM/kg/day potassium and phosphate each. Thus 3 ml/kg/day added would provide 3 mM potassium and 1.8 mM phosphate. These quantities should not be given on the first day of life when fluid volumes are limited. Care must also be exercised if the infusing catheter is in or near the right atrium. A preparation of sodium phosphate may be similarly prepared.

INDEX